Differential Diagnosis in Neuro-oncology

Differential Diagnosis in Neuro-oncology

J. Hildebrand and M. Brada

Illustrated in collaboration with D. Balériaux

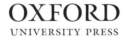

OXFORD
UNIVERSITY PRESS

OXFORD

UNIVERSITY PRESS

Great Clarendon Street, Oxford OX2 6DP
Oxford University Press is a department of the University of Oxford.
It furthers the University's objective of excellence in research, scholarship,
and education by publishing worldwide in
Oxford   New York

Athens   Auckland   Bangkok   Bogotá   Buenos Aires   Calcutta
Cape Town   Chennai   Dar es Salaam   Delhi   Florence   Hong Kong   Istanbul
Karachi   Kuala Lumpur   Madrid   Melbourne   Mexico City   Mumbai
Nairobi   Paris   São Paulo   Singapore   Taipei   Tokyo   Toronto   Warsaw

with associated companies in
Berlin   Ibadan

Oxford is a registered trade mark of Oxford University Press
in the UK and in certain other countries

Published in the United States
by Oxford University Press Inc., New York

© Oxford University Press, 2001

The moral rights of the author have been asserted

Database right Oxford University Press (maker)

First published 2001

A catalogue record for this title is available from the British Library

Library of Congress Cataloging in Publication Data
Hildebrand, J. (Jerzy)
Differential diagnosis in neuro-oncology/J. Hildebrand and M. Brada; illustrated in
collaboration with D. Balériaux.
Includes bibliographical references.
1. Nervous system–Cancer × Diagnosis   2. Metastasis   3. Diagnosis, Differential.
I. Brada, M. (Michael)   II. Title.
RC280.N4 H54 2001   616.99948075–dc21   00-050161
ISBN 0 19 263213 2 (HBK)

1 3 5 7 9 10 8 6 4 2

Typeset by EXPO Holdings, Malaysia

Printed in Great Britain on acid free paper by
Biddles Ltd.
Guildford & King's Lynn.

Introduction

Neurological disorders are common in cancer patients. They are a consequence not only of primary tumours of the central and peripheral nervous system but also of systemic malignancy. One in five patients with disseminated malignancy develop neurological complications other than neurogenic pain. The majority of neurological problems in patients with systemic malignancy are the direct consequence of metastatic disease or the result of metabolic disorders. Neurological disorders may be due to anti-neoplastic treatments or the administration of drugs frequently used in cancer patients. The incidence of CNS infections and Vascular lesions is also increased in malignant disease, and the causes often differ from those seen in general population. In addition, a small proportion of neurological disorders seen in cancer patients are paraneoplastic resulting from a remote effect of cancer on the nervous system. All the causes may also contribute to neurological deficit seen in patients with primary tumours of the nervous system although direct effect of the tumour is clearly of primary importance.

Most neurological lesions in cancer patients are rapidly progressive and potentially life threatening, and have a profound effect on the quality of life. The initial steps in management require a rapid identification of the nature and location of the pathogenic process. The treatment outcome frequently depends as much on the speed of diagnosis as on the subsequent therapy.

While modern neuroimaging provides invaluable clues to the diagnosis of nervous system lesions they need to be interpreted in the light of clinical data. Clinical examination therefore remains a cornerstone of the differential diagnosis of neurological lesions affecting the cancer patient.

The aim of this book is to help the clinician to reach the correct diagnostic and therapeutic decision. It takes as the starting point the most common neurological syndromes occurring in cancer patients. Each chapter then follows an identical sequence with the causes of the neurological deficit considered in a standard order of (a) neoplastic, (b) treatment related, (c) infectious, (d) vascular and (e) paraneoplastic lesions, and is concluded with a section on treatment. The final chapter deals with the management of the most common primary and metastatic CNS tumours.

Contents

Abbreviations

AA	anaplastic astrocytoma
ACTH	adrenocorticotrophic hormone
ADH	antidiuretic hormone
AL	acute leukaemia
ALL	acute lymphoblastic leukaemia
ALS	amyotrophic lateral sclerosis
AML	acute myeloblastic leukaemia
Ara-C	cytosine arabinoside
AZQ	diaziquone
BAEP	brainstem auditory evoked potentials
BBB	blood-brain barrier
BCNU	carmustine
BNCT	boron neutron capture therapy
BPA	p-boromophenylalanine
BTCG	brain tumour cooperative group
BUdR	5-bromodeoxyuridine
CAR	cancer-associated retinopathy
CCG	Children's Cancer Group
CCNU	[1-(2-chloroethyl-3-cyclohexyl-1-nitzosourea (Lomustine®)
CCSG	children cancer study group
CHOP	cyclophosphamide, Adriamycin·, vincristine, and prednisone
CIDP	chronic inflammatory demyelinating polyneuropathy
CK	creatinine kinase
CMAP	compound muscle action potential
CMV	cytomegalovirus
CNS	central nervous system
CR	complete response
CRF	corticotrophin-releasing factor
CSF	cerebrospinal fluid
CT	computed tomography
CUSA	cavitron ultrasound aspiration
DIC	disseminated intravascular coagulation
DTPA	diethylenetriaminepentaacetic acid
EBV	Epstein-Barr virus
EEG	electroencephalograph
EMG	electromyograph(y)
FLAIR	fluid attenuation inversion recovery
FSH	follicle-stimulating hormone
GBM	glioblastoma
GH	growth hormone

GnLH	gonadotrophin
GnRH	gonadotrophin-releasing hormone
hCG	human chorionic gonadotrophin
HeCNU	(1-(2-hydroxyethyl)-3-(2 chloroethyl)-3-nitrosourea (no trade name)
5-HIAA	5-hydroxyindole acetic acid
HRS	high-rate stimulation
ICHT	intracranial hypertension
IGF-1	insulin growth factor 1
im	intramuscular(ly)
IPS	inferior petrosal sinuses
IUdR	5-iododeoxyuridine
iv	intravenous(ly)
Ivt	intraventricular
LDH	lactate dehydrogenase
LET	linear energy transfer (radiation)
LH	luteinizing hormone
MDP	methyldiphosphonate
MGUS	monoclonal gammopathy of undetermined significance
MMSE	Mini-Mental State Examination
MND	motor neuron disease
MOPP	Mechlorethamine (= $N+1_2$; O_2 nitrogen mustard) vincristine, procarbazine, prednisone
MRI	magnetic resonance imaging
MTX	methotrexate
NBTE	non-bacterial thrombotic endocarditis
NCI	National Cancer Institute
NF1	type 1 neurofibromatosis
NF2	type 2 neurofibromatosis
NSCLC	non-small-cell lung cancer
PALA	N-phosphoacetyl-L-aspartate
PCD	paraneoplastic cerebellar degeneration
PCNSL	primary non-Hodgkin's CNS lymphoma
PCNU	1-(2-chloroethyl)-3 (2,6- dioxo-3-piperidyl-1-nitrosourea)
PCR	polymerase chain reaction
PCV	procarbazine, CCNU, vincristine
PET	positron emission tomography
PML	progressive multifocal leucoencephalopathy
PNET	primitive neuroectodermal tumour
PNS	peripheral nervous system
po	orally
POG	Paediatric Oncology Group
PR	partial response
PRF	prolactin-releasing factor
PSA	prostate specific autigen

PTHrp	parathyroid-hormone-related peptide
RNS	repetitive nerve stimulation
RTOG	Radiation Therapy Oncology Group
SCLC	small-cell lung cancer
SIOP	International Society of Pediatric Oncology
T_3	triiodothyronine
T_4	thyroxine
TRH	thyrotrophin-releasing hormone
TSH	thyroid-stimulating hormone
VHL	von Hippel–Lindau (disease)
WBRT	whole-brain radiation therapy
WI	weighted image

1 Altered consciousness

Introduction

This chapter is concerned with impairment of consciousness due to an *altered state of arousal ranging from somnolence to coma but not to a deficit of cognitive or mental function*. The latter situation, where patients are fully awake but demonstrate cognitive disorders such as impairment in memory, disorientation in time and space, or global dementia, is considered separately (Chapter 2).

Such a distinction between arousal and cognitive changes is justified for two reasons. The cause and mechanism of the two conditions are usually different. Altered arousal is a medical emergency requiring a rapid diagnosis and therapy, while most cognitive disorders, including progressive global dementia, generally do not require immediate intervention.

The distinction between altered consciousness and impaired cognitive function is not easy, and sometimes not even possible. A typical example is the **confusional state** which combines reduced wakefulness, perhaps including irritability and hyperexcitability (delirium), with cognitive disorder such as lack of attention, short-term memory deficit, and disorientation in time and space. The causes of confusional state are similar to those of more pronounced alteration of wakefulness. They present the same diagnostic and therapeutic challenge and degree of emergency, and will be considered in this chapter.

The clinical approach to a patient with altered state of consciousness followed here is largely based on the principles described by Plum and Posner in their book *The diagnosis of stupor and coma* (1). The arousal mechanism requires a non-specific stimulation of the cerebral cortex by an activating system. The most important activating structure, the **reticular formation**, is located in the rostral part of the brainstem and receives collateral input from major somatic and sensory pathways. Wakefulness (consciousness) may be altered either by a diffuse insult or dysfunction of the cerebral cortex, or by a focal lesion injuring the reticular formation. Metabolic or toxic extraneural pathological processes alter consciousness by affecting the entire cerebral cortex. Focal, cerebral lesions usually interfere with the ascending stimulation of the cerebral cortex.

Infratentorial lesions damage the reticular formation either through direct damage by an ischaemic, haemorrhagic, demyelinating, infectious, or tumoral process, or by compression. The majority of structural **supratentorial** lesions produce stupor and coma through a mass effect causing displacement and herniation of cerebral structures. Consequently, any asymmetry or focal abnormality on neurological examination in a patient with altered consciousness favours a focal primary brain lesion. A neurological examination without focal deficit favours a metabolic or a toxic aetiology. The principal aim of the neurological examination of a comatose patient is therefore to try to distinguish

Table 1.1　Main points of the neurological examination allowing differentiation between primary neurological and metabolic or toxic causes of altered consciousness

Clinical feature	Primary brain lesion		Metabolic or toxic disorder
	Occurrence	Location	
Respiration			
Cheyne-Stokes type		Bilateral deep-hemispheric or diencephalon	Uraemia Hypoxia
Hyperpnoea (hyperventilation)	Rare	Hypothalamus (pulmonary oedema)	Metabolic acidosis Respiratory alkalosis Regular
Rate	May be irregular		
Apneustic			
Cluster breathing		Pons	
Ataxic		Pons	
Needs voluntary control		Medulla	
Eye examination			
Conjugate horizontal deviation	Ipsilateral	Frontal Pons	Absent (eyes staight ahead)
Oculocephalic caloric response	Present or ╱	Hemispheres	Brisk or ╱
	Absent	Midbrain	
Skew deviation		Dorsal pons	Absent
Pupillary size	May be unequal	IIIrd nerve, ipsilateral dilatation	Equal
Pupillary light reflex	Absent	Midbrain	Present
Motor activity (spontaneous or to pain)			
Muscle tone	May be asymmetric	Corticospinal tract	Symmetric
Tendon and cutaneous reflexes			
Babinski sign	Uni- or bilateral		Rarely present (hypoglycaemia)

╱, Decreased or difficult to elicit.

a metabolic from a primary neurological cause of altered consciousness. The main points of this examination are summarized in Table 1.1.

Before performing the neurological examination it is important to ensure that brain is supplied with adequate oxygen and glucose. It is also essential to obtain a detailed history from carers, particularly concerning drug consumption and possible metabolic disorders.

Clinical presentation

Metabolic and toxic encephalopathies

The clinical manifestation of altered consciousness due to metabolic or toxic changes ranges from mild confusional state to coma. Occasionally patients may be delirious and irritable, with reactions of fear and hallucinations. With the possible exception of unilateral or bilateral upgoing plantar response, focal neurological deficit is not found. Alteration of arousal is, next to pain, the second most common symptom in patients referred to the Neurology Service of the Memorial Sloan Kettering Cancer Center (2). Of 132 such patients, metabolic or drug-related encephalopathy was present in 80 (61%) and was the most frequent non-metastatic neurological manifestation of systemic cancer.

Structural intracranial lesions

Supratentorial space-occupying lesions

Supratentorial space-occupying lesions alter consciousness though intracranial hypertension (ICHT) and inadequate adjustment to the growing intracranial mass resulting in displacement of cerebral structures, herniation, and hydrocephalus.

The cardinal manifestations of ICHT are headache, vomiting, and papilloedema. **Headache** is the most common presenting symptom. It tends to be frontal (Vth nerve territory) in supratentorial, and occipital (IXth and Xth territory) in posterior fossa space-occupying lesions. It is exacerbated at night, by coughing, straining or Valsalva manoeuvre. **Vomiting** may be sudden and may occur without nausea. **Papilloedema** is a classical sign of ICHT in older children and adults. Patients may also complain of transient obscuring of vision. Prolonged ICHT may produce bradycardia and systemic hypertension. Sixth nerve palsy is common in ICHT but has no localizing value. Brain lesions causing uniformly distributed ICHT are associated with little clouding of consciousness, but focal expanding processes with structural displacement and herniation lead to altered consciousness.

Herniation can occur at three sites: the falx cerebri, the incision of the tentorium cerebelli, and the foramen magnum (Fig. 1.1). In **subfalcine herniation**, seen principally in unilateral frontal lesions, the cingulate gyrus herniates beneath the lower edge of the falx. This displacement often remains asymptomatic. Neurological deficit occurs when the ipsilateral anterior cerebral artery is compressed. Lateral displacement of midline is associated with alteration of consciousness, which is proportional to the magnitude of the shift (3).

Lateral transtentorial herniation is caused by mass lesion of the temporal fossa. The median edge of the temporal lobe (uncus or hippocampal gyrus) herniates through the tentorial hiatus, causing compression of the midbrain. The usual initial sign is ipsilateral unresponsive dilated pupil followed by IIIrd nerve palsy, contralateral hemiparesis, and depression of consciousness. The herniating structure may push the midbrain against the opposite edge of the tentorium, causing false localizing signs such as ipsilateral weakness or Babinski sign. Central diencephalic or diffuse hemispheric lesions may cause vertical displacement through the tentorial hiatus, leading to a **central transtentorial herniation** where hemispheres and basal nuclei are displaced caudally, compressing the structures of the

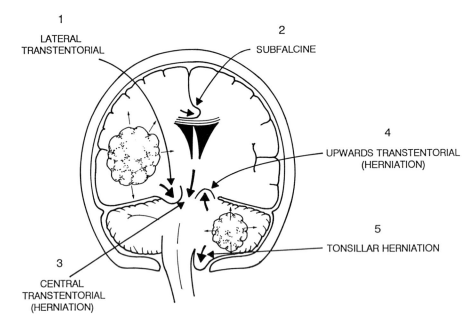

Fig. 1.1 Coronal section of the brain schematically showing the five types of herniation described in the text.

diencephalon and the brainstem. Clinically, pupils evolve from small and reactive to symmetrically dilated and fixed. Respiration gradually changes from periodic Cheyne–Stokes pattern to an ataxic breathing, irregular in amplitude and rate, and consciousness is progressively lost.

Expanding posterior fossa lesions

Expanding posterior fossa lesions may cause an upwards transtentorial **herniation** of the brainstem and cerebellar structures. Acute displacement starts with loss of upward gaze and may evolve into loss of consciousness and death. Upwards transtentorial herniation is often complicated by obstructive hydrocephalus.

Posterior fossa tumours may cause **tonsilar herniation**, which also complicates central transtentorial herniation. Tonsilar displacement in the foramen magnum produces neck stiffness, head tilt, and, less commonly, ataxia and nystagmus. Eventually pressure results in compression of the medulla, causing respiratory irregularities, apnoea, and death. Tonsilar herniation may be accelerated by inappropriate lumbar puncture.

The main aim of the neurological examination performed in patients with impaired consciousness is to determine whether the cause is systemic (i.e. metabolic or toxic) or primarily neurological. While focal deficit may help to localize the brain lesion, in stuporous or comatose patients the neurological examination is fragmentary. In addition ICHT, displacement of brain structures, and herniations frequently cause 'false localizing' signs.

It is important to emphasize that, unlike the supratentorial lesions, most posterior fossa lesions impair consciousness by destroying or directly compressing the reticular formation. They do not need to displace brainstem structures to alter arousal, although both the upwards transtentorial and the tonsilar herniation may contribute to loss of consciousness.

Meningeal syndrome

The search for meningeal signs is important in any patient with impaired consciousness but particularly in patients with cancer. Even though rare (about 0.4% of all cancer patients), subarachnoid bleeding or CNS infections are more common in cancer patients than in the general population. In addition, neoplastic meningitis, occurring in about 5% of patients with cancer, may alter consciousness.

The clinical presentation of leptomeningeal diseases in cancer patients may be misleading. In leptomeningeal metastases, signs of meningeal irritation and altered consciousness may be combined with cranial nerve and spinal root palsies. In meningeal infections in immuno-suppressed and severely leucopenic patients, typical meningitic symptoms and signs, including neck stiffness, may be very mild or even absent. In this category of patients even fever may not be a prominent feature, and cerebrospinal fluid (CSF) analysis may show surprisingly low leucocyte counts. Signs of meningeal irritation may also disappear in deeply comatose patients.

Main aetiologies

The main causes of consciousness alteration in cancer patients are summarized in Table 1.2.

Neoplastic lesions

1. Primary brain tumours and brain metastases

Impaired consciousness is rarely a presenting feature in patients with primary or metastatic cerebral tumours. However, this may occur in intracerebral or intratumoral haemorrhage, post-ictal state, pituitary apoplexy, or sterile meningitis.

Symptomatic **bleeding** may occur in patients with primary tumours, mainly glioblastoma (Fig. 1.2.) and oligodendroglioma, and in patients with brain metastases. The distribution of the main primary cancers giving rise to brain metastases is shown in Table 1.3. Brain metastases are, next to coagulation abnormalities, the most common cause of intracerebral bleeding in patients with systemic cancer (5). Metastases most frequently associated with intracerebral haemorrhage originate from germ-cell tumours (haemorrhagic in 59%) or melanoma (31%). Bleeding is uncommon in lung cancer metastases (5%) and breast cancer brain metastases (0.9%).

Seizure may be an early manifestation of primary and metastatic brain tumours (see Chapter 3). Post-ictal state may occasionally present as a **coma** of unknown origin.

Pituitary apoplexy has been reported in 5% of patients (14 out of 300) with pituitary tumours (6). In 1.6% of patients (5 out of 300), pituitary apoplexy was the presenting symptom of pituitary adenoma. In pituitary apoplexy infarction or haemorrhage cause an acute enlargement of the pituitary tumour (Fig. 1.3). The clinical presentation is sudden, with

Table 1.2   Main causes of altered consciousness in cancer patients

Lesions	Causes
Neoplastic	1. Primary or metastatic
	Intratumoural haemorrhage
	Post-ictal state
	Pituitary apoplexy
	Aseptic meningitis
	2. Leptomeningeal metastases
	3. Systemic (extraneural) metastases
Treatment related	1. Chemotherapy, mainly in high dose or intra-CSF
	2. Radiation therapy; acute or early delayed manifestations
	3. Neurosurgery, aseptic meningitis
	4. Supportive treatments: analgesics, sedative agents, anti-epileptics, antidepressants, antipsychiatric drugs, cyclosporin A
Infectious	Abscess, meningitis, meningoencephalitis, encephalitis
Vascular	Intracerebral haemorrhage
	Subarachnoid haemorrhage
	Non-bacterial thrombotic endocarditis
	Disseminated intravascular coagulation
Paraneoplastic	Paraneoplastic opsoclonus without antibody (rare)
	Endocrinopathies

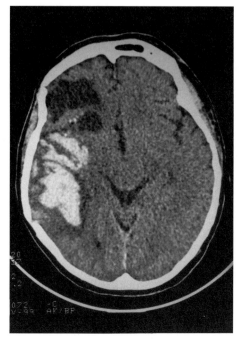

Fig. 1.2   CT scan showing intracerebral bleeding causing declined consciousness in a patient with recurrent glioblastoma.

Table 1.3 Distribution of primary tumours in brain metastases

Primary tumour	Rate	
	Average (%)	Range (%)
Lung	39	22–65
Breast	19	6–39
Melanoma	6	2–16
Digestive tract	5	1–7
Kidney	5	3–9
Unknown	13	6–19

Adapted from J. Hildebrand (4).

severe headache, visual loss attributed to optic chiasma compression, ocular nerve palsy, stupor, and coma. While fever and CSF hypertension and pleocytosis may suggest infectious meningitis, the syndrome is due to chemical irritation by tumour-released lipid material.

Acute sterile meningitis seen in pituitary apoplexy has also been described following a rupture of epidermoid cysts (7) or craniopharyngiomas.

2. *Leptomeningeal metastases*
Despite CNS prophylaxis, leptomeningeal metastases are seen in less than 10% of patients with acute leukaemia (see Chapter 12, p. 264). The distribution of solid tumours causing leptomeningeal metastases, reported in four studies published between 1960 and 1990, is shown

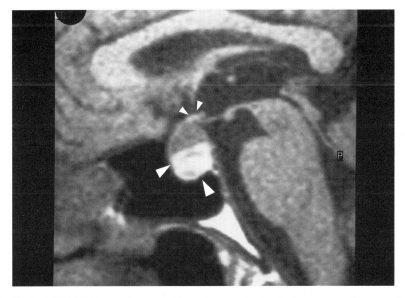

Fig. 1.3 Sagittal T_1WI MR scan demonstrating a haemorrhagic pituitary macroadenoma. The bleeding involves the lower part of the pituitary (large arrows); the optic chiasma is compressed (small arrows).

Table 1.4 Distribution of primary tumours in leptomeningeal metastases

Authors (reference)	Number of cases	Percentage occurrence						
		Lung	Breast	Digestive tract (stomach only)	Melanoma	Lymphoma	Unknown	Other
Brucher and Cervos-Navaro, 1960 (8)	48	33	6	43 (33)	–	0	4	13
Little et al., 1974 (9)	29	24	31	17 (14)	–	0	7	21
Olson et al., 1974 (10)	50	16	36	4	10	28	2	4
Drlicek et al., 1990 (11)	102	37	28	–	14	–	–	23

in Table 1.4. The apparent variation between the studies is due to differences in referral patterns and the declining incidence of gastric carcinoma in the West. Leptomeningeal metastases also occur in primary brain tumours, particularly medulloblastomas (12),
ependymomas (13), and germ-cell tumours (14). The clinical presentation is a widespread
multifocal involvement of the central and peripheral nervous system, causing raised intracranial pressure, confusional state, seizures, meningeal signs and spinal root and cranial nerve
palsies (15). Out of 102 patients studied by Grisold *et al.*, 16 had a decreased level of consciousness, often at diagnosis (15).

Leptomeningeal metastases may be demonstrated by contrast-enhanced magnetic resonance
imaging (MRI) in about 70% of patients (Fig. 1.4). The diagnosis is confirmed by the presence
of neoplastic cells in the CSF, and this may be accompanied by low glucose and high protein.
Biological markers, such as human chorionic gonadotrophin or α-fetoprotein, are useful in the
diagnosis of germ-cell tumour dissemination (see Chapter 6, p. 108). The CSF concentrations of
β-glucoronidase and lactate dehydrogenase (LDH) isoenzyme are frequently elevated in leptomeningeal metastases. However, their practical use is limited by the lack of specificity.

3. Systemic metastases

Systemic metastases may cause metabolic encephalopathy and alter consciousness by damaging the function of several vital organs. The main metastatic locations causing

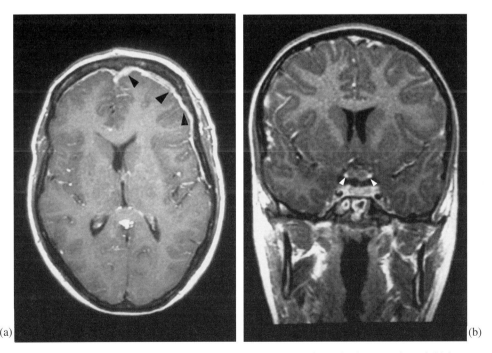

(a)   (b)

Fig. 1.4 T_1WI gadolinium-enhanced MR scans, showing: (a) an irregular leptomeningeal thickening (arrows) in a patient with widespread meningeal carcinomatosis originating from prostate cancer;
(b) a leptomeningeal acute leukaemia infiltrating the optic nerves (arrow).

encephalopathies are summarized in Table 1.5. They include bones (causing hypercalcaemia), digestive tract and mesenteries (causing vitamin deficiency, malabsorption, hypocalcaemia), urinary tract obstruction (uraemia), lung (anoxia) and liver (hepatic encephalopathy and hyperammonaemia).

Treatment-related complications

1. Chemotherapy

Cancer patients frequently receive multimodal therapy, and it is frequently difficult to identify a single factor responsible for the observed neurotoxicity. Both additive and synergistic toxicities are possible. But synergism between radiation and chemotherapy has been clearly demonstrated, mainly for methotrexate (see Fig. 2.3). All cytotoxic agents used in anticancer therapy have demonstrated neurotoxicity when in direct contact with the CNS. However, CNS complications are infrequent because very few agents cross the blood–brain barrier. Therefore, most CNS neurotoxicities are observed when the blood–brain barrier is either circumvented (when the drugs are administrated in the CSF) or overwhelmed by high systemic doses or intra-arterial administration.

Methotrexate may be used for intra-CSF injection or in systemic high doses, and is the most frequent agent causing chemotherapy-induced encephalopathy. About half of the treated patients will develop a transient meningeal reaction after either prophylactic or therapeutic intra-CSF injection of methotrexate. However, only a few will progress to a confusional state. Symptoms and signs of encephalopathy usually start within few hours following treatment initiation and resolve within 72 hours (16). CSF pleocytosis is frequent. Concomitant radiation therapy and overt meningeal leukaemia increase the risk of methotrexate encephalopathy. Acute encephalopathy has also been observed in a few patients following high-dose methotrexate. The patients present with altered consciousness, ranging from somnolence to coma, which in most cases clears spontaneously within 48 hours (17).

Cytosine arabinoside and **5-fluorouracil** are two antipyrimidines known primarily to cause cerebellopathy (see Chapter 4) although both (18–20) may also cause acute encephalopathy. The CNS toxicity of 5-fluorouracil may be enhanced by **levamizole** (21).

Cisplatin is highly neurotoxic. Focal and diffuse cortical disorders are frequent after intra-arterial administration (22), but rare after systemic chemotherapy. The neurotoxic effect of the drug must be differentiated from electrolyte imbalance, such as hypomagnesaemia due to renal toxicity or excessive hydration.

Vincristine encephalopathy is rare when the drug is used intravenously (23,24). However, vincristine is extremely neurotoxic for the CNS, invariably causing death after erroneous intrathecal injection. It has been postulated that the CNS toxicity of intravenous vincristine may be due to local destruction of the blood–brain barrier. In rare cases, encephalopathy has been attributed to secretion of antidiuretic hormone as a result of the direct action of vincristine on the hypothalamus or the peripheral volume receptors, causing hyponatraemia (25).

Symptoms of usually mild encephalopathy, such as lassitude, sedation, or drowsiness, may be seen when **procarbazine**, a monoamine oxidase inhibitor, is given orally at a daily dose of 150 mg or more (26,27). The drug also has a synergistic sedative effect when combined with barbiturates and phenothiazines. Severe encephalopathy is the main limiting factor for the intravenous use of procarbazine.

Table 1.5 Acute metabolic enceophalopathies in cancer patients

Metabolic disorder	Paraneoplastic production	Other causes related to cancer	Treatment
Hypercalcemia	Parathyroid hormone-related peptide, 1,25–hydroxy vitamin D	Bone metastases, multiple myeloma	Bisphosphonates, saline infusion corticosteroids
Hypocalcemia		Malabsorption postradiation lesions, mesenteric metastases renal wasting of Mg and Ca caused by cisplatin	Intravenous or oral calcium Intravenous oral magnesium 1,25 di OH vitamin D
Hypophosphatemia	Deficit in 1,25-hydroxy vitamin D (?): other unknown factors, PTHrp	Cachexia, excesive glucose perfusion Respiratory alkalosis	K phosphate < 60 mEq /24h
Hypernatremia	ACTH (moderate)	Hemoconcentration, posterior pituitary metastases, cisplatin nephrotoxicity	Hydration, antidiuretic hormone
Hyponatremia	Inappropriate secretion of antidiuretic hormone	Vincristine, cyclophosphamide Excessive hydration + chemotherapy Adrenal insufficiency (metastases): rare	Urea, demeclocycline, water restriction, NaCl + furosemide, anti AVP (V_2) receptor, hydrocortisone (adrenal insufficiency)
Hypomagnesemia		Nephrotoxic chemotherapy (cisplatin)	
Hypoglycemia	Insulin, insulinlike products	Excessive consumption by tumour cells (?), insulinoma	Glucose infusion, somatostatin analogs, diazoxide
Hyperglycemia	ACTH, glucagon, somatostatin	Glucocorticosteroid therapy	
Uremia		Urinary tract obstruction Nephrotoxic chemotherapy	
Anoxia, anoxemia		Severe anemia, heart failure (doxorubicin) Primary or metastatic lung tumours, lung infections or thrombo-emboli Interstitial lung diseases (pneumocystis, CMV, carcinomatous lymphangitis)	
Hepatic failure		Liver primary or matastatic tumours I-Asparaginase	
Carcinoid syndrome	Serotonine ↑ in serum, ↓ in brain (?) ↑ 5OH indol. acet. ac. in urine	Carcinoid tumours	Somatostatine, interferon α
A vitamin deficiency [Wernicke's encephalopathy]	Anorexia due to tumour necrotic factor and other cytokines	Digestive tract tumours Treatment related anorexia & vomiting	
Hyperviscosity syndrome	IgM hyperproduction		Plasmapheresis

L-**Asparaginase** may produce alteration in consciousness ranging from confusion to coma. This is caused primarily by hepatic failure (28,29) or, much less frequently, by thrombosis of intracranial venous sinuses (30).

Acute, usually reversible, encephalopathy has been reported with several **alkylating agents**, including nitrogen mustard (31), chlorambucil (32), high-dose nitrosoureas (33), and ifosfamide (34). High-dose **etoposide** therapy has produced an acute confusion, somnolence and papilloedema in patients treated for malignant melanoma (35). **Interferons**, whether administered intrathecally or systemically, may produce emotional lability, delirium, and clouding of consciousness (36).

2. Radiation therapy

A syndrome combining headaches, nausea, drowsiness, and somnolence may occur within 2 weeks of the onset of radiation therapy, or shortly after its completion, in patients treated for brain tumours. The syndrome is more severe in patients with pre-existing ICHT and high daily doses (37).

A transient somnolence of varying degree has been reported (38) in leukaemic children after prophylactic cranial irradiation. Younger children tend to have more severe symptoms. This syndrome occurs 6–8 weeks after the completion of radiation therapy.

3. Neurosurgery

An aseptic meningitis with alteration in consciousness has been reported occasionally after neurosurgery. The pathogenesis of this syndrome remains poorly understood (39).

4. Supportive treatments

Among drugs currently used in supportive care of cancer patients, sedatives and benzodi-azepines, analgesics (morphine and its derivatives), antidepressants (amitriptyline, doxepine, trazodone, and others), neuroleptics (phenothiazines, butyrophenones), and anti-epileptics (especially phenobarbital at high serum concentrations, 20 μg/ml or more, vigabatrin, and sodium valproate) may cause or aggravate somnolence. In patients treated with valproate, encephalopathy with severe decline of consciousness may also be related to an elevated ammonium level without hepatic dysfunction (40). **Cyclosporin A** has been reported to cause mild encephalopathy, in the form of a confusional state, in up to 30% of patients (41). Oral administration may decrease cyclosporin neurotoxicity (42).

Infections

In cancer patients, many factors contribute to the increased incidence of CNS infections. Patients with malignant diseases are frequently immuno- and myelosuppressed, due to tumour involve-ment (bone marrow disease), anticancer therapy (chemotherapy, bone marrow transplantation, radiation), glucocorticosteroid administration, and neurosurgical intervention (shunt, reservoir). Most CNS infections are due to opportunistic pathogens (Table 1.6). Opportunistic CNS infec-tions are seen particularly in patients with Hodgkin's and non-Hodgkin's lymphoma, and leukaemia. Impairment of consciousness may be the presenting feature in all CNS infections, especially acute bacterial meningoencephalitis and herpes simplex encephalitis.

Table 1.6 Main opportunistic organisms causing CNS infections

Most common nervous infection	Agent	Predisposing factors	Frequency
Radiculomyelitis	Herpes zoster-varicella	T-lymphocyte, mononuclear defect	Very frequent
Meningitis and meningoencephalitis	*Listeria monocytogenes*	T-lymphocyte, mononuclear defect	Frequent
	Enteric bacilli	Neutropenia, surgery	
	Staphylococcus aureus	Head and neck surgery	
	Staphylococcus epidermidis	CSF shunt, Ommaya reservoir	
	Streptococcus pneumoniae	Splenectomy	
	Cryptococcus neoformans	T-lymphocyte, mononuclear defect	Frequent
Abscess	*Nocardia asteroides*	T-lymphocyte, mononuclear defect	
	Enteric bacilli	Neutropenia, neurosurgery	
	Staphylococcus aureus	Neutropenia, neurosurgery	
	Aspergillus sp.	Neutropenia, bone-marrow transplantation	
	Cryptococcus neoformans	T-lymphocyte, mononuclear defect	
	Toxoplasma gondii	T-lymphocyte, mononuclear defect	
Encephalitis	Papovavirus (progressive multifocal leucoencephalopathy)	T-lymphocyte, mononuclear defect	
	Herpes simplex	Possibly immunodepression	
	Toxoplasma gondii	T-lymphocyte, mononuclear defect	

Vascular lesions

The most frequent cause of intracerebral bleeding in cancer patients, mainly in acute leukaemia, are coagulation abnormalities. The second most common cause is intratumoral bleeding, which may mimic haemorrhagic stroke and lead to rapid loss of consciousness. As in the general population, intracerebral haemorrhage may be caused by systemic hypertension (5). Subdural or subarachnoid bleeding may alter consciousness. It occurs preferentially in leukaemic and thrombocytopenic patients.

Alteration of consciousness is uncommon following ischaemic stroke involving supratentorial structures. It may occur in very large lesions surrounded by cytogenic oedema causing herniation and developing 48–72 hours following the onset of stroke. In cancer patients, ischaemic lesions are often multiple and alteration of consciousness is more frequent. The main causes of ischaemic lesions in cancer patients are non-bacterial thrombotic endocarditis (NBTE, also called marantic endocarditis), and disseminated intravascular coagulation (DIC). The pathogenesis of NBTE and DIC may not differ fundamentally, but they differ statistically in their neurological presentation. In NBTE the most common presentation is with abrupt focal deficit and seizures, although diffuse encephalopathy and decreased arousal may be eventually seen. Cerebral infarcts caused by DIC are multiple and smaller and, when symptomatic, tend to produce a diffuse encephalopathy with altered consciousness.

Paraneoplastic diseases

Altered consciousness is not a common feature of neurological paraneoplastic disorders, including the early stages of limbic encephalitis (see Chapter 2, p. 37, 38). The only exception are adults with paraneoplastic opsoclonus without anti-Ri antibodies (see Chapter 6, p. 108). The majority of these patients have underlying small-cell lung cancer and up to 25% progress to stupor or coma (43).

Paraneoplastic endocrinopathies, resulting from the production of excess hormone or hormone-like substances by the tumour cells (mainly small-cell lung carcinoma) may cause metabolic encephalopathy with alteration in consciousness. Several examples are listed in Table 1.5. Production of parathyroid-hormone-related peptide or of 1,25-hydroxy-vitamin D cause hypercalcaemia. Adrenocorticotrophic hormone (ACTH) production may cause hypernatraemia or hyperglycaemia. Hypoglycaemia may be due to the production of insulin or insulin-like products, and inappropriate secretion of antidiuretic hormone may be responsible for hyponatraemia.

Investigations

Figure 1.5 shows the diagnostic algorithm in cancer patients developing alteration of consciousness. The differential diagnosis of altered consciousness is first based on neurological examination, which allows the distinction of three groups of patients:

(1) without focal neurological or meningeal signs;

(2) with meningeal signs; and

(3) with focal neurological deficits.

1. Absence of focal signs

Absence of focal signs, or of clinical features listed in Table 1.1, suggests a toxic or metabolic encephalopathy.

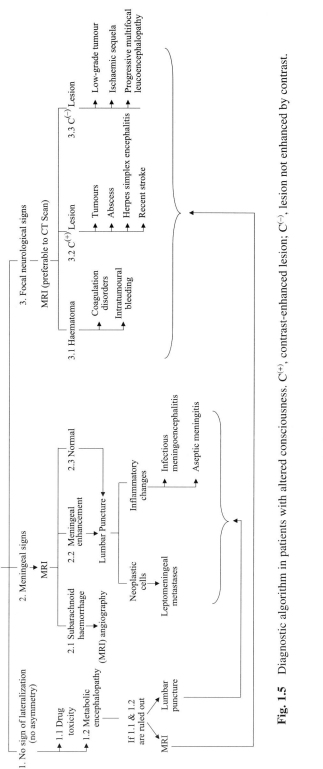

Fig. 1.5 Diagnostic algorithm in patients with altered consciousness. $C^{(+)}$, contrast-enhanced lesion; $C^{(-)}$, lesion not enhanced by contrast.

1.1 Drug toxicity Toxic, mainly drug-induced, encephalopathy is often suggested by the patient's history and may be confirmed for certain drugs by the determination of serum concentration. Many patients with cancer are on chemotherapy and only a few develop drug-related encephalopathy, as most antineoplastic agents do not cross the blood–brain barrier. Diagnosis of a decline in consciousness due to chemotherapy at conventional doses should be accepted with great caution and should be considered the diagnosis of exclusion.

1.2 Metabolic encephalopathy Suspicion of metabolic changes requires a rapid determination of arterial Po_2 and Pco_2 levels, and of blood glucose, urea, creatinine, sodium, ammonia, calcium, phosphorus, and magnesium.

Absence of focal signs does not rule out the possibility of a primary structural brain lesion causing alteration of consciousness, but it makes it less likely. Therefore, when the diagnosis of a toxic or metabolic encephalopathy becomes unlikely, brain MRI or computed tomography (CT) scan and, if necessary, a lumbar puncture should be performed without delay. In many centres these examinations will probably be initiated in parallel with the investigations of metabolic disorders.

2. *Presence of meningeal signs*

Signs of meningeal irritation may be caused by subarachnoid haemorrhage, leptomeningeal metastases, or infection. Brain MRI or CT scan is the first examination in patients with meningeal signs, before performing a lumbar puncture. This precaution will decrease the risk of tonsilar herniation and avoid unnecessary lumbar puncture, for example in patients with subarachnoid haemorrhage, as lumbar puncture in thrombocytopenic patients may cause symptomatic spinal subdural haematoma (44).

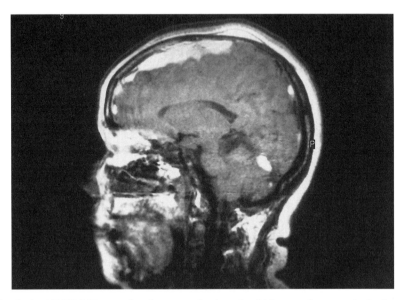

Fig. 1.6 Sagittal T_1WI MR scan showing several subarachnoid haemorrhages at the brain convexity and in the posterior fossa, and a subcutaneous haematoma, in a child with acute lymphoblastic leukaemia.

2.1 Subarachnoid haemorrhage   In cancer patients, the most common causes of subarachnoid haemorrhage are acute leukaemia and coagulation disorders (Fig. 1.6). The decision to perform angiography or MRI angiography to rule out an aneurysm should be considered in patients without a tendency to bleed (thrombocytopenia, DIC, anticoagulant therapy, or sepsis), and in patients without leptomeningeal or cortical brain metastases. Aneurysms are not an uncommon cause of subarachnoid haemorrhage, even in cancer patients (5).

2.2 Meningeal enhancement   In the presence of a meningeal contrast enhancement on CT or MRI, lumbar puncture should be performed. The presence of neoplastic cells is diagnostic of leptomeningeal metastases. However, the identification of the neoplastic cells may need repeated examinations (45), which are indicated especially when the CSF levels of glucose are low and proteins are elevated. While the identification of metastatic carcinoma cells is not difficult, inflammatory, predominantly T lymphocytes may be difficult to distinguish from lymphoma cells (usually of B type). The identification of cells from primary brain tumour may also pose difficult diagnostic problems (46).

CNS infections in cancer patients are often associated with immunosuppression and neutropenia. Inflammatory meningeal reaction and the clinical presentation, including fever and meningeal irritation, may therefore be subtle.

CSF examination is critical to the diagnosis of meningeal infection. It is advisable to collect CSF volumes in the region of 10 ml, as larger volumes increase the chance of detecting micro-organisms. The examination of centrifuged sediment, by appropriate staining for bacteria, mycobacteria, and fungi, also increases the diagnostic yield of CSF examination. *Cryptococcus neoformans* can be visualized by adding Indian ink to the sediment because the dye is excluded by the capsule that surrounds the organism. The CSF supernatant can then be used for the determination of glucose, protein, lactic acid, and detection of specific antigens. The CSF should be cultured unless the responsible agent is clearly identified. The polymerase chain reaction (PCR) is a sensitive method in the identification of herpes virus.

An inflammatory CSF reaction may follow intrathecal injection of various agents, including methotrexate, cytosine arabinoside, antibiotics, analgesic or anaesthetic drugs, or contrast dye. Aseptic meningitis may also complicate pituitary apoplexy and ruptured epidermoid cysts or craniopharyngiomas (6,7). It has also been described following neurosurgery (39). Aseptic meningitis mimics infectious meningitis clinically by producing signs of meningeal irritation and fever.

2.3 Normal MRI   In patients with normal MRI and meningeal signs, CSF analysis needs to be performed, as MRI is normal in about 30% of patients with leptomeningeal metastases and at least half of the cases with bacterial meningitis.

3. *Presence of focal neurological signs*
In the majority of patients with altered consciousness and focal neurological deficit, brain MRI and, in many patients CT scan, will show one or several lesions, which fall into three broad categories.

3.1 Haematoma   In the presence of intracranial haematomas coagulopathy and thrombocytopenia should be considered, particularly in patients with haematopoietic malignancy. In the absence of clotting disorders, intratumoral haemorrhage becomes the most likely diagnosis, particularly in patients with germ-cell tumours, melanoma, glioblastoma, or oligodendroglioma.

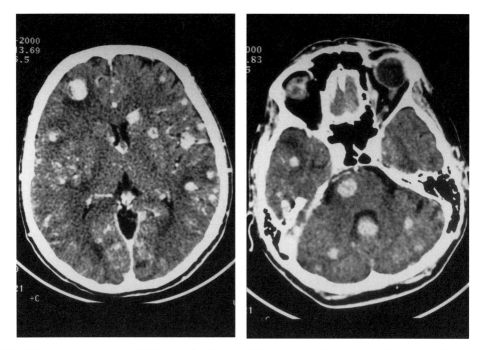

Fig. 1.7 Contrast-enhanced CT scan, showing multiple supra- and infratentorial breast carcinoma brain metastases.

3.2 C$^{(+)}$ lesion Focal contrast-enhanced single or multiple lesions, with or without mass effect, first evoke the diagnosis of primary or secondary tumours (Fig. 1.7). When such lesions are resectable, operation will be performed not only in patients in whom there is no evidence of a systemic primary cancer but also in patients known to harbour a systemic malignant disease who satisfy operability criteria such as a good general condition and reduced or controlled systemic cancer (see Chapter 12, p. 257). Operation will allow the definite diagnosis and may represent the first therapeutic step.

When to perform a diagnostic biopsy in patients with multiple or inoperable brain lesions suggesting malignant disease largely remains a matter of clinical judgement. In this situation, biopsy may reveal an unexpected pathology in up to 10% of patients. We tend to perform this procedure when:

1. The primary cancer has not been proven, particularly in patients with a normal chest radiograph and CT scan, which are the most contributive examinations in the search of primary tumour in patients with brain metastases of unknown origin (47). In such patients we do not perform lengthy investigations to find a putative primary tumour, which often unduly delays diagnosis and treatment, whereas brain biopsy may contribute to the identification of the primary tumour.

2. The location, the pathology, and the lack of progression of the primary tumour make the development of brain metastases unlikely.

3. The radiological aspect of the lesion suggests another pathology. Indeed, not all multiple neoplastic lesions are metastatic. Glioblastomas are multiple in about 5% of the

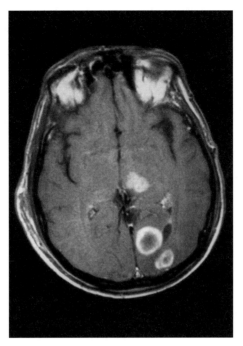

Fig. 1.8 Multiple bacterial abscesses demonstrated by gadolinium-enhanced T_1WI MR scan. The figure illustrates a late capsule stage, characterized by a complete capsule surrounding liquefied necrotic and inflammatory debris. At this mature stage brain oedema and mass effect may be discrete.

cases. Half of the patients with primary CNS lymphomas have multiple lesions at presentation. Typical radiological features may suggest the diagnosis of primary brain lymphoma (Fig. 2.2.) and biopsy should be performed before the administration of glucocorticosteroids as they produce a rapid and complete disappearance of the lesion (48) and jeopardize the chances of correct diagnosis.

The neoplastic nature of contrast-enhanced lesions should be questioned in patients with an increased risk for infection, because both the systemic and CNS manifestations of infection may be suppressed in immunodepressed or leucopenic cancer patients. Radiologically, brain abscesses may resemble brain metastases, as they are often multiple, may be surrounded by oedema, and show a ring-shaped contrast enhancement (Fig. 1.8). In immunosuppressed patients, an expanding temporal contrast-enhanced or unenhanced lesion, often surrounded by oedema raises the possibility of herpes simplex encephalitis (Fig. 1.9). The diagnosis can be confirmed rapidly by PCR performed on a CSF sample. High suspicion of brain abscess or herpes encephalitis should lead to appropriate medical treatment, and confirmation of the diagnosis in the case of a response to antibiotics. Biopsy should be performed if the treatment fails.

The diagnosis of ischaemic stroke should be considered in patients with risk factors such as bacterial or marantic endocarditis, DIC, or diffuse atherosclerosis. The uptake of contrast

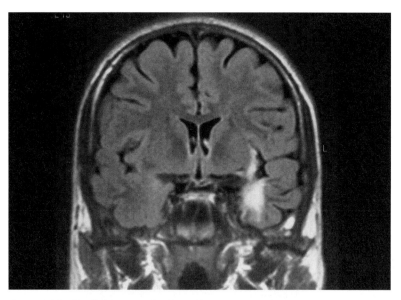

Fig. 1.9   Coronal FLAIR (fluid attenuation inversion recovery) MR scan showing a hyperintense lesion corresponding to herpes simplex virus encephalitis. The lesion typically predominates in the temporal lobe. In this case, the mass effect is mild and the lesion is unilateral.

medium parallels the breakdown of the blood–brain barrier and may persist for up to 2 months. In supratentorial ischaemic stroke, mass effect is necessary to cause consciousness disorders. This occurs in massive lesions with cytotoxic oedema, unresponsive to glucocor-ticosteroids (Fig. 1.10). Occasionally even smaller ischaemic lesions may be transiently expansive or space occupying and may be mistaken for tumoral lesions (Fig 1.11).

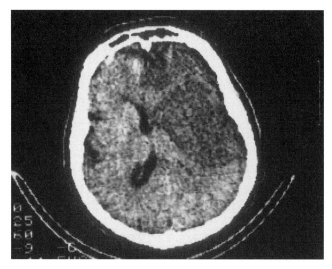

Fig. 1.10   Contrast-enhanced CT scan performed 3 days following stroke in a comatose patient. The ischaemic lesion involves the anterior and middle cerebral artery territories. Note the mass effect due to cytogenic oedema.

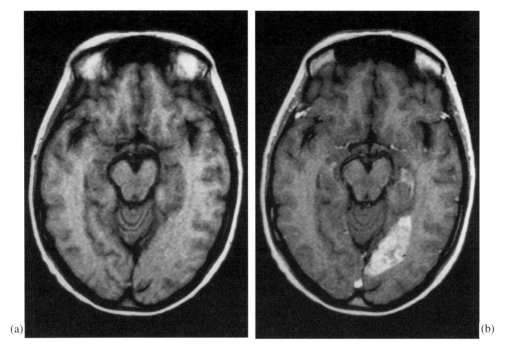

(a)   (b)

Fig. 1.11 Axial T₁WI MR scan of a recent ischaemic stroke involving the left temporal lobe (terminal territory of the posterior cerebral artery). (a) Before gadolinium administration the lesion produces a moderate mass effect. Note the vanishing of cortical sulci. (b) Enhancement of the infarcted area after gadolinium injection. Tumour diagnosis has been considered in this patient.

3.3 C$^{(-)}$ lesion Non-enhancing brain lesions usually represent low-grade tumours or the sequelae of ischaemic stroke. Low-grade tumours often produce mass effects, whereas old stroke lesions tend to cause adjacent cortical and subcortical atrophy (Fig. 2.10). Both pathologies rarely present with a decreased level of consciousness, unless cortically located, when they may cause seizures (see Chapter 3, p. 49, 50) and post-ictal stupor or coma.

Lesions due to progressive multifocal leucoencephalopathy (PML) generally do not enhance on CT or MRI (Fig. 1.12). PML usually presents with focal deficits, and in its early stages rarely causes altered consciousness.

Therapy

In cancer patients treatment intensity needs to take into account the overall prognosis. Just how intensive should be the management of a comatose patient with malignant disease depends on the extent of underlying malignancy, the availability and efficacy of anticancer treatment, age, and performance status prior to alteration of consciousness. Patients' and carers' wishes also need to be taken into account. Assuming reasonable life expectancy and recovery, the management of comatose patients consists of two phases: a prompt correction of the mechanism directly responsible for the declined consciousness (emergency treatment), and the treatment of the underlying malignant disease.

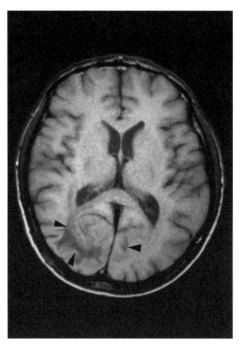

Fig. 1.12   Axial T₁WI MR scan in a lymphoma patient with progressive multifocal leucoencephalopathy. Confluent hypointense white matter lesions (arrows) predominate in the right occipital
lobe. Typically there is no mass effect and no gadolinium enhancement in most patients. The lesions
are hyperintense on T₂WI.

   The therapeutic algorithm proposed in Fig 1.13 is based on the initial distinction between
patients in whom consciousness alteration is caused by intracranial parenchymal or
meningeal lesions and those with toxic or metabolic encephalopathy. This algorithm is concerned only with the emergency treatment of altered level of consciousness.

1. Lesion with mass effect

The main causes of focal non-haemorrhagic intracranial lesions with mass effect are
tumours, abscess, or herpes encephalitis. In all these lesions, mass effect may be largely
due to surrounding vasogenic oedema, which usually responds to glucocorticosteroids
within 24 hours. In case of emergency it may be appropriate to use an intravenous bolus
of 100 mg dexamethasone followed by a daily dose of 16 mg. When glucocorticosteroids
cannot be used, osmotic diuretics (mannitol in a dose of 1 g/kg in 30-minute infusion
repeated several times a day, or glycerol 1.5 g/kg/day in six doses) effectively reduce vasogenic oedema surrounding brain tumours. Specific treatment of the underlying brain
tumour is considered in Chapter 12. If hydrocephalus participates to alteration in consciousness, external or internal ventricular drainage should be performed.
Glucocorticosteroids can also be used in conjunction with appropriate antibiotics or aci-
clovir in early treatment of bacterial abscess or herpes encephalitis when oedema appears
to be the major component of the mass effect.

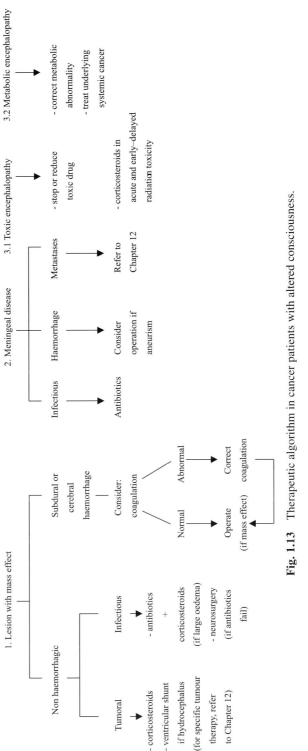

Fig. 1.13 Therapeutic algorithm in cancer patients with altered consciousness.

If a brain abscess does not respond to antibiotics, a stereotactic biopsy may be justified to identify the responsible organism and its antibiotic sensitivity. In patients with symptomatic mass effect, open surgery may be required.

In subdural or intracerebral haematoma, the use of glucocorticosteroids or osmotic diuretics remains unproven. Excision of haemorrhagic tumour may restore consciousness. In patients where thrombocytopenia or coagulation disorders cause the intracranial bleeding but preclude operation, the prognosis is very poor unless the coagulation disorder is corrected rapidly.

2. Meningeal disease

Suspected infectious meningeal disease requires rapid treatment with broad-spectrum antibiotics or antifungal drugs prior to definite identification of the organism. The treatment of the main opportunistic agents is given in Table 1.7. When subarachnoid haemorrhage is due to an aneurysm, operation should be considered in patients in good general condition and long life expectancy.

3. Toxic or metabolic encephalopathy

In patients with normal neuroimaging, the most likely cause of altered consciousness is toxic or metabolic encephalopathy.

Table 1.7   First-line treatment of main opportunistic CNS infections in cancer patients

Infectious agent	Therapy (empirical)[a]
Herpes simplex	Aciclovir, 10 mg/kg/t.i.d. for 14–21 days
Herpes zoster	Aciclovir, 10 mg/kg/t.i.d. for 14–21 days
Listeria monocytogenes	Ampicillin, 2 g × 6/day±gentamicin 1.5 mg/kg × 3/day for 3–6 weeks
E. coli	Third- or fourth-generation cephalosporins
Staphylococcus aureus	Vancomycin, 15 mg/kg b.i.d. for 6 weeks (abscess)
	Oxacillin, 2 g × 6/day (if sensitive)
Coagulase-negative staphylococci	
Streptococcus pneumoniae	Ceftriaxone, 2 g b.i.d. or t.i.d.; cefotaxime 2–4 g × 6/day[b]
	Penicillin G, 12×10^6 to 18×10^6 U/day for 10 days (if sensitive)
Cryptococcus neoformans	Amphotericin B, 0.5–1 mg/kg every 24 h plus fluorocytosine 40 mg/kg every 6 h until response, then fluconazole 400 mg × 2/day to 6–10 weeks
Aspergillus	Amphotericin B, 1 mg/kg every 24 h for 21 days (total dose 1–2 g)
Nocardia asteroides	Sulfadiazine, 1.5–3 g × 4/day for several months to 1 year
Toxoplasma gondii	Sulfadiazine, 1–2 g × 4/day plus pyrimethamine day 1: 100 mg total dose then 50 mg/day for 3–6 weeks plus folinic acid

a Antibiotic regimens must be adapted according to the sensitivity of the pathogen.
[b] Combination of vancomycin with the third-generation cephalosporin should be used in many geographical areas (see the local sensitivities of *Strep. pneumoniae*).
b.i.d, Twice a day; t.i.d., three times a day.

3.1 Toxic encephalopathy When consciousness alteration is attributed to chemotherapy, drug administration should be discontinued. Methylene blue may reverse the encephalopathy caused by ifosfamide (49). In L-asparaginase-induced encephalopathy or in side-effects attributed to several drugs used in supportive treatment, dose reduction may suffice. Corticosteroids are useful in acute and early delayed neurotoxicity of radiation therapy, probably by restoring the integrity of the blood–brain barrier.

3.2 Metabolic encephalopathy The management of metabolic encephalopathies combines treatment of the underlying neoplasia and a rapid symptomatic correction of the metabolic abnormality. Both the dysfunction of vital organs caused by systemic metastases, and the paraneoplastic endocrinopathies may respond to the treatment of neoplastic disease. However, even if successful, recovery is slow. The main symptomatic treatments of metabolic encephalopathies are summarized in Table 1.5. Rehydration and biphosphonates are the first-line therapy for hypercalcaemia. In patients with myeloma or lymphoma, hypercalcaemia responds to glucocorticosteroids, usually after a delay of 2–3 days. Hyponatraemia lasting for less than 48 hours may be corrected rapidly, but in chronic forms the increase in serum sodium should not exceed 15 mEq/litre per 24 hours to avoid brain oedema and osmotic demyelinating syndrome.

References

(1) Plum F, Posner JB. The diagnosis of stupor and coma. Davis, *Philadelphia*, 1987.
(2) Clouston PD, De Angelis LM, Posner JB. (1992). The spectrum of neurological disease in patients with systemic cancer. *Ann Neurol*, **31**, 268–273.
(3) Ropper AH. (1986). Lateral displacement of the brain and level of consciousness in patients with an acute hemispheral mass. *N Engl J Med*, **314**, 953–958.
(4) Hildebrand J. Lesions of the nervous system in cancer patients, Raven Press. New York, 1978.
(5) Graus F, Rogers LA, Posner JB. (1985). Cerebrovascular complications in patients with cancer. *Medicine (Baltimore)*, **64**, 16–35.
(6) Weisberg LA. (1977). Pituitary apoplexy. *Am J Med*, **63**, 109–115.
(7) Becker WJ, Watters GV, de Chadarevian JP, Vanasse M. (1984). Recurrent aseptic meningitis secondary to intracranial epidermoids. *Can J Neurol Sci*, **3**, 387–389.
(8) Brucher JM, Cervos-Navarro J. (1960). La carcinomatose méningée – Etude anatomoclinique de 11 cas. *Acta Neurol Psychiatr Belg*, **60**, 368–395.
(9) Little JR, Dale AJD, Okazaki H. (1974). Meningeal carcinomatosis. Clinical manifestations. *Arch Neurol*, **30**, 138–143.
(10) Olson ME, Chernik NL, Posner JB. (1974). Infiltration of leptomeninges by systemic cancer. A clinical and pathologic study. *Arch Neurol*, **30**, 122–137.
(11) Drlicek M, Liszka U, Grisold W *et al.* (1990). Clinical manifestations of meningeal carcinomatosis. *J Neurol (suppl)*, **237**, S4.
(12) Deutsch M, Reigel DH. (1981). Myelography and cytology in the treatment of medullobastoma. *Int J Radiat Oncol Biol Phys*, **7**, 721–725.
(13) Salazar OM. (1983). A better understanding of CNS seeding and a brighter outlook for post-operatively irradiated patients with ependymomas. *Int J Radiat Oncol Biol Phys*, **9**, 1231–1234.

(14) Bjornsson J, Scheithauer BW, Okazaki H, Leech RW. (1985). Intracranial germ cell tumors: Pathobiological and immuno-histological aspects of 70 cases. *J Neuropathol Exp Neurol*, **44**, 32–46.

(15) Grisold W, Drlicek M, Setinek U. (1998). LC: Clinical syndrome in different primaries. *J Neurooncol*, **38**, 103–110.

(16) Geiser CF, Bishop Y, Jaffe N *et al.* (1975). Adverse effects of intrathecal methotrexate in children with acute leukemia in remission. *Blood*, **45**, 189–195.

(17) Walker RW, Allen JC, Rosen G, Caparros B. (1986). Transient cerebral dysfunction secondary to high-dose methotrexate. *J Clin Oncol*, **4**, 1845–1850.

(18) Gottlieb D, Bradstock K, Koutts J *et al.* (1987). The neurotoxicity of high-dose cytosine arabinoside is age-related. *Cancer*, **60**, 1439–1441.

(19) Hwang TL, Yung WK, Estey EH, Fields WS. (1985). Central nervous system toxicity with high-dose Ara-C. *Neurology*, **35**, 1475–1479.

(20) Lynch HT, Droszcz CP, Albano WA, Lynch JF. (1981). Organic brain syndrome secondary to 5-fluorouracil toxicity. *Dis Colon Rectum*, **24**, 130–131.

(21) Hook CC, Kimmel DW, Kvols LK *et al.* (1992). Multifocal inflammatory leukoencephalopathy with 5-fluorouracil and Levamisole. *Ann Neurol*, **31**, 262–267.

(22) Feun LG, Wallace S, Stewart DJ *et al.* (1984). Intracarotid infusion of cis-diamminedichloroplatinum in the treatment of recurrent malignant brain tumors. *Cancer*, **54**, 794–799.

(23) Whittaker JA, Parry DH, Bunch C, Weatherall DJ. (1973). Coma associated with vincristine therapy. *Br Med J*, **4**, 335–337.

(24) Lôo LM, Zittoun R. (1969). Intoxication aiguë è forme comateuse par la vincristine. *Gaz Med Fr*, **76**, 2693–2698.

(25) Slater LM, Wainer RA, Serpick AA. (1969). Vincristine neurotoxicity with hyponatremia. *Cancer*, **23**, 122–124.

(26) Brunner KW, Young CW. (1965). A methylhydrazine derivative in Hodgkin's disease and other malignant neoplasms: Therapeutic and toxic effects studied in 51 patients. *Ann Intern Med*, **63**, 69–86.

(27) Stolinsky DC, Solomon J, Pugh RP *et al.* (1970). Clinical experience with procarbazine in Hodgkin's disease, reticulum cell sarcoma, and lymphosarcoma. *Cancer*, **26**, 984–989.

(28) Land VJ, Sutow WW, Fernbach DJ *et al.* (1972). Toxicity of l-asparaginase in children with advanced leukemia. *Cancer*, **30**, 339–347.

(29) Oettgen HF, Stephenson PA, Schwartz MK *et al.* (1970). Toxicity of *E. coli* l-asparaginase in man. *Cancer*, **25**, 253–278.

(30) Feinberg WM, Swenson MR. (1988). Cerebrovascular complications of l-asparaginase therapy. *Neurology*, **38**, 127–133.

(31) Bethlenfalvay NC, Bergin JJ. (1972). Severe cerebral toxicity after intravenous nitrogen mustard therapy. *Cancer*, **29**, 366–369.

(32) Wolfson S, Olney MB. (1957). Accidental ingestion of a toxic dose of chlorambucil. *JAMA*, **165**, 239–240.

(33) Burger PC, Kamenar E, Schold SC *et al.* (1981). Encephalomyelopathy following high-dose BCNU therapy. *Cancer*, **48**, 1318–1327.

(34) Gieron MA, Barak LS, Estrada J. (1988). Severe encephalopathy associated with ifosfamide administration in two children with metastatic tumors. *J Neurooncol*, **6**, 29–30.

(35) Leff RS, Thompson JM, Daly MB. (1988). Acute neurologic dysfunction after high-dose Etoposide therapy for malignant glioma. *Cancer*, **62**, 32–35.

(36) Adams F, Fernandez F, Mavligit G. (1988). Interferon-induced organic mental disorders associated with unsuspected pre-existing neurologic abnormalities. *J Neurooncol*, **6**, 355–359.

(37) Young DF, Posner JB, Chu F, Nisce L. (1974). Rapid-course radiation therapy of cerebral metastases : Results and complications. *Cancer*, **34**, 1069–1076.

(38) Freeman JE, Johnston PG, Voke JM. (1973). Somnolence after prophylactic cranial irradiation in children with acute lymphoblastic leukemia. *Br Med J*, **4**, 523–525.

(39) Ross D, Rosegay H, Pons V. (1988). Differentiation of aseptic and bacterial meningitis in post-operative neurosurgical patients. *J Neurosurg*, **65**, 669–674.

(40) Zaret BS, Beckner RR, Marini AM *et al.* (1982). Sodium valproate-induced hyperamonemia without clinical hepatic dysfunction. *Neurology*, **32**, 206–208.

(41) Hughes RL. (1990). Cyclosporine-related central nervous system toxicity in cardiac transplantation. *N Engl J Med*, **323**, 420–421.

(42) Wijdicks EF, Dahlke LJ, Wiesner RH. (1999). Oral cyclosporine decreases severity of neurotoxicity in liver transplant recipients. *Neurology*, **52**, 1708–1710.

(43) Dalmau J, Graus F. (1997). Paraneoplastic syndromes of the nervous system. In: Cancer of the nervous system. Black McLP, Loeffler JS (eds). *Blackwell Science*, pp. 674–700.

(44) Edelson RN, Chernik NL, Posner JB. (1979). Spinal subdural hematomas complicating lumbar puncture. *Arch Neurol*, **31**, 134–137.

(45) van Oostenbrugge RJ, Twijnstra A. (1999). Presenting features and value of diagnostic procedures in leptomeningeal metastases. *Neurology*, **53**, 382–385.

(46) Kolmel HW. (1998). Cytology of neoplastic meningosis. *J Neurooncol*, **38**, 121–125.

(47) van de Pol M, van Aalst VC, Wilmink JT, Twijnstra A. (1996). Brain metastases from an unknown primary tumour: which diagnostic procedures are indicated? *J Neurol Neurosurg Psychiatry*, **61**, 321–323.

(48) Pirotte B, Levivier M, Goldman S *et al.* (1997). Glucocorticoid induced long-term remission of lymphoma: Case report and review of the literature. *J Neurooncol*, **38**, 238–253.

(49) Kupfer A, Aeschlimann C, Cerny T. (1996). Methylene blue and the neuro-toxic mechanisms of ifosfamide encephalopathy. *Eur J Clin Pharmacol*, **50**, 249–252.

2 Cognitive and behavioural disorders

Introduction

Intellectual and behavioural disorders can be assessed reliably only in fully aroused patients. Cognitive disorders range from isolated deficits, such as aphasia, amnesia, agnosia, and apraxia, to global dementia. The most common behavioural abnormalities in cancer patients are anxiety and depression.

There is a growing interest in the recognition of these abnormalities. Cognitive function abnormalities may result from anticancer treatment and are potentially avoidable. Impaired cognitive function significantly impairs quality of life if left untreated.

Clinical presentation of selected syndromes

Clinical examination of patients with cognitive and behavioural disorders is often difficult. In patients with dementia, amnesia, mutism, aphasia, marked attentional disorders, or psychotic behaviour, medical history is either impossible or unreliable. Relatives and carers are often poor judges when it comes to evaluation of intellectual decline in closely related family members, although performance at work provides useful information. In children, changes in school marks are a sensitive criterion for detecting a change.

Examination and quantitative evaluation of many cognitive disorders requires the help of an experienced neuropsychologist. It is beyond the scope of this chapter to review the details of the neuropsychological examination. Instead, we concentrate on the most common neuropsychological problems encountered in cancer patients.

Aphasia is an acquired impairment or loss of language generally due to focal lesions located in the so-called dominant hemisphere. There are many syndromes of aphasia, numerous classifications and nomenclatures. Non-fluent aphasia (also known as Broca's aphasia) is characterized by an impaired output but a relatively preserved comprehension. It is often associated with right hemiplegia and is caused by a left frontal opercular lesion which may be associated with deep-lying lesions, particularly in severe cases. Non-fluent aphasia may be mistaken for dysarthria, a purely motor disorder of articulation without any linguistic deficit. Most neurological lesions causing dysarthria are anatomically distant from Broca's area. Fluent aphasia (also named Wernicke's aphasia) is characterized by fluent verbal output, paraphrasia, neologisms, and comprehension defect. Fluent aphasia is usually caused by a left posterior temporal lesion. Fluent aphasia may be mistaken for a confusional state, usually caused by more diffuse brain damage.

Aphasia, which is accompanied by efforts to communicate must be distinguished from **mutism**, where such efforts are not seen. Mutism is often associated with akinesia and is seen typically in frontal lesions.

Many physicians continue to use the term of **frontal lobe syndrome** despite the fact that:

(1) neuropsychological manifestations due to frontal lobe injury differ according to the site, and the number of lesions; and

(2) lesions located outside the frontal lobes may produce features resembling the so-called frontal syndrome.

In brain tumours, however, where the correspondence between the anatomical site of the lesion and its clinical expression is made less precise by mass effect and oedema, the concept of frontal syndrome has some practical use. It refers to a not uncommon situation where more-or-less subtle, behavioural and mental changes precede more conspicuous motor or sensory deficits. Behavioural changes, of which the patient often remains unaware, may consist of abnormal social conduct, inability to adjust emotional reactions, aggressiveness, or depression. These disorders seem to be more common in left frontal tumours. Cognitive defects associated with frontal tumours often consist in inappropriate planning and decision making, apathy, distractibility, poor attention, and inability to organize the future. Working (short-term) memory, which is vulnerable to interference, is disturbed. But long-term memory and intelligence, when tested by Wechsler scales, are often better preserved. However, these patients may demonstrate a striking discrepancy between a preserved IQ and inadequate behaviour in real life.

Bilateral frontal lesions, especially slowly growing tumours such as meningioma, may cause dementia. **Dementia** is defined as loss of memory and loss of at least one other cognitive ability. Changes in memory have been reported mainly in frontal, left temporal, and thalamic tumours, and in lesions located around the third ventricle. Despite the existence of diagnostic criteria (1), diagnosis of dementia may be difficult in everyday practice. Dementia is a syndrome. Before considering the long list of differential diagnoses, it is important to exclude severe depression, a treatable condition that is frequent in cancer patients.

The Mini-Mental State Examination (MMSE) has become the most widely used bedside test to evaluate dementia. MMSE is a 30-point scale that tests orientation (10 points), attention (3 points), mental calculation (5 points), recall (3 points), and mostly language (9 points). The MMSE was originally designed by Folstein *et al.* (2) to distinguish normal from pathological cognitive decline in the elderly. A score below 24/30 is pathological. However, MMSE has not been validated in cancer patients. In addition, because it is simple and short, learning effect limits the use of MMSE during follow-up, especially when memory is reasonably preserved. MMSE is also sensitive to the patient's level of education. Despite these limitations, MMSE is used increasingly worldwide; this includes the longitudinal assessment of cognitive functions in therapeutic trials in neuro-oncology.

There are several patterns of dementia. **Subcortical dementia**, which is seen frequently in neuro-oncology, is characterized by slowness of thinking (bradyphrenia), poor attention, and impaired memory, while cortical cognitive disorders such as aphasia, apraxia, or agnosia are less prominent.

Depression and **anxiety** are the most common psychiatric problems in cancer patients. Depression occurs in one-quarter of hospitalized cancer patients (3). In patients with primary

Table 2.1   Main causes of cognitive and mood disorders in cancer patients

Lesions	Causes
Neoplastic	1. Brain tumours
	Extrinsic: frontal, olfactory meningioma
	Intrinsic:
	single: gliomas
	multiple: primary lymphomas
	metastases
	2. Leptomeningeal metastases
Treatment related	1. Late-delayed leucoencephalopathy
	2. Focal radiation necrosis
	3. Psychiatric disorders caused by drugs
Infectious	1. Abscess
	2. Progressive multifocal leucoencephalopathy
Vascular	1. Subdural and epidural haematomas
	2. Vascular dementia
Paraneoplastic	Limbic encephalitis (Hu, CV_2 and Ma2 antibodies)
Emotional reactions	1. Depression
	2. Anxiety

brain tumours, depression is frequent with frontal tumours (4), particularly slowly growing meningioma. It also occurs in patients with tumours in other locations including infratentorial tumours (5,6). In pituitary prolactinoma depression has been attributed to hyperprolactinaemia (7).

Anxiety and panic attacks are mostly emotional reactions, but they may be associated with temporal lobe tumours (8).

Main aetiologies

The main causes of cognitive and behavioural disorders in cancer patients are summarized in Table 2.1.

Neoplastic lesions

1. Primary brain tumours and brain metastases

Cognitive and behavioural disorders are frequently the presenting signs in prefrontal and frontal tumours, where lateralized motor and sensory deficits may be absent or delayed. Psychological signs may, however, be associated with non-lateralized signs, such as abnormality of posture and gait or incontinence. The most frequent **extrinsic** tumours causing these features are frontal (Fig. 2.1) or olfactory groove meningiomas. The most common **intrinsic** tumours are high- or low-grade gliomas, or metastatic tumours. Personality and mental changes, with gait disorders, are the most common presenting signs in patients with multiple brain metastases (9).

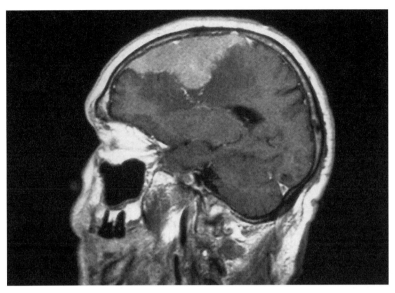

Fig. 2.1 Sagittal T_1WI MR scan, after gadolinium administration, of a frontal meningioma in a woman presenting with cognitive disorders. The tumour was isointense with grey matter before gadolinium injection (see also Fig. 4.3). Note the extensive peritumoural oedema seen as a hypointense, poorly defined area.

Tumours of the sellar region and posterior fossa are also associated with personality and cognitive changes, such as emotional lability or decline in school performance. The pathogenesis of these manifestations is poorly understood as not all of these patients present with hydrocephalus.

Primary non-Hodgkin's CNS lymphomas (PCNSL) are multiple in about half the patients (Fig. 2.2). Mental disorders, ranging from behavioural changes to dementia of subcortical type, were the most frequent single symptom at first presentation in the review by Herrlinger *et al.*, ranging from 24 to 73% of the patients (10).

2. Leptomeningeal metastases

Primary tumours most commonly causing leptomeningeal carcinomatosis are listed in Table 1.4. Mental changes are the most frequent initial manifestation of leptomeningeal metastases (11). Careful clinical examination, however, will often disclose features of meningeal irritation or other central and peripheral nervous system deficit.

Treatment-related complications

1. Late-delayed leucoencephalopathy

Cognitive decline, ranging from mild neuropsychological impairment to profound dementia of subcortical type, was first observed **in children** after CNS prophylaxis of acute leukaemia. Terms used in the literature such as (disseminated) necrotizing leucoencephalopathy, suba-

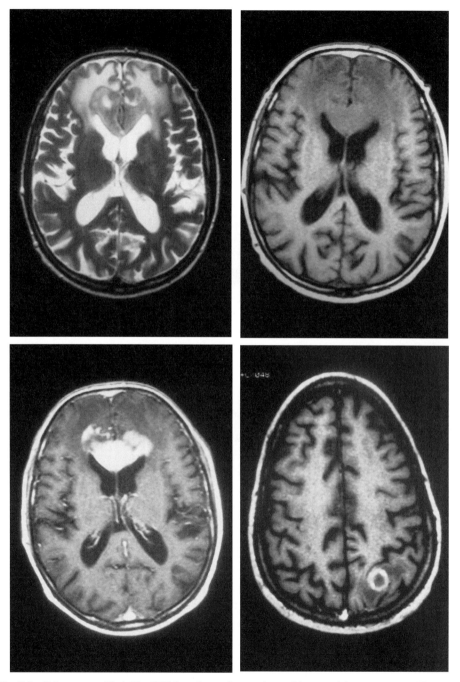

Fig. 2.2 Primary non-Hodgkin CNS lymphoma in a patient with normal immune status. The tumour is multifocal and infiltrates periventricular areas. It is moderately hyperintense on T_2WI (Upper Left), and enhances strongly and homogeneously on T_1WI (Lower left). The tumour is hypointense on T_1WI (Upper Right). Ring-shaped enhancement typically seen in primary brain lymphomas occurring in immunodepressed individuals, in this case an AIDS patient (Lower right). (By courtesy Dr K. Hoang-Xuan)

Table 2.2 Leucoencephalopathies in patients treated for CNS leukaemia

Encephalopathy	Number of cases	Main symptoms and signs	Pathology: main features	Reference
Encephalopathy in AL associated with MTX	7	Confusion, tremor, ataxia, irritability, drooling, somnolence, coma	Infarcted areas (1 case examined)	12
Encephalopathy following CNS prophylaxis	6 (of 33)	Lethargy, somnolence, irritability, seizures, tremor, ataxia		13
Parenchymatous degeneration of CNS in leukaemia	1 (of 23)	Dementia, seizures, ataxia, spasticity	Fibrillary gliosis	14
Disseminated g necrotizin leuco-encephalopathy	5	Lethargy, dysphagia, irritability, focal deficit	Multifocal coagulative necroses in white matter	15
Subacute leuco-encephalopathy in childhood leukaemia	13	Mental changes, seizures, ataxia, spasticity, focal deficits	Multiple necrotic pain, astrocytosis in white matter	16
	4 (of 23)	Dementia, seizures, spastic quadriplegia or paraplegia	White matter gliosis	17

Adapted from Hildebrand (18).
AL, ; MTX, methotrexate.
AL: acute leukemia

cute leucoencephalopathy, or encephalopathy of childhood leukaemia probably refer to the same pathological entity (Table 2.2). The CNS injury results from therapy combining cranial irradiation, systemic and intrathecal methotrexate. As illustrated by the Venn diagram of Bleyer and Griffin (19) (Fig. 2.3), cognitive impairment is rare (1–2%) when either treatment is used alone. Its incidence increases when two treatments are combined, and is seen in almost half the children when all three treatment modalities are used. Other risk factors are young age, overt meningeal leukaemia at the time of treatment, and high doses of methotrexate and radiation therapy. Pathologically the disease is characterized by a multi-focal coagulation necrosis of the white matter surrounding the lateral ventricles and centrum ovale.

Clinically the disease begins insidiously 6 months to several years after treatment, with irritability, personality changes, and learning difficulties, and gradually evolves to dementia. Although mood and cognitive changes are early and prominent features, other symptoms and signs develop in the course of the disease, including tremor, gait ataxia, slurred speech, and seizures (see Table 2.2 for references).

Late-delayed leucoencephalopathy with mental retardation has also been observed in children irradiated for brain tumours, especially medulloblastoma (20,22,23). Most children develop radiation encephalopathy from 6 months to 2 years after irradiation. Encephalopathy has been observed 28 and 33 years after brain tumour therapy and has been ascribed to late effects of radiation (24).

Late-delayed leucoencephalopathy occurs **in adults** up to 4 years after the completion of radiation therapy. De Angelis *et al.* (25) reported 12 patients cured of their brain metastases

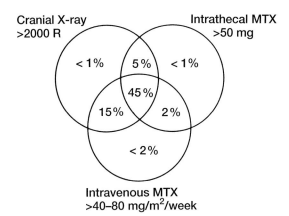

Fig. 2.3 Diagram illustrating the combined CNS toxicity of cranial irradiation, intrathecal and systemic (intravenous) methotrexate (MTX). Leucoencephalopathy occurred in only 1–2% of patients treated with one modality, whereas 45% of leukaemic children treated with all three modalities developed the complication. (From Blayer and Griffin ref. 19, with permission.)

by radiation therapy, and possibly concomitant chemotherapy, who developed progressive dementia 5–36 months following brain irradiation. Similar observations were made in patients with small-cell lung cancer (SCLC) after prophylactic brain irradiation (usually 3000 cGy in 10 fractions) combined with systemic chemotherapy (26). Dementia has been observed in 40% of patients with primary CNS lymphoma (PCNSL) aged over 50 years treated with high-dose methotrexate shortly before cranial irradiation. The typical course of the disease in adults is progressive dementia of subcortical type characterized by slowness of ideation, severe memory impairment, difficulties in focusing attention, apathy, and emotional lability. Progressive gait ataxia and incontinence are common associated signs. Radiation leucoencephalopathy usually leads to death, but in a minority of patients cognitive decline may stabilize. MRI shows a widespread increased signal on T_2-weighted images involving the white matter, widening of cortical sulci, and ventricular dilatation (Fig. 2.4). The extent of white matter changes correlates with cognitive decline, but the correlation of cortical and subcortical atrophy to cognitive decline is less clear. Using a quantitative MRI technique Mulhern *et al.* (27) have found a positive correlation between full-scale IQ and normal white-matter volume in medulloblastoma survivors treated with cranial irradiation with or without chemotherapy. In addition, medulloblastoma patients had a statistically lower full-scale IQ and smaller white-matter volume than matched survivors treated for low-grade astrocytoma by tumour resection only (27). Although a CT scan may show diffuse white-matter abnormalities after brain irradiation, it is less sensitive than MRI, and a normal CT does not rule out a neuropsychological impairment due to radiation therapy. An overall lowering of IQ and poorer ability to retrieve information from long-term memory was observed in adults irradiated for nasopharyngeal carcinoma, and most patients had a normal brain CT scan (28).

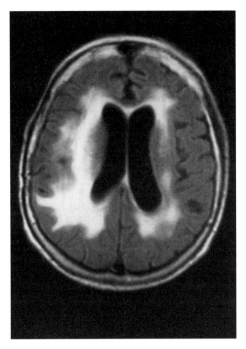

Fig. 2.4 Late-delayed radiation-induced leucoencephalopathy in a patient presenting with progressive dementia of subcortical type. The FLAIR MR scan demonstrates a widespread hyperintense signal, involving selectively the white matter and sparing the basal ganglia.

2. *Focal radiation necrosis*

The risk of focal radiation necrosis is related to total dose and dose per fraction. It occurs rarely following doses of 6000 cGy or less, at 200 cGy or less per fraction. Giving radiation more than once a day (hyperfractionation, see Chapter 12, p. 234) increases the risk of radiation damage, as the time between doses does not allow for the full recovery of repairable radiation damage (29). In most patients with tumour recurrence following conventional irradiation, pathological examination will demonstrate radiation-induced changes in addition to tumour infiltration. In such patients, the clinical deficit is most likely to be due to progressive tumour growth, with little or no contribution from irradiation.

Focal necrosis is a very frequent complication of brachytherapy, particularly when given in addition to conventional irradiation. About 40% of these patients need surgical resection of the necrotic mass (30). Pathologically the lesion consists of a coagulative necrosis and thickening and necrosis of vessel walls. Focal necrosis is observed mainly during the second year following external irradiation. The delay is shorter after brachytherapy. Clinical manifestations of focal radiation necrosis differ from diffuse radiation leucoencephalopathy and closely resemble tumour recurrence. Isolated cognitive disorders such as aphasia or apraxia may occur, but global dementia is less common. Radiologically, radiation necrosis also

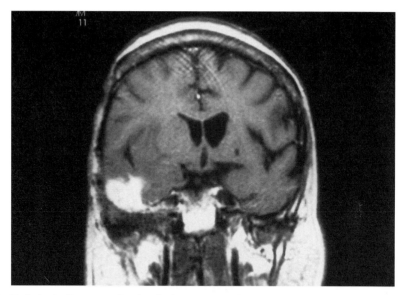

Fig. 2.5 Pathologically proven focal radiation necrosis of the right temporal lobe that developed 5 years after resection and irradiation of a sphenoid ridge meningioma. The coronal T_1WI MR scan shows a gadolinium-enhanced lesion surrounded by oedema and producing a moderate mass effect.

mimics tumour recurrence (Fig. 2.5) Focal necrosis may respond transiently to cortico-steroids. Radiation necrosis appears hypometabolic on positron emission tomography (PET) scans using fluorodeoxyglucose (Fig. 2.6), allowing the differential diagnosis with tumour regrowth (31). However, hypermetabolic foci have been reported in pathologically proven post-radiation necrosis (32).

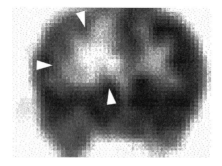

Fig. 2.6 Positron emission tomography after injection of [^{18}F]fluorodeoxyglucose. Coronal slice at the level of the temporal poles in a patient with radionecrosis in the right frontal lobe. Note the frontal cortical and subcortical hypometabolism (arrows). (By courtesy Dr S. Goldman.)

3. Psychiatric disorders caused by medical treatments

Most drugs used in cancer chemotherapy occasionally cause encephalopathy and confusional state (see Chapter 1, p. 10, 11). The administration of **glucocorticosteroids** produces mainly behavioural disorders. Mental disturbances are less frequent with methylprednisolone or dexamethasone than with natural corticosteroids or ACTH. Behavioural and personality changes such as anxiety, nervousness, insomnia, or euphoria are fairly common, but serious psychiatric manifestations, including depression and acute psychotic and delirious reactions, occur in no more than 3% of cases (33). Depression may be seen in the early stages of glu- cocortisteroid therapy or during drug tapering. It usually resolves after the drug is disconti- ued. Acute psychotic and delirious reactions are characterized by paranoid behaviour, often associated with visual or auditory hallucinations.

Interferon (34) and **interleukin-2** (35) occasionally cause depression and cognitive changes. **Tamoxifen** administration has been associated with hallucinations and increased aggressivity (36). Hallucinations may also be caused by **dopamine agonists** (bromocriptine) used in the treatment of prolactinoma (see Table 11.3).

Infections

Frontal abscess may produce cognitive and behavioural disorders similar to tumours at this location. The differential diagnosis between abscess (Fig. 1.8), primary brain tumours, and metastases (Fig. 1.7) may be difficult on clinical and radiological grounds, as systemic fea- tures of infection and CSF inflammatory changes may be missing when the infection is confined to brain parenchyma.

Progressive multifocal leucoencephalopathy caused by a papovavirus is a rare disease that mainly occurs in immunodepressed patients, particularly those with lymphoma or chronic lymphocytic leukaemia. The most prominent clinical features are multiple focal deficits, often preceded by mood changes and mental disorders (37).

Vascular lesions

Frontal, epidural, or subdural haematoma (Fig. 1.6) may cause the so-called frontal syn- drome or dementia, especially when bilateral. In cancer patients, subdural bleeding is mainly associated with thrombocytopenia with or without disseminated intravascular coagulation.

Repeated haemorrhagic or ischaemic strokes may lead to vascular dementia. Multiple vascular brain lesions are more common in cancer patients than in the general population, and are therefore more likely to produce cognitive disorders, including dementia. Multiple strokes are mainly due to septic or non-bacterial endocarditis, disseminated intravascular coagulation, or thrombocytopenia. Vascular dementia is often associated with focal neuro- logical signs.

Paraneoplastic diseases

Limbic encephalitis

Amongst various paraneoplastic neurological disorders, mood and cognitive changes are consistently present only in limbic encephalitis. Limbic encephalitis has been reported mainly in patients with small-cell lung cancer (SCLC) (38) in whom high serum and CSF titres of anti-Hu antibodies may be present, and less frequently in patients with other cancers, usually without anti-Hu antibodies. Limbic encephalitis has also been reported in association with CV_2 antibody, mostly in SCLC patients (39) and Ma2 antibody in testicular cancer (40). Of 13 patients with testicular cancer studied by Voltz *et al.*, 10 had serum and CSF Ma2 antibodies, and of these 10 patients 8 had limbic encephalitis which occurred either in isolation or in combination with other neurological deficits, such as brainstem encephalomyelitis or cerebellar syndrome (40).

In its pure form, limbic encephalitis is characterized by behavioural changes such as anxiety, agitation or depression, and sleep disorders, and by cognitive disorders (primarily memory disturbances) evolving in weeks to months, then reaching a plateau with severe neurological abnormalities (38). Neocortical functions are relatively preserved, at least during the early stages of the disease. The pathological lesions, consisting of inflammatory infiltrate, predominate in limbic, temporal, and hypothalamic regions. Limbic encephalitis may be part of a more diffuse disease which combines signs of brainstem involvement (see Chapter 6, p. 108), cerebellar ataxia (see Chapter 4, p. 68 to 71), low motor neuron lesions, and sensory neuronopathy (see Chapter 8, p. 160, 161). MRI and CT scans are normal in most patients with limbic encephalitis, but in some patients median temporal abnormalities may be found (Fig. 2.7).

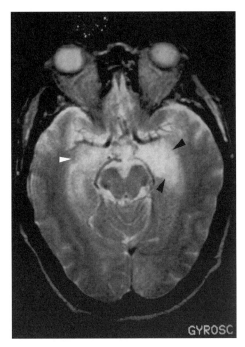

Fig. 2.7 Paraneoplastic limbic encephalitis producing a hyperintense bitemporal (arrows) signal on axial T_2WI MR scan. (By courtesy Dr F. Graus.)

Emotional reactions

Not all mood disorders encountered in cancer patients are caused by organic brain lesions. Anger, anxiety, insomnia, and depression are common emotional reactions to disease and fear for the future.

Prolonged episodes of depression are frequent in cancer patients (3). They often remain undiagnosed because they are considered as appropriate reactions to the situation and because various physical manifestations accompanying depression, such as anorexia, weight loss, fatigue, or loss of libido, are assigned to the neoplastic disease and therapy.

Investigations

In patients with cognitive and behavioural disorders, brain MRI, and in many patients contrast-enhanced CT scan, will guide the differential diagnosis. The algorithm shown in Fig. 2.8 is based on four distinct MRI or CT scan patterns:

(1) focal brain lesions;

(2) meningeal enhancement;

(3) diffuse white matter changes; and

(4) normal.

1. Intracranial focal lesions

Focal brain lesions may be either extrinsic or intrinsic.

1.1 Extrinsic   The main extrinsic lesions are meningiomas (Fig. 2.1) and subdural or sub-arachnoid haematomas (Fig. 1.6). Both have a fairly typical radiological configuration and their identification is seldom problematic.

1.2 Intrinsic   Intrinsic brain lesions are either haemorrhagic or non-haemorrhagic. Lesions may or may not enhance with contrast.

The main causes of intracerebral bleeding in cancer patients are coagulation abnormalities or intratumoural haemorrhage. Coagulation disorders are common in haematological malignancies, mainly acute leukaemias. Tumours most likely to bleed are glioblastoma, oligodendroglioma, primary germ-cell tumours, and metastases originating from systemic germ-cell tumours, melanoma, and, less frequently, lung carcinoma (see Chapter 1, p. 5). When coagulation disorders and intratumour haemorrhage are excluded, hypertension becomes the most likely cause of cerebral bleeding, as in the general population.

The differential diagnosis of non-haemorrhagic contrast-enhanced lesions, which includes primary and metastatic tumours, abscess, and recent ischaemic stroke, is considered in Chapter 1 (p. 17 to 20). The most common locations for lesions causing cognitive disorders are frontal and temporal lobes, or structures surrounding the third ventricle.

Lesions that do not enhance with contrast and present with mass effect usually correspond to low-grade primary tumours, and diagnostic biopsy is considered appropriate. In low-grade gliomas, PET scans using [^{18}F]fluorodeoxyglucose commonly demonstrate an uniformly hypometabolic lesion. Hypermetabolic foci (Fig. 2.9) may guide the stereotactic

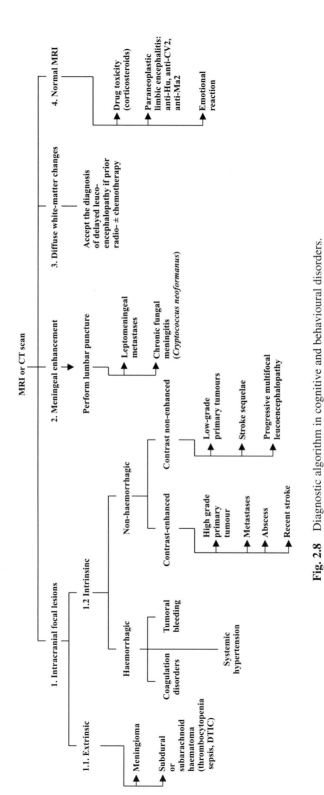

Fig. 2.8 Diagnostic algorithm in cognitive and behavioural disorders.

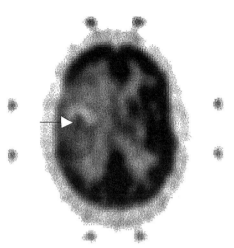

Fig. 2.9 Positron emission tomography with [^{18}F]fluorodeoxyglucose performed in stereotactic condition (note the fiducials surrounding the brain) in a patient with histologically verified low-grade astrocytoma of the right hemisphere. Stereotactic biopsy of a recent hypermetabolic spot (arrow) showed focal anaplastic degeneration. (By courtesy Dr S Goldman)

biopsy towards regions of anaplasia (41). In the absence of a mass effect, non-enhanced lesions most likely represent the sequelae of stroke, especially if they are associated with focal cortical and subcortical atrophy (Fig. 2.10) or if they occur in patients with risk factors or a history of cerebrovascular disease. Progressive multifocal leucoencephalopathy produces non-enhancing lesions (Fig. 1.12). The diagnosis of this rare disease should be considered primarily in patients with lymphoma or chronic leukaemia.

2. *Meningeal enhancement*
In cancer patients with mental disorders, focal or diffuse meningeal enhancement (Fig. 1.4) is highly suggestive of leptomeningeal metastases. MRI abnormalities are found in up to 70% of patients with proven leptomeningeal carcinomatosis. Definite diagnosis of leptomeningeal carcinomatosis requires the identification of neoplastic cells in the CSF, which may necessitate repeated lumbar punctures. Although MRI is a sensitive examination in the diagnosis of meningeal carcinomatosis, it is not specific. The differential diagnosis of the meningeal syndrome is described in detail in Chapter 1 (p. 17).

Infectious meningitis usually causes altered consciousness and confusional state rather than cognitive changes. However, in chronic forms of cryptococcal meningitis, cognitive and behavioural disorders may occur in patients with normal arousal state.

3. *Diffuse white-matter changes*
In cancer patients presenting with cognitive disorders, particularly dementia of subcortical type, widespread white-matter changes (Fig. 2.4.) are virtually diagnostic of late treatment-related encephalopathy in patients previously treated by cranial irradiation, with or without chemotherapy.

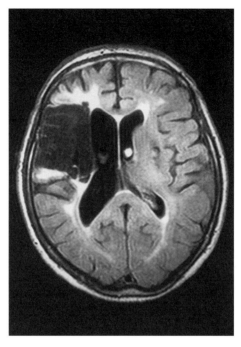

Fig. 2.10   Axial FLAIR MR scan showing the sequela of an ischaemic stroke. Note the enlargement of the adjacent lateral ventricle, resulting from subcortical atrophy.

4. *Normal MRI*

Normal MRI does not rule out neoplastic or infectious meningeal disease. Patients with normal MRI and cognitive disorder should therefore have a CSF examination, especially if the history does not favour drug-induced or reactive affective disorder.

Moderate inflammatory changes are found in the CSF in limbic encephalitis where MRI is normal in most patients. This diagnosis should be considered particularly in patients with SCLC, and may be confirmed by high serum and CSF levels of anti-Hu antibodies. CV2 (39) or Ma2 (40) antibodies may help to establish the diagnosis of paraneoplastic encephalitis in patients with SCLC or testicular cancer, respectively.

Despite the fact that reactive behavioural disorders are common in cancer patients, they should be considered only when all organic lesions have been ruled out with reasonable certainty.

Therapy

Cognitive and behavioural disorders caused by tumours may regress when the underlying neoplasia is effectively treated. The therapy of the most frequent forms of intrinsic primary brain tumours, brain and meningeal metastases is considered in Chapter 12.

In cerebral convexity, olfactory groove, and anterior sagittal sinus meningiomas, which are most frequently associated with cognitive disorders, complete surgical resection can be achieved and leads to an improvement of cognitive functions (42). Conventional fractionated irradiation with up to 5500 cGy may follow incomplete removal and improves tumour control, although this is unlikely to lead to further improvement in cognitive function (43,44). Late radiation toxicity is an additional problem which may aggravate cognitive deficit, and focused techniques of irradiation of small residual tumours (3–4 cm in diameter) may reduce the risks of late damage (45).

Abscesses due to *Toxoplasma gondii, Nocardia* sp. or *Listeria* sp. are first treated by appropriate antibiotics (Table 1.7). Surgery is seldom used because they are often multiple and deeply located, and many cancer patients are in poor general condition.

There is no available effective therapy for most patients with delayed radiation-induced leucoencephalopathy. However, improvement was reported following ventriculoperitoneal shunting in 24 of 30 patients with radiation-therapy-induced leucoencephalopathy and progressive ventriculomegaly, in whom other causes of hydrocephalus were excluded. Incontinence and gait disorders were more likely to improve than cognitive deficits, which were present in all patients before operation (46). Focal radiation necrosis may be treated conservatively by corticosteroids (47) and possibly by heparin (48). More severe forms with mass effect may require surgical resection (49).

The use of immunosuppressive therapy has not been shown to be effective in limbic encephalitis (50). However, complete response of the underlying tumour seems to have a favourable effect on anti-Hu-associated encephalomyelitis (51). Spontaneous improvement has been reported occasionally (52).

Not all mental manifestations seen in cancer patients need to be treated. Disorders due to glucocorticosteroids as well as other drugs may respond to dose tapering or drug discontinuation. In patients with persistent and severe behavioural disorders, the use of tranquillizers, antidepressants, or antipsychotic drugs may be necessary. Prophylactic administration of lithium carbonate to avoid psychotic episodes in patients treated with glucocorticosteroids is based on rare single-case observations (53) and is not recommended.

Reactive depression in cancer patients is generally undertreated probably because it is too often considered to be an 'appropriate' reaction. Yet, despite its reactive component, it responds to antidepressants. Antidepressive therapy can commence with inhibitors of serotonin reuptake because these drugs are well tolerated at optimal therapeutic dose. We use tricyclic antidepressants such amitriptyline, imipramine, or nortriptyline (up to 125–150 mg taken in one dose before sleep) when the therapeutic effect of serotonin reuptake inhibitors is insufficient or in patients where neuropathic pain is prominent. The analgesic effect of tricyclic antidepressants is usually seen at a daily dose lower than required for antidepressive effect. Alongside medication, all patients should be offered psychological support.

Acute and chronic anxiety states are best treated with benzodiazepines, which also have an anti-emetic and anti-epileptic effect. Unfortunately, they are also sedative and contribute to somnolence and falls in the elderly. Benzodiazepines should be discontinued slowly to avoid seizures precipitated by abrupt withdrawal.

References

(1) Diagnostic Statistical Manual of Mental Disorders, 4th edn. APA, Washington DC, 1994.
(2) Folstein MF, Folstein SE, McHugh PR. (1975). 'Mini-mental state'. A practical method for grading the cognitive state of patients for the clinician. *J Psychiatr Res*, **12**, 189–198.

(3) Bukberg J, Penman D, Holland JC. (1984). Depression in hospitalized cancer patients. *Psychosom Med*, **46**, 199–212.

(4) Direkze M, Bayliss SG, Cutting JC. (1971). Primary tumours of the frontal lobe. *Br J Clin Pract*, **25**, 207–213.

(5) Cairns H. (1950). Mental disorders with tumors of the pons. *Folia Psychiat Neerl*, **53**, 193–203.

(6) Keschner M, Bender MB, Strauss I. (1937). Mental symptoms in cases of subtentorial tumor. *Arch Neurol Psychiatry*, **37**, 1–18.

(7) Gangbar R, Swinson RP. 1983. Hyperlactinemia and psychiatric illness. *Am J Psychiatry*, **140**, 790–791.

(8) Strobos RR. 1953. Tumors of the temporal lobe. *Neurology*, **3**, 732–760.

(9) Hildebrand J. (1973). Early diagnosis of brain metastases in unselected population of cancerous patients. *Europ J Cancer*, **9**, 621–626.

(10) Herrlinger U, Schabet M, Bitzer M *et al.* (1999). Primary central nervous system lymphoma: From clinical presentation to diagnosis. *J Neurooncology*, **43**, 219–226.

(11) Grisold W, Drlicek M, Setinek U. (1998). LC: Clinique syndrome in different primaries. *J Neurooncology*, **38**, 103–110.

(12) Kay HE, Knapton JP, O'Sullivan JP *et al.* (1972). Encephalopathy in acute leukaemia associated with methotrexate therapy. *Arch Dis Child*, **47**, 344–354.

(13) McIntosh S, Aspnes GT. (1973). Encephalopathy following CNS prophylaxis in childhood lymphoblastic leukemia. *Pediatrics*, **52**, 612–615.

(14) Hendin B, DeVivo DC, Torack R *et al.* (1974). Proceedings: parenchymatous degeneration of the central nervous system in childhood leukemia. *Cancer*, **33**, 468–482.

(15) Rubinstein LJ, Herman MM, Long TF, Wilbur JR. (1975). Disseminated necrotizing leukoencephalopathy: A complication of treated central nervous system leukemia and lymphoma. *Cancer*, **35**, 291–305.

(16) Price RA, Jamieson PA. (1975). The central nervous system in childhood leukemia. II. Subacute leukoencephalopathy. *Cancer*, **35**, 306–318.

(17) Meadows AT, Evans AE. (1976). Effects of chemotherapy on the central nervous system. A study of parenteral methotrexate in long-term survivors of leukemia and lymphoma in childhood. *Cancer*, **37**, 1079–1085.

(18) Hildebrand J. (1978). Lesions of the nervous system in cancer patients. Raven Press, New York, p. 52.

(19) Bleyer WA, Griffin TW. (1980). White matter necrosis, mineralizing microangiopathy, and intellectual abilities in survivors of childhood leukemia: Associations with central nervous system irradiation and methotrexate therapy. In: Radiation damage to the nervous system. A delayed therapeutic hazard. Gilbert HA, Kagan AR (eds). Raven Press, New York, p. 154–174.

(20) Radcliffe J, Packer RJ, Atkins TE *et al.* (1992). Three- and four-year cognitive outcome in children with noncortical brain tumours treated with whole-brain radiotherapy. *Ann Neurol*, **32**, 551–554.

(21) Duffner PK, Cohen ME, Brecher ML *et al.* (1984). CT abnormalities and altered methotrexate clearance in children with CNS leukemia. *Neurology*, **34**, 229–233.

(22) Hirsch JF, Renier D, Czernichow P *et al.* (1979). Medulloblastoma in childhood. Survival and functional results. *Acta Neurochir*, **48**, 1–15.

(23) Duffner PK, Cohen ME, Thomas P. (1983). Late effects of treatment on the intelligence of children with posterior fossa tumors. *Cancer*, **51**, 233–237.

(24) Duffey P, Chari G, Cartlidge NE, Shaw PJ. (1996). Progressive deterioration of intellect and motor function occurring several decades after cranial irradiation. *Arch Neurol*, **53**, 814–818.

(25) DeAngelis LM, Delattre JY, Posner JB. (1989). Radiation-induced dementia in patients cured of brain metastases. *Neurology*, **32**, 789–796.

(26) So NK, O'Neill BP, Frytak S *et al.* (1987). Delayed leukoencephalopathy in survivors with small cell lung cancer. *Neurology*, **37**, 1198–1201.

(27) Mulhern RK, Reddick WE, Palmer SL *et al.* (1999). Neurocognitive deficits in medulloblastoma survivors and white matter loss. *Ann Neurol*, **46**, 834–841.

(28) Lee PW, Hung BK, Woo EKW *et al.* (1989). Effects of radiation therapy on neuropsychological functioning in patients with nasopharyngeal carcinoma. *J Neurol Neurosurg Psychiatr*, **52**, 488–492.

(29) Safdari H, Fuentes JM, Dubois JB *et al.* (1985). Radionecrosis of the brain: Time of onset and incidence related to total dose and fractionation of radiation. *Neuroradiology*, **27**, 44–47.

(30) Gutin Ph, Leibel SA, Wara WM *et al.* (1987). Recurrent malignant glioma: Survival following interstitial brachytherapy with high activity iodine-125 source. *J Neurosurg*, **67**, 864–873.

(31) Di Chiro G, Oldfield E, Wright DC *et al.* (1988). Cerebral necrosis after radiotherapy and/or intraarterial chemotherapy for brain tumors: PET and neuropathologic studies. *Am J Roentgenol*, **150**, 189–197.

(32) O'Neill A, Macalpinlac H, DeAngelis L. (1996). Positron emission tomography (PET), hypermetabolism with cerebral radionecrosis. *J Neurooncology*, **28**, 88(abstract).

(33) Boston Collaboration Drug Surveillance Program. (1972). Acute adverse reaction to prednisolone in relation to dosage. *Clin Pharmacol Ther*, **13**, 694–698.

(34) Kirkwood JM, Ernstoff MS, Davis CA *et al.* (1985). Comparison of intramuscular and intravenous recombinant alpha-2 interferon in melanoma and other cancers. *Ann Intern Med*, **103**, 32–36.

(35) Denicoff KD, Rubinow DR, Papa MZ *et al.* (1987). The neuropsychiatric effects of treatment with interleukin-2 and lymphokine-activated killer cells. *Ann Inter Med*, **107**, 293–300.

(36) Love RR. (1989). Tamoxifen therapy in primary breast cancer: Biology, efficacy and side effects. *J Clin Oncol*, **7**, 803–815.

(37) Vanderhaeghen JJ, Perier O. (1965). Leuco-encéphalite multifocale progressive. Mise en évidence de particules virales par microscopie électronique. *Acta Neurol Psychiatr Bel*, **65**, 816–837.

(38) Dalmau J, Graus F, Rosenblum MK, Posner JB. (1992). Anti-Hu-associated paraneoplastic encephalomyelitis/sensory neuronopathy: a clinical study of 71 patients. *Medicine*, **71**, 59–72.

(39) Honnorat J, Antoine JC, Derrington E *et al.* (1996). Antibodies to a subpopulation of glial cells and a 66 kDa developmental protein in patients with paraneoplastic neurological syndromes. *J Neurol Neurosurg Psychiatry*, **61**, 270–278.

(40) Voltz R, Gultekin SH, Rosenfeld MR *et al.* (1999). A serologic marker of paraneoplastic limbic and brain-stem encephalitis in patients with testicular cancer. *N Engl J Med*, **340**, 1788–1795.

(41) Levivier M, Goldman S, Pirotte B *et al.* (1995). Diagnostic yield of stereotactic brain biopsy guided by positron emission tomography with [^{18}F]fluorodeoxyglucose. *J Neurosurg*, **82**, 445–452.

(42) Chee CP, David A, Galbraith S, Gillham R. (1985). Dementia due to meningioma: outcome after surgical removal. *Surg Neurol*, **23**, 414–416.

(43) Taylor BW Jr, Marcus RB Jr, Friedman WA *et al.* (1988). The meningioma controversy: postoperative radiation therapy. *Int J Radiat Oncol Biol Phys*, **15**, 299–304.

(44) Fick J, Wilson CB, Fuller GN. (1996). Meningiomas. In: Cancer in the nervous system. Levin VA (ed). Churchill Livingstone, New York, pp. 187–198.

(45) Loeffler JS, Alexander E 3rd. (1990). The role of stereotactic radiosurgery in the management of intracranial tumors. *Oncology*, **4**, 21–31.

(46) Thiessen B, DeAngelis LM. (1998). Hydrocephalus in radiation leukoencephalopathy: results of ventriculoperitoneal shunting. *Arch Neurol*, **55**, 705–710.

(47) Shaw PJ, Bates D. (1984). Conservative treatment of delayed cerebral radiation necrosis. *J Neurol Neurosurg Psychiatry*, **47**, 1338–1341.

(48) Glantz MJ, Burger PC, Friedman AH *et al.* (1994). Treatment of radiation-induced nervous
        system injury with heparin and warfarin. *Neurology*, **44**, 2020–2027.
(49) Gutin PH. (1991). Treatment of radiation necrosis of the brain. In: Radiation injury to the
        nervous system. Gutin PH, Leibel SA, Sheline GE (eds). Raven Press, New York, pp. 271–282.
(50) Graus F, Vega F, Delattre JY *et al.* (1992). Plasmapheresis and antineoplastic treatment in CNS
        paraneoplastic syndromes with antineuronal autoantibodies. *Neurology*, **42**, 536–540.
(51) Keime-Guibert F, Graus F, Broët P *et al.* (1999). Clinical outcome of patients with anti-
        Hu-associated encephalitis after treatment of the tumor. *Neurology*, **53**, 1719–1723.
(52) Byrne T, Mason WP, Posner JB, Dalmau J. (1997). Spontaneous neurological improvement in
        anti-Hu associated encephalomyelitis. *J Neuro Neurosurg Psychiatry*, **62**, 276–278.
(53) Falk WE, Mahnke MW, Poskanzer DC. (1979). Lithium prophylaxis of corticotropin-induced
        psychosis. *JAMA*, **241**, 1011–1012.

3 Epileptic seizures

Introduction

This chapter deals only with epileptic seizures which appear during the course of neoplastic diseases or lead to their diagnosis. Causes of epilepsy antedating or unrelated to the neoplastic process will not be considered. However, the severity of pre-existing seizures may be affected by the course of the malignant disease through CNS infections, metabolic changes, or administration of antineoplastic drugs, which may be either directly neurotoxic or interfere with serum concentrations of anti-epileptic agents.

Clinical presentation and electroencephalograms

Focal and secondary generalized epileptic seizures

The majority of cancer-related seizures are focal. In some patients, however, secondary generalization may occur quickly, so that the focal phase of the epileptic seizure may pass unnoticed. A careful history, recording the characteristics of a focal seizure, is helpful in localizing the epileptogenic brain lesion. Motor focal seizures are characterized by clonic jerks beginning in one limb or in the face. They may spread progressively to the entire ipsilateral side of the body (Jacksonian progression). A sensation of numbness or paraesthesia in one part of the body points to the post-rolandic area. Olfactory or gustatory (often unpleasant) hallucinations, a feeling of 'déjà vu', fear, or pleasure, suggest a temporal location of the epileptic focus. Simple visual hallucinations most commonly indicate an occipital lesion.

In patients with brain tumours, focal deficits such as aphasia or unilateral weakness (Todd's hemiparesis) which follow focal seizures are more frequent and tend to last longer (over 24 hours), than in other pathological conditions. These slowly reversible focal signs must be differentiated from focal deficits caused by the underlying brain tumour or the surrounding oedema.

Rapid succession of focal seizures may lead to **epilepsia partialis continua**. Although, in this situation, consciousness is fully preserved, many consider this condition to be a variant of status epilepticus and treat accordingly. Repeated complex partial (psychomotor) seizures may lead to a **non-convulsive status epilepticus**, characterized by intermittent episodes of confusion, automatisms, and unusual behaviour, which may last for hours. Non-convulsive status epilepticus may be mistaken for confusional state or psychotic behaviour. Its diagnosis requires an electroencephalographic (EEG) epileptic pattern (Fig. 3.1). The epileptogenic focus is mostly located in the temporal lobe. Clinical signs and EEG abnormalities of non-convulsive status epilepticus may be alleviated by intravenous diazepam, and this therapeutic response strengthens the diagnosis.

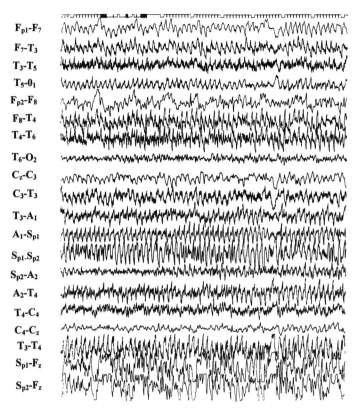

Fig. 3.1 Non-convulsive complex partial status. The EEG shows bilateral spikes predominating in the left mesotemporal region (A_1–SP_1 and SP_1–SP_2). (Courtesy of Dr B. Legros.)

All focal seizures may generalize, producing tonic–clonic epilepsy followed by a post-ictal state, which may be unusually durable in patients with an underlying organic brain lesion, especially a brain tumour (see Chapter 1, p. 5).

Primary generalized epileptic seizures

Cancer-related primary generalized seizures are relatively uncommon. If they occur, they are mostly due to toxic or metabolic disorders and drug withdrawal. In cancer patients, primary generalized seizures may occur either in isolation or as part of the metabolic or toxic encephalopathies listed in Table 1.5.

Electroencephalogram (EEG)

The diagnosis of epileptic seizures is based on EEG and clinical information. EEG is diagnostic of epilepsy when ictal epileptiform activity is recorded during a clinical seizure. However, inter-ictal recording of spikes (20–70 ms in duration) or sharp waves (70–200 ms in duration) (Fig. 3.2) is a strong argument in favour of epilepsy in patients with appropriate

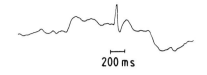

200 ms

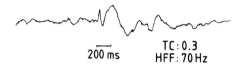

200 ms

TC: 0.3
HFF: 70 Hz

Fig. 3.2 An example of a spike (upper trace) and of a spike followed by a slow wave (lower trace). The recording was performed using a time constant of 0.3 s and a high-frequency filter of 70 Hz. (Courtesy of Dr P. Tugendhaft.)

history and clinical ictal manifestations. Because epileptic discharges are paroxysmal, it may be necessary to repeat EEG recording. Sleep recording using chloral hydrate increases the frequency of epileptiform discharges and makes their identification easier. Following a primary or secondary generalized seizure, the EEG recording will first undergo a diffuse flattening, followed by a diffuse slowing of cortical electric activity (Fig. 3.3). Another useful indicator of a recent seizure is the rise of serum prolactin concentration, which peaks around 30 minutes following seizure (1). The change of serum prolactin level is marked and frequent after generalized seizures, it is less important in complex partial seizures, and is rare in simple focal seizures. Unfortunately, the rise in serum prolactin may also follow a syncope, thus limiting the diagnostic value of this examination.

Main aetiologies

The main causes of seizures occurring in cancer patients are summarized in Table 3.1.

Neoplastic lesions

Primary or metastatic tumours in the brain and leptomeningeal metastases are the most common causes of epilepsy in patients with cancer.

1. Primary brain tumours

At least one-third of patients with intrinsic supratentorial primary tumours suffer epileptic seizures (2). Deeply located supratentorial and infratentorial tumours are less epileptogenic than cortical neoplasia. For similar pathology and location, the incidence of epileptic seizures tends to be higher in children than in adults. The incidence is also higher in the more benign forms, such as low-grade glioma where seizures occur in two patients out of three (range 30–90%), than in high-grade glioma (anaplastic astrocytoma or glioblastoma). However,

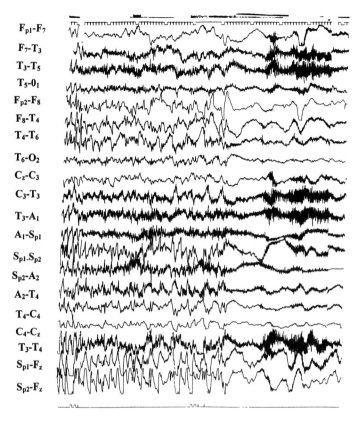

F_{p1}-F_7

F_7-T_3

T_3-T_5

T_5-0_1

F_{p2}-F_8

F_8-T_4

T_4-T_6

T_6-O_2

C_z-C_3

C_3-T_3

T_3-A_1

A_1-S_{p1}

S_{p1}-S_{p2}

S_{p2}-A_2

A_2-T_4

T_4-C_4

C_4-C_z

T_3-T_4

S_{p1}-F_z

S_{p2}-F_z

Fig. 3.3   Post-ictal EEG showing abrupt cessation of bilateral spike discharges followed by low-voltage slow activities (flattening of the EEG). (Courtesy of Dr B. Legros.)

Table 3.1   Main causes of epileptic seizures in cancer patients

Lesions	Causes
Neoplastic	1. Primary intrinsic and extrinsic brain tumours
	2. Brain metastases
	3. Leptomeningeal metastases
Treatment related	1. Chemotherapy, mainly in high dose, intra-CSF, or intracarotid injection
	2. Radiation therapy
	3. Supportive treatments
Infectious	In all CNS infections
Vascular	Cortical stroke
Paraneoplastic	1. Limbic encephalitis
Metabolic	Hyponatraemia, hypoglycaemia, hypocalcaemia hypomagnesaemia

patients with low-grade tumours survive longer and this factor, by itself, increases the risk of seizure. Temporal and frontal tumours are more epileptogenic than occipital tumours (3). Seizures are often the presenting features, leading to earlier diagnosis of small primary brain tumours. This possibly explains why in many studies (4,5) the presence of seizures is a favourable prognostic factor for survival. Seizures may be, for years, the only manifestation of slowly growing tumours such as low-grade astrocytoma, ganglioglioma, or dysembryogenic neuroepithelial tumours. Gangliogliomas are almost always associated with seizures, often refractory to medical treatment. They are primarily paediatric tumours with a predilection for temporal and frontal lobes (6). Dysembryonic neuroepithelial tumour is a rare neoplasia found in patients operated for intractable epilepsy (7). Two-thirds are located in the temporal and one-third in the frontal lobe. Meningioma, the most common extrinsic brain tumour, causes seizures in about 20% of patients bearing this neoplasia.

2. *Brain metastases*

Brain metastases are one of the most common neurological complications of systemic cancer. Their overall incidence ranges from 12 to 35% of all patients with generalized cancer (8). The most frequent primary tumours are listed in Table 1.3.

Seizures, mostly of focal type, are present in 20–40% of patients with brain metastases, and may be the presenting feature. They occurred as the first manifestation of brain metastases in 16% of patients studied by Paillas *et al.* (9) and 25% of patients reported by Simionescu (10). Seizures tend to occur more often in patients with multiple metastases and are particularly frequent in melanomas, where brain metastases are usually multiple.

3. *Leptomeningeal metastases*

Meningeal and brain metastases often coexist, but purely meningeal metastases may also be epileptogenic. Seizures were recorded in 10–14% of patients with leptomeningeal carcinomatosis (11,12) and in 10% of children with acute lymphoblastic leukaemia (13), although not all had an overt meningeal leukaemia. Metastases attached to the dura are also epileptogenic.

Treatment-induced seizures

1. *Chemotherapy*

Most anticancer agents do not cross the blood–brain barrier and they are seldom epileptogenic when administrated systemically at conventional doses. Seizures occur in less than 1% of patients treated with systemic chemotherapy (14). However, chemotherapy is more epileptogenic when it is administered in high dose, directly into the CSF or by intracarotid injection, where the blood–brain barrier is either overwhelmed or absent. The protective role of the blood–brain barrier against epileptic seizures is suggested by the observation that patients with brain metastases may present seizures when having a contrast-enhanced brain CT scan. It is assumed that the neurotoxic product is able to reach the cortex because the blood–brain barrier is disturbed around brain metastases.

Table 3.2 Drug-induced epileptic seizures

Drug	Treatment modality	Comments
Methotrexate	IV high dose, intra-CSF (16,17)	Also related to radiation therapy in late-delayed leucoencephalopathy
Cisplatin	IA(18), IV(19) (very rare)	
Vincristine	IV (very rare)	Putative focal destruction of blood–brain barrier (20,21)
		Hyponatraemia (inappropriate secretion of ADH) (22)
Nitrogen mustard	IV high dose (23)	
Nitrosoureas	BCNU (24), IA HeCNU (25)	
Ifosfamide	IV	Non-convulsive status epilepticus (26)
Cytosine arabinoside	IV high dose	Concomitant CNS acute leukaemia (27)
Etoposide (VP16)	High dose (28)	
Thiotepa	IV high dose (29)	In bone-marrow transplant
Busulfan	High dose (30)	In posterior leucoencephalopathy syndrome (31,36)
Asparaginase		Through hepatic encephalopathy (32)
Interferon-α	Low dose (33)	
Metronidazole	High dose (34)	
Cyclosporin A		Partially through hypomagnesaemia (15,35)
		In posterior leucoencephalopathy syndrome (36)
Antibiotics		β-Lactams (37), quinolones (38)
Antidepressants		Mainly tricyclic, even newer drugs (39)
Neuroleptics		Phenothiazines, butyrophenones (40)
Anti-epileptics	High dose	Mainly phenytoin (41)
Withdrawal		Tranquillizers (benzodiazepines), alcohol (42)

Abbreviations : ADH, antidiuretic hormone; BCNU, ; HeCNU, ; IV, intravenous; IA, intracarotid.

Disruption of the blood–brain barrier by hypertonic mannitol or glycerol, or by a bradykinin analogue, may cause seizure, even before the injection of antineoplastic drugs (see Chapter 12, p. 231).

Chemotherapeutic agents are believed to cause epileptic seizures mainly by direct CNS toxicity, although the mechanism is poorly understood. They may also produce epileptogenic metabolic changes (considered in table 3.2). The drugs used in cancer chemotherapy that have been associated with epileptic seizures are listed in Table 3.2. The issue of how often these drugs produce seizures is confounded by concomitant use of potentially epileptogenic supportive treatments (also listed in Table 3.2), by the presence of malignant brain and meningeal lesions, and by prior or concomitant neurosurgery or radiation therapy.

Posterior leucoencephalopathy syndrome is an example of a disease where epilepsy pathogenesis is multifactorial. This syndrome, characterized by headaches, seizures, cortical blindness, and systemic hypertension, has been mainly reported in leukaemic patients after allogenic bone-marrow transplantation. High doses of cyclosporin A probably play a key pathogenic role (15,31,35,36), but these patients also received cranial irradiation and treatment with other drugs, including busulfan, platinum derivatives, or cyclophosphamide, which are all potentially epileptogenic.

2. Radiation therapy

Brain irradiation is regarded as a potential cause of seizures. However, its contribution to epileptogenesis is difficult to assess quantitatively as it is often combined with other epileptogenic factors.

In **acute radiation-induced encephalopathy**, seizures may occur within hours following initial cranial irradiation (43). Their occurrence is probably favoured by putative breakdown of the blood–brain barrier. However, this has not been demonstrated following small doses of irradiation received in the initial phases of a protracted course of radiotherapy.

Seizures have been reported in 20–30% of patients with **late-delayed necrotizing leucoencephalopathy**. However, these figures may be biased by the presence of neoplastic brain lesions in number of patients.

Focal radiation lesions due to high doses of irradiation are also epileptogenic. Complex partial seizures have been observed in patients without malignant CNS lesions after radiotherapy for nasopharyngeal tumours (44), where the inferomedial aspects of the temporal lobes received high irradiation doses.

3. Supportive treatments

Several drugs currently used in the management of cancer patients are epileptogenic (Table 3.2). **Cyclosporin A** causes seizures, at least partially through hypomagnesaemia. **Antibiotics**, mainly quinolones, β-lactams, and penicillin, **antidepressants**, mainly tricyclics, and **neuroleptics**, such as phenothiazines and butyrophenones (also used as antiemetics), are potentially epileptogenic. Paradoxically, several anti-epileptics, mainly phenytoin, may become epileptogenic at high serum concentration. Acute withdrawal of all tranquillizers causes seizures in chronically treated patients.

Infections

All CNS infections listed in Table 1.6 are highly epileptogenic.

Vascular lesions

Cancer patients have an increased risk of both ischaemic and haemorrhagic stroke (45). Epileptogenic vascular lesions involve the cerebral cortex and the majority of stroke-related seizures have a delayed onset (46). Embolic and haemorrhagic strokes are thought to be more epileptogenic than thromboses. For instance, epileptic seizures occur frequently in marantic endocarditis. Thrombosis of the cerebral venous sinus and cortical veins, which is highly epileptogenic in the general population, seldom causes seizures in cancer patients (47).

Paraneoplastic diseases

Paraneoplastic encephalomyelitis, which includes limbic encephalitis (see Chapter 2, p. 37, 38), is the only neurological paraneoplasia to cause seizures. Seizures are rarely the presenting manifestation of paraneoplastic encephalomyelitis. They almost always occur during the course of the disease (48) and may present as epilepsia partialis continua (49).

Metabolic disorders

Metabolic disorders seen in cancer patients are caused either by neoplastic destruction of vital organs or by paraneoplastic production of biologically active proteins. The most common metabolic disorders causing epileptic seizures with or without encephalopathy include the following.

Hyponatraemia which, in cancer patients, is a feature of inappropriate antidiuretic hormone (ADH) secretion. This syndrome may result from tumour production of ADH or ADH-like products, from hypothalamic damage by primary or metastatic tumours, surgery, or irradiation, and from administration of carbamazepine, vincristine, or cyclophosphamide. Hyponatraemia may also result from excessive hydration.

Hypoglycaemia, which may be due to paraneoplastic production of insulin-like products, excess insulin produced by insulinomas, excessive consumption of glucose by tumour cells, or malnutrition.

Hypocalcaemia and **hypomagnesaemia**, which may be caused by renal loss due to cisplatin treatment, or by malabsorption.

Investigations

The differential diagnosis of paroxysmal attacks is based primarily on their clinical presentation (Fig. 3.4).

1. Epileptic nature clinically certain

When the epileptic nature of a seizure is clinically evident, an EEG confirmation may not be necessary. A brain MRI and, if not available, a CT scan may reveal either meningeal or parenchymal pathology, or it may be normal.

1.1 Meningeal lesion Most meningeal lesions causing epileptic seizures in cancer patients are either neoplastic (meningioma, dural or leptomeningeal metastases) or infectious. The radiological aspect of meningioma is fairly typical (Figs 2.1 and 4.3). Usually its diagnosis does not require further investigation and will be confirmed by surgery.

In patients with leptomeningeal metastases MRI will demonstrate meningeal contrast enhancement (Fig. 1.4) in about 70% of the cases. The diagnosis needs to be confirmed by the identification of neoplastic cells in the CSF, which may require repeated lumbar punctures. Infectious meningitis may also demonstrate an abnormal meningeal signal on MRI. The main infectious agents causing meningitis or meningoencephalitis in cancer patients are reviewed in Chapter 1 (see Table 1.6).

1.2 Parenchymal brain lesion Epileptogenic parenchymal lesions are mostly cortical or cortico-subcortical. They may be neoplastic, infectious, or vascular. In patients with proven cancer, the diagnosis of brain metastases causing seizures may be accepted when single or multiple contrast-enhanced lesions (Fig. 1.7), surrounded by oedema, are found in individuals, without increased risk of infectious or vascular lesions. The decision to perform a diagnostic biopsy and the differential diagnosis are considered in Chapter 1 (p. 18).

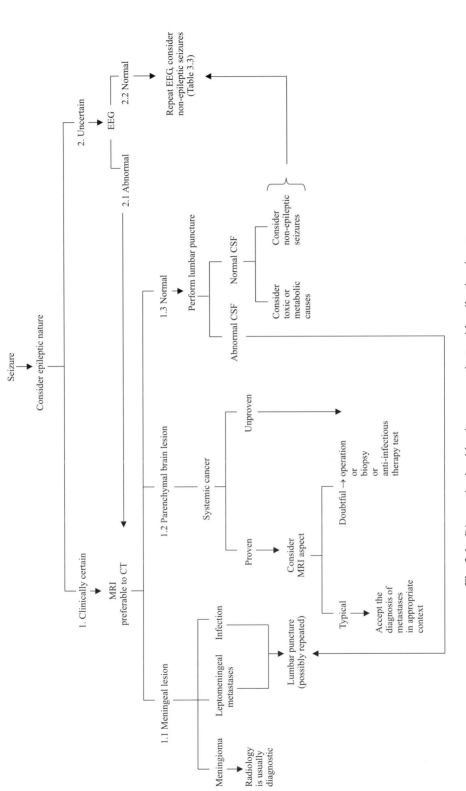

Fig. 3.4 Diagnostic algorithm in cancer patients with epileptic seizures.

Table 3.3 Differential diagnosis of generalized seizures

Clinical features	Generalized epileptic seizure	Syncope	Pseudo-seizure
Prodrome	Primary: none Secondary: epileptic aura	Faint feeling Light-headedness	Variable
Trauma due to falling	Frequent	Rare	Uncommon
Duration of myoclonic jerks	30–60 seconds	Absent or few jerks	Prolonged myoclonic phase
Post-ictal somnolence or coma	Present	Absent	Absent
Post-ictal EEG changes	Always present	Absent	Absent
Post-ictal elevation of serum prolactin	Frequent in generalized epileptic seizures	Rare but possible	Absent

1.3 Normal MRI In patients with normal MRI, metabolic causes such as hypoglycaemia, hyponatraemia, hypocalcaemia, or hypomagnesaemia should be excluded. These disorders are the most frequent metabolic causes of seizures and, because they are easy to diagnose and to treat blood glucose, sodium, calcium, and magnesium should also be measured and corrected in patients with potentially epileptogenic structural lesions. Subsequently, a lumbar puncture should be performed, as in 30% of patients with leptomeningeal metastases, and in about 50% of patients with infectious meningitis, MRI shows no meningeal enhancement. When both MRI and CSF are normal, other metabolic or toxic disorders are the most likely cause of seizures, either in isolation or as part of an encephalopathy (see Tables 1.5 and 3.2). Toxic causes are usually determined by history. Systemic chemotherapy administered at standard doses seldom causes epileptic seizures.

2. Epileptic nature uncertain

When the epileptic nature of a seizure is uncertain, EEG recording should be performed and, if necessary, repeated. The elevation of serum prolactin levels shortly after a seizure suggests the epileptic nature of the attacks (see Table 3.3).

2.1 EEG abnormal When an EEG shows focal epileptic features or other abnormalities, MRI or CT scan is indicated to demonstrate or rule out a structural lesion.

2.2 EEG normal When repeated EEGs are normal, the diagnosis of non-epileptic seizures may be considered, although in epileptic seizures caused by withdrawal or metabolic disorders, intercritical EEG does not usually show epileptogenic features. The differential diagnosis, which may be difficult, includes syncope and pseudo-seizures. Table 3.3 summarizes the main points on which the differential diagnosis is based. Syncope is defined as a transient loss of consciousness due to impaired cerebral blood flow; the most common cause in cancer patients is orthostatic hypotension. Pseudo-seizures refer to psychogenic paroxysmal events, which are involuntary and may mimic epileptic seizures. Pseudo-seizures frequently occur in the presence of a witness, and are more common in patients with a history of genuine epileptic seizures than in the general population.

Therapy

Prophylactic anti-epileptic treatment in patients with primary or metastatic brain tumours is no longer advocated. Its benefit has not been proven in a prospective study (50) and retrospective analyses yield contradictory results. However, the role of anti-epileptic prophylaxis is not entirely clear, particularly in relation to neurosurgery and in patients with melanoma brain metastases where seizures are particularly frequent. Prophylactic diazepam (5–10 mg iv) can be used at the time of a contrast-enhanced CT scan (but not MRI plus gadolinium) in patients with brain metastases.

Not all epileptic seizures require prolonged administration of anti-epileptic drugs. When seizures are caused by metabolic, toxic, or infectious disorders, prolonged treatment with anti-epileptic drugs is seldom necessary. Their administration may usually be discontinued when the epileptogenic disorder is corrected. Prolonged administration of anticonvulsants to patients who no longer have seizures after the appropriate treatment of a tumour should be considered on an individual basis. For example, in patients considered to be cured, anticonvulsants may be discontinued with little risk of subsequent seizures. Patients with residual tumour, considered to be at risk of further seizures, should continue anti-epileptic medication. In patients with brain tumours, carbamazepine and phenytoin are the most commonly used drugs to control seizures. The consensus is to use these as monotherapy at maximally tolerated doses, rather than in combination. Phenytoin, which can be given intravenously, has the advantage that it may be used to treat status epilepticus and is not myelotoxic. Carbamazepine may lower the white cell count and (exceptionally) cause agranulocytosis.

Several factors complicate the use of anti-epileptic drugs in cancer patients. Epilepsy caused by brain tumours tends to be relatively refractory to medical treatment. Concomitant administration of chemotherapy or glucocorticosteroids makes it difficult to maintain stable blood therapeutic levels, which therefore need to be monitored and adjusted. Conversely, anti-epileptics may lower serum concentrations of anticancer agents. This mechanism also explains why the toxicity of drugs that need to be metabolized into an active form in the liver (such as cyclophosphamide) is enhanced by anti-epileptics metabolized in the liver.

Anticonvulsants themselves are neurotoxic. At high serum levels they may produce neurological symptoms and signs, such as ataxia and nystagmus (phenytoin) or drowsiness and diplopia (carbamazepine), which mimic tumour progression. In addition, both phenytoin and carbamazepine have been reported to increase the risk of skin reaction to brain irradiation (51). If carbamazepine, phenytoin, or their association fail, other anti-epileptics may be used or added. These include valproic acid, or more recent drugs such as gabapentin or lamotrigine. Phenobarbital is best avoided in patients with brain tumours because it produces sedation, and 10–20% of patients with brain tumour develop a painful shoulder–hand syndrome, usually contralateral to the side of tumour (52).

Status epilepticus is a severe, life-threatening condition and requires urgent treatment. Prolonged epilepsia partialis continua, caused by brain metastases, may also lead to permanent neurological damage in the hemisphere where the epileptogenic lesion is located.

Table 3.4   Treatment algorithm in status epilepticus (adapted from Lowenstein and Alldredge, ref. 53)

1. Start intravenous administration of:
lorazepam 0.1 mg/kg at 2 mg/min or diazepam 2 mg/min up to 10 mg total dose
2. If seizures continue:
phenytoin 20 mg/kg at 50 mg/min or valproate 10–15 mg/kg iv bolus (3–5 min)
3. If seizures continue:
add phenytoin 5–10 mg/kg, and proceed immediately to anaesthesia if status epilepticus develops in an intensive care unit, lasts for more than 60–90 minutes or if there is severe hyperthermia
4. If seizures continue:
phenobarbital 20 mg/kg at 50–75 mg/min, add phenobarbital 5–10 mg/kg if seizure continuous
5. General anaesthesia with midazolam or propofol

A therapeutic algorithm for status epilepticus has been proposed by Lowenstein and Alldredge (53) and it is appropriate to follow it in patients with malignant disease (Table 3.4).

References

(1) Yerby MS, van Belle G, Friel PN, Wilensky AJ. (1987). Serum prolactins in the diagnosis of epilepsy: sensitivity, specificity and predictive value. *Neurology*, **37**, 1224–1226.

(2) McKeran RO, Thomas DGT. (1980). The clinical study of gliomas. In: Brain tumours, scientific basis, clinical investigation and current therapy. Thomas DGT, Graham DI (eds). Butterworth, London, pp. 194–230.

(3) Scott GM, Gibberd FB. (1980). Epilepsy and other factors in prognosis of glioma. *Acta Neurol Scand*, **61**, 227–239.

(4) MRC Brain Tumour Working Party. Prognostic factors in high-grade malignant glioma: Development of a prognostic index. *J Neurooncology*, **9**, 47–55.

(5) Smith DF, Hutton JL, Sandemann D *et al.* (1991). The prognosis of primary intracerebral tumours presenting with epilepsy: The outcome of medical and surgical management. *J Neurol Neurosurg Psychiatry*, **54**, 915–920.

(6) Haddad SF, Moore SA, Menezes AH, Van Gilder JC. (1992). Ganglioglioma: 13 years of experience. *Neurosurgery*, **31**, 171–178.

(7) Daumas-Duport C, Scheithauer BW, Chodkiewicz JP *et al.* (1988). Dysembryoplastic neuroepithelial tumour: a surgically curable tumor of young patients with intractable partial seizures. *Neurosurgery*, **23**, 545–556.

(8) Arbit E, Wronski M. (1996). Clinical decision making in brain metastases. *Neurosurg Clin N Am*, **7**, 447–457.

(9) Paillas JE, Soulayrol R, Combalbert A *et al.* (1966). Etude sur les métastases Cérébrales solitaires des cancers viscéraux. *Neurochirurgie*, **12**, 337–360.

(10) Simionescu ME. (1960). Metastatic tumors of the brain. A follow-up study of 195 patients with neurosurgical considerations. *J Neurosurg*, **17**, 361–373.

(11) Grisold W, Drlicek M, Setinek U. (1998). LC: Clinical syndrome in different primaries. *J Neurooncol*, **38**, 103–110.

(12) Kaplan JG, DeSouza TG, Farkash A *et al.* (1990). Leptomeningeal metastases: comparison of clinical features and laboratory data of solid tumors, lymphomas and leukemias. *J Neurooncology*, **9**, 225–229.

(13) Ochs JJ, Bowman WP, Pui CH *et al.* (1984). Seizures in childhood lymphoblastic leukaemia patients. *Lancet*, **ii**, 1422–1424.

(14) Flowers A. (1995). Seizures and syncope. In: Cancer in the nervous system. Levin VA (ed.). Churchill Livingstone, pp. 314–324.

(15) Hinchey J, Chaves C, Appignani B *et al.* (1996). A reversible posterior leukoencephalopathy syndrome. *N Engl J Med*, **334**, 494–500.

(16) Jaffe N, Takaue Y, Anzai T, Robertson R. (1985). Transient neurological disturbances induced by high-dose methotrexate treatment. *Cancer*, **56**, 1356–1360.

(17) Kay HE, Knapton PJ, O'Sullivan JP. (1972). Encephalopathy in acute leukaemia associated with methotrexate therapy. *Arch Dis Child*, **47**, 344–354.

(18) Newton HB, Page MA, Junck L, Greenberg HS. (1989). Intra-arterial cisplatin for the treatment of malignant gliomas. *J Neurooncol*, **7**, 39–45.

(19) Berman IJ, Mann MP. (1980). Seizures and transient cortical blindness associated with cis-platinum (II) diamminedichloride (PDD) therapy in a thirty-year-old man. *Cancer*, **45**, 764–766.

(20) Kleinknecht D, Jacquillat C, Weil M. (1967). Les accidents neurologiques centraux de la vincristine. *Nouv Rev Hematol Fr*, **7**, 132–136.

(21) Johnson FL, Bernstein ID, Hartmann JR, Chard RL Jr. Seizures associated with vincristine sulfate therapy. *J Pediatr*, **82**, 699–702.

(22) Slater LM, Wainer RA, Serpick AA. (1969). Vincristine neurotoxicity with hyponatremia. *Cancer*, **23**, 122–125.

(23) Bethlenfalvay NC, Bergin JJ. (1972). Severe cerebral toxicity after intravenous nitrogen mustard therapy. *Cancer*, **29**, 366–369.

(24) Burger PC, Kamenar E, Schold SC *et al.* (1981). Encephalomyelopathy following high-dose BCNU therapy. *Cancer*, **48**, 1318–1327.

(25) Poisson M, Chiras J, Fauchon F. (1990). Treatment of malignant recurrent glioma by intra-arterial, infra-ophtalmic infusion of HeCNU 1-(2-chloroethyl)-1-nitroso-3-(2-hydroxyethyl)urea. *J Neurooncology*, **8**, 255–262.

(26) Wengs WJ, Talwar D, Bernard J. (1993). Ifosfamide-induced nonconvulsive status epilepticus. *Arch Neurol*, **50**, 1104–1105.

(27) Hwang TL, Yung AWK, Estey EH, Fields WS. (1985). Central nervous system toxicity with high-dose Ara-C. *Neurology*, **35**, 1475–1479.

(28) Leff RS, Thompson JM, Daly MB *et al.* (1988). Acute neurologic dysfunction after high-dose etoposide therapy for malignant glioma. *Cancer*, **62**, 32–35.

(29) Lazarus HM, Reed MD, Spitzer TR *et al.* (1987). High-dose IV thiotepa and cryopreserved autologous bone marrow transplantation for therapy of refractory cancer. *Cancer Treat Rep*, **71**, 689–695.

(30) Marcus RE, Goldman JM. (1984). Convulsions due to high-dose busulphan. *Lancet*, **2**, 8417–8418.

(31) Hartmann O, Banhamou E, Beaujean F *et al.* (1986). High-dose busulfan and cyclophosphamide with autologous bone marrow transplantation support in advanced malignancies in children: a phase-II study. *J Clin Oncol*, **12**, 1804–1810.

(32) Land VJ, Sutow WW, Fernbach DJ *et al.* (1972). Toxicity of L-asparaginase in children with advanced leukemia. *Cancer*, **30**, 339–347.

(33) Janssen HL, Berk L, Vermeulen M, Schalm SW. (1990). Seizures associated with low-dose alpha-interferon. *Lancet*, **ii**, 1580.

(34) Frytak S, Moertel CG, Childs DS, Albers JW. (1978). Neurologic toxicity associated with high-dose metronidazole therapy. *Ann Intern Med*, **88**, 361–362.
(35) Walker RW, Brochstein JA. (1988). Neurologic complications of immuno-suppressive agents. *Neurol Clin*, **6**, 261–278.
(36) Ghany AM, Tutschka PJ, McGhee RB Jr *et al.* (1991). Cyclosporine-associated seizures in bone marrow transplant recipients given busulfan and cyclosporine. *Transplantation*, **52**, 310–315.
(37) Schliamser SE, Broholm KA, Liljedahl AL, Norrby SR. (1988). Comparative neurotoxicity of benzylpenicillin, imipenem/cilastatin and FCE 22101, a new injectible penem. *J Antimicrob Chemother*, **22**, 687–695.
(38) Walton GD, Hon JK, Mulpur TG *et al.* (1997). Ofloxacin-induced seizures. *Ann Pharmacother*, **31**, 1475–1477.
(39) Blackwell B, Simon JS. (1988). Antidepressant drugs. In: Meyler's side effects of drugs, (11th edn). Dukes MNG (ed.). Elsevier, Amsterdam, pp. 27–70.
(40) Oliver AP, Luchins DJ, Wyatt RJ. (1982). Neuroleptic-induced seizures: an in vitro technique for assessing relative risk. *Arch Gen Psychiatry*, **32**, 206–209.
(41) Perucca E, Gram L, Avanzini G, Dulac O. (1998). Antiepileptic drugs as a cause of worsening seizures. *Epilepsia*, **39**, 5–17.
(42) Sellers EM. (1988). Alcohol, barbiturate and benzodiazepine withdrawal syndromes: Clinical management. *CMAJ*, **139**, 113–120.
(43) Oliff A, Bleyer WA, Poplack DG. (1978). Acute encephalopathy after initiation of cranial irradiation for meningeal leukaemia. *Lancet*, **ii**, 13–15.
(44) Woo E, Lam K, Yu YL *et al.* (1988). Temporal lobe and hypothalamic–pituitary dysfunction after radiotherapy for nasopharyngeal carcinoma: A distinct clinical syndrome. *J Neurol Neurosurg Psychiatry*, **51**, 1302–1307.
(45) Graus F, Rogers LR, Posner JB. (1985). Cerebrovascular complications in patients with cancer. *Medicine (Baltimore)*, **64**, 16–35.
(46) Olsen TS, Hogenhaven H, Thage O. (1987). Epilepsy after stroke. *Neurology*, **37**, 1209–1211.
(47) Posner JB. (1995). In: Neurologic complications of cancer. Davis, Philadelphia, p. 225.
(48) Dalmau J, Graus F, Rosenblum MK, Posner JB. (1992). Anti-Hu–associated paraneoplastic encephalomyelitis/sensory neuronopathy. A clinical study of 71 patients. *Medicine (Baltimore)*, **71**, 59–72.
(49) Shavit YB, Graus F, Probst A *et al.* (1999). Epilepsia partialis continua: A new manifestation of anti-Hu–associated paraneoplastic encephalomyelitis. *Ann Neurol*, **45**, 255–258.
(50) Foy PM, Chadwick DW, Rajgopalan N *et al.* (1992). Do prophylactic anticonvulsivant drugs alter the pattern of seizures after craniotomy? *J Neuro Neurochir Psychiatry*, **55**, 753–757.
(51) Delattre JY, Safai B, Posner JB. (1988). Erythema multiforme and Stevens–Johnson syndrome in patients receiving cranial irradiation and phenytoin. *Neurology*, **38**, 194–198.
(52) Taylor LP, Posner JB. (1989). Phenobarbital rheumatism in patients with brain tumor. *Ann Neurol*, **25**, 92–94.
(53) Lowenstein DH, Alldredge BK. (1998). Status epilepticus. *N Engl J Med*, **338**, 970–976.

4 Cerebellar dysfunction

Introduction

The cerebellar disorders considered in this chapter result from functional or intrinsic structural cerebellar lesions. They may present either with purely cerebellar symptoms and signs or may be combined with clinical manifestations due to the involvement of neighbouring, or even distant, nervous structures. For example, toxic or paraneoplastic cerebellopathies may occur as part of a more widespread encephalopathy or encephalomyelitis.

Structural lesions arising in the proximity of the cerebellum, such as brainstem gliomas or ependymomas of the floor of the fourth ventricle, may cause cerebellar deficits, and are discussed in Chapter 6.

Clinical manifestations

Cerebellar lesions cause clinical manifestations either due to intrinsic cerebellar damage or as a result of a mass effect. The principal features of **intrinsic** cerebellar lesions include:

1. **Gait ataxia**, often combined with **truncal ataxia**, is the most frequent and the most conspicuous sign of cerebellar dysfunction. It is due to midline cerebellar injury and is characterized by gait unsteadiness, wide-based, jerky steps, and uneven stride length.

2. **Dysarthria**, consisting of scanning speech, **saccadic hypermetria**, and **saccadic ocular pursuit**, also results largely from midline cerebellar lesion.

3. **Dysmetria**, sometimes referred to as **appendicular ataxia**, is due to cerebellar hemisphere lesion and may be unilateral. Dysmetria usually consists of hypermetric movements, where movement first overshoots the target, or, less commonly, of hypometria, where the movement stops before reaching the target. Cerebellar dysmetria is elicited by the finger/nose or heel/knee test.

4. **Nystagmus**, seen in cerebellar lesions, is either spontaneous or evoked by gaze, and changes direction with change of gaze. In unilateral cerebellar hemispheric lesions, nystagmus may be present only when gazing in one direction, thereby appearing similar to a nystagmus caused by peripheral lesions.

5. Cerebellar **tremor** is typically slow, intention tremor, with a maximum amplitude at the end of the movement. Cerebellar tremor is caused by hemispheric lesions and may be unilateral.

The main manifestations of posterior fossa lesions due to **mass effect** are hydrocephalus, intracranial hypertension, upwards transtentorial herniation, or tonsilar herniation, described in Chapter 1 (p. 4, Fig. 1.1).

Pancerebellopathy refers to a clinical syndrome combining signs of midline and cerebellar hemisphere lesions.

Main aetiologies

Clinical signs suggestive of cerebellar lesions, such as mild gait ataxia, are common in cancer patients. From the reported literature it is not always clear whether these changes reflect a cerebellar dysfunction or are the result of disability in chronically ill patients. Nevertheless, signs of cerebellar atrophy on CT scans have been found by Wessel *et al.* in 15 out of 50 patients with lung cancer (1), and loss of Purkinje cells is often found at autopsy in cancer patients. These observations suggest a particular sensitivity of Purkinje cells to metabolic changes such as hypoxia or hypoglycaemia, or to toxic agents including alcohol. The cerebellar diseases listed in Table 4.1 have been selected because a clear link to cerebellar damage has been demonstrated.

Table 4.1   Main causes of cerebellar lesions in cancer patients

Lesions	Causes
Neoplastic	1. Primary tumours:
	medulloblastoma
	astrocytoma, mainly pilocytic
	meningioma
	dermoid tumours
	haemangioblastoma (von Hippel–Lindau disease)
	Lhermitte–Duclos disease
	2. Metastases
Treatment related	1. Chemotherapy
	5-fluorouracil
	cytosine arabinoside
	rarely, other antineoplastic agents
	2. Supportive treatments
	phenytoin
	lithium
	cyclosporin A
Vascular and infectious	Haematoma, embolic stroke
	Abscess
Paraneoplastic	1. Anti-Yo syndrome
	2. Anti-Hu syndrome
	3. Anti-Ri syndrome
	4. Anti-CV2 syndrome
	5. Associated with Hodgkin's diseases (anti-Tr)
	6. Anti-Ma (anti-Ta) syndrome

Neoplastic lesions

The main causes of cerebellar dysfunction in cancer patients are primary or metastatic tumours.

1. Primary tumours

The main intrinsic primary tumours originating in the cerebellum are medulloblastomas and astrocytomas, which primarily occur in children. Dermoid tumours, haemangioblastoma, Lhermitte–Duclos disease, and extrinsic meningiomas may also occur in this site.

Medulloblastoma is the most common type of primitive neuroectodermal tumour (PNET) and represents 20% of primary brain tumours in children, with peak incidence between 7 and 12 years (2). In children, they typically arise from the vermis. Medulloblastomas are rare after the age of 15 years (3) and represent less than 4% of primary brain tumours in adults, where their origin tends to be more lateral. Medulloblastomas are fast-growing tumours with a tendency to invade the fourth ventricle, the brainstem, and the meninges, with a propensity for distant CSF seeding (4,5). Direct extension accounts for cranial nerve palsies which, alongside intracranial hypertension and gait ataxia, are the most common presenting features. The main radiological characteristics of medulloblastoma are illustrated in Fig. 4.1.

Cerebellar astrocytomas range from benign juvenile pilocytic astrocytomas, which are most common in children, to grade 2 infiltrating fibrillary astrocytoma and grade 4 glioblastoma (6,7). Pilocytic astrocytoma, which represents 80–90% of cerebellar astrocytomas (6–9), must be recognized because of its favourable prognosis, with over 90% of patients alive at 10 years (9). Histologically the tumours are formed by fascicles of elongated bipolar astrocytes. Microvascular proliferation is common in pilocytic astrocytoma and probably accounts for the enhancement characteristic on MRI and CT scans (Fig. 4.2), which does not indicate malignancy. The presence of vascular proliferation and nuclear atypia occasionally lead to overgrading of juvenile pilocytic astrocytoma, but they are not associated with adverse prognosis. Pilocytic astrocytomas may metastatize through the CNS even though they remain histologically benign (10). Compared to medulloblastomas, astrocytomas arise more frequently in the cerebellar hemispheres (Fig. 4.2) and unilateral appendicular dysmetria may be an early sign which is overshadowed by gait ataxia and signs of intracranial hypertension as the tumour progresses.

Meningiomas originating from the cerebellar tentorium or cerebellar convexity (Fig. 4.3) cause cerebellar signs, often associated with cranial nerve lesions and intracranial hypertension. Most meningiomas are diagnosed after the age of 50 years, more frequently in women.

Dermoid tumours are rare midline tumours that occupy the region of the vermis and may extend into the fourth ventricle. Radiologically they appear as a lobulated, well-defined cystic mass that is hyperintense on T_1WI MR scan. They are most commonly diagnosed during the first two decades of life, presenting with intracranial hypertension or acute aseptic meningitis following cyst rupture.

Haemangioblastomas are rare tumours arising most commonly in the paramedian region of the cerebellum in young and middle-aged adults (11). Some may produce erythropoietin or erythropoietin-like substance, causing polycythemia and hyperviscosity. Haemangioblastomas may be a manifestation of von Hippel–Lindau (VHL) disease, which combines retinal angiomatosis and cerebellar ataxia caused by haemangioblastoma. VHL

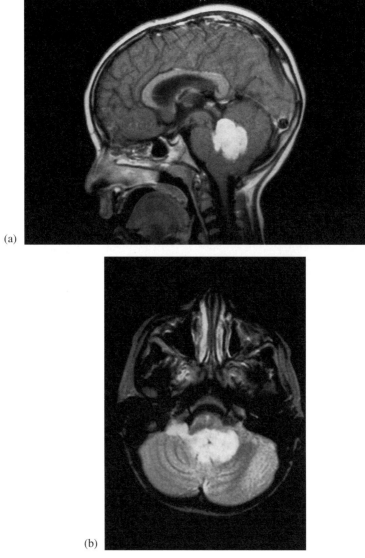

(a)

(b)

Fig. 4.1   (a) Sagittal MR scan of a medulloblastoma. The tumour that was hypointense on T_1WI is intensely enhanced by gadolinium injection. (b) An axial view shows tumour expansion into the pontocerebellar angle, causing cranial nerve palsy and a central cyst, a common radiological feature in medulloblastoma. Medulloblastoma intensity is variable on T_2WI.

disease also predisposes to the development of other neoplasms, such as endolymphatic sac tumours, renal cell carcinoma or renal cysts, phaeochromocytoma, and pancreatic tumours or cysts (12). The disease has an autosomal dominant inheritance pattern. The severity of clinical expression varies considerably within families. The VHL gene has been located on chromosome 3p. Cerebellar haemangioblastoma presents a fairly typical aspect both on CT and MRI (Fig. 4.4).

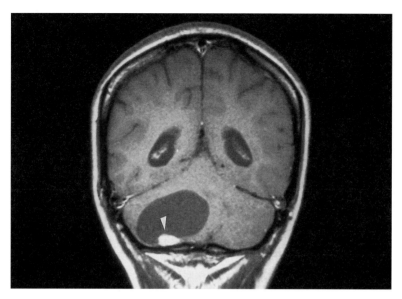

Fig. 4.2 Coronal T_1WI MR scan of a cerebellar pilocytic astrocytoma. The tumour is typically formed by a small mural nodule (arrow), intensely enhanced by gadolinium, and a large well-delineated cyst. Pilocytic astrocytomas are hyperintense on T_2WI.

Lhermitte–Duclos disease, also known as dysplastic cerebellar gangliocytoma, presents as an expanding cerebellar lesion (Fig. 4.5). The disease may recur after surgical resection and is seen in association with Cowden's syndrome. For these reasons, some authors classify this condition in the category of neoplastic gangliocytoma (13), whereas others regard it as a malformation.

2. Metastases

Metastases are the most common malignant cerebellar tumours in adults. Ten per cent of patients with brain metastases have posterior fossa symptoms. Although there is a suggestion that abdominal and pelvic primary cancers preferentially cause cerebellar metastases (14), the distribution may be similar to that shown in Table 1.3. If untreated, cerebellar metastases tend to grow rapidly and cause gait disability, intracranial hypertension, and death within a few weeks.

Treatment-related complications

1. Chemotherapy

Cerebellar injury related to anticancer chemotherapy is mainly caused by **5-fluorouracil** and **cytosine arabinoside**. High doses of 5-fluorouracil are associated with a pancerebellar syndrome, characterized by gait ataxia, limb dysmetria, nystagmus, and dysarthria (15,16). PALA (*N*-phosphoacetyl-L-aspartate) inhibits pyrimidine synthesis and is used to enhance 5-fluorouracil cytotoxicity; besides being neurotoxic by itself, it increases the cerebellar toxic-

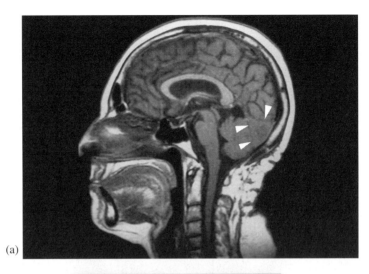

(a)

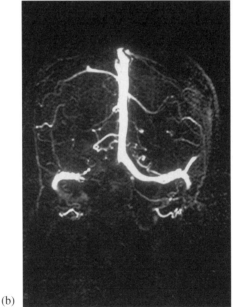

(b)

Fig. 4.3 Meningioma of the cerebellar tentorium. (a) The tumour presents typically as a mass almost isointense with grey matter (arrows) on the sagittal T_1WI MR scan. The tumour was intensely enhanced by gadolinium (see also Fig. 2.1). (b) Angio-MRI showing right lateral sinus invasion in the same patient.

ity of 5-fluorouracil (17). Single doses of cytosine arabinoside above 3 g/m^2 may produce a florid pancerebellar syndrome, which usually follows an episode of somnolence and encephalopathy. Cerebellar disorder due to cytosine arabinoside has also been observed, mainly in older patients, after cumulative doses exceeding 30 g (18,19).

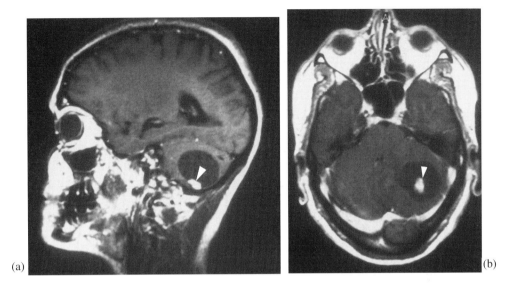

(a)   (b)

Fig. 4.4   Typical post-constrast T₁WI MR scan of a cerebellar haemangioblastoma in two different patients. Note the enhanced nodule (arrow) and the well-delineated cystic lesion.

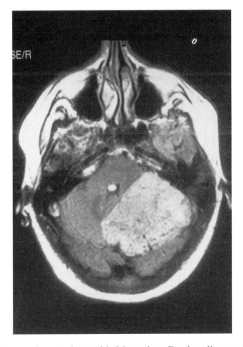

Fig. 4.5   Axial T₂WI MR scan in a patient with Lhermitte–Duclos disease. Note the characteristic folial, tigroid pattern of increased signal intensity and the mass effect caused by the lesion.

Procarbazine, hexamethylmelamine or **mitotane** (20) have also been reported to cause ataxia. However, it is not certain whether this results from cerebellar dysfunction, or from peripheral neuropathy producing sensory gait ataxia. Reversible cerebellar dysfunction has been also observed in patients treated with **tamoxifen** (21).

2. *Supportive treatments*

Phenytoin is the most common anti-epileptic drug used in neuro-oncology. Dose-related reversible nystagmus and ataxia are seen in patients with serum concentrations above 20 μg/ml (22,23). Cerebellar atrophy has been observed after prolonged administration, and is less likely to be seen in cancer patients. **Lithium** salt is used in the treatment of psychotic disorders and lithium toxicity may cause cerebellar degeneration, especially when it is given to patients with pyrexia or it is combined with the administration of neuroleptics or carbamazepine (24). Cerebellar dysarthria and ataxia are rare complications of **cyclosporin A** therapy and have been observed in patients who have undergone liver transplantation (25).

Vascular and infectious lesions

The issue of cerebellar stroke or infection has not been addressed specifically in cancer patients. Assuming that the causes of vascular and infectious CNS complications are those generally seen in cancer patients, there may be an increased incidence of :

(1) **haematomas** in patients with coagulation abnormalities (mainly acute leukaemias) or haemorrhagic metastases (mainly originating from germ-cell tumours or melanoma);

(2) **ischaemic strokes** in patients with disseminated intravascular coagulopathy, bacterial or non-bacterial endocarditis; and

(3) cerebellar **abscesses** caused by opportunistic organisms such as *Nocardia asteroides, Aspergillus* sp., *Cryptococcus neoformans*, or *Toxoplasma gondii* in immunosuppressed patients.

Paraneoplastic diseases

Paraneoplastic cerebellar degenerations (PCDs) are among the most common, most typical, and best defined paraneoplastic syndromes involving the central nervous system. They are often identified by antibodies present in the serum and the CSF. These antibodies are characteristic not only of the paraneoplastic syndrome but also of the underlying cancer (Table 4.2). In the majority of patients, the development of the paraneoplastic syndrome precedes the diagnosis of the underlying malignancy, which tends to follow a more indolent course. The neurological deficit often dominates the clinical picture. Six types of PCD have been identified (Table 4.2).

1. *Anti-Yo syndrome*

Anti-Yo antibodies are associated with isolated subacute PCD. The disorder usually starts as gait ataxia, followed by limb and truncal dysmetria, dysarthria, and intention tremor. Patients may complain of nystagmus-related oscillopsia. The neurological signs are purely cerebellar, evolve in weeks to months and remain stable thereafter. Only CT and MRI scans performed

Table 4.2 Paraneoplastic cerebellar degeneration (PCD) syndromes

Antibody	Antigen	PNS other than PCD	Associated tumour(s)	Comments
Anti-Hu, Anna-1, Type-IIa	Neuronal nuclear protein, 35–40 kDa	Limbic encephalitis, encephalomyelitis, sensory neuronopathy	SCLC, neuroblastoma (R), non-SCLC (R), prostate carcinoma (R)	Anti-Hu titres must be high; Antigen present in all tumours
Anti-Yo, PCA-1, APCA-1, Type 1	Purkinje cell cytoplasmic protein, 34 kDa and 62 kDa		Ovarian or breast carcinoma, other gynaecological carcinomas	Antigen found in the tumour only if PNS present
Anti-Ri, Anna-2, or Type IIb	Mainly nuclear neuronal protein, 55 kDa and 80 kDa	Opsoclonus, myoclonus, encephalomyelitis (R)	Breast carcinoma, gynaecological carcinoma	Antigen found in the tumour only if PNS present
CV$_2$	Oligodendrocyte cytoplasmic protein, 66 kDa	Limbic encephalitis, encephalomyelitis, sensory neuropathy	Miscellaneous, predominantly SCLC	
Anti-Tr	Purkinje cell protein		Hodgkin's disease (HD)	Tr-antibody levels may fall at HD treatment
Anti-Ma1, Anti-Ma2	Nuclei and cytoplasm, 37 kDa (Ma1) and 40 kDa (Ma2)	Brainstem dysfunction (Ma1); limbic, brainstem encephalitis (Ma2)	Miscellaneous (Ma1); testicular cancer (Ma2)	Anti-Ta recognizes Ma2 epitope

Abbreviations: SCLC, small-cell lung carcinoma; PNS, paraneoplastic neurological syndrome; (R), rare.

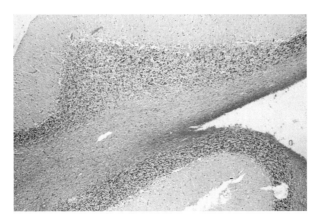

Fig. 4.6 Complete disappearance of Purkinje cells in the cerebellar hemisphere in subacute paraneoplastic cerebellar degeneration diagnosed in a woman with carcinoma of the ovary (please see plate section). Hematoxylin eoside stain (Courtesy of Professor J.J. Vanderhaeghen.)

late in the course of the disease may reveal cerebellar atrophy. CSF shows inflammatory changes, and occasionally oligoclonal bands. Pathological lesions consist of diffuse loss of Purkinje cells (Fig. 4.6.) and thinning of granular and molecular layers.

Anti-Yo antibodies are directed against cytoplasmic proteins of molecular mass 34 and 62 kDa, found only in the Purkinje cells. Indirect immunostaining reveals a characteristic coarse pattern. Yo antigens are expressed in ovary and breast carcinomas only in patients with PCD (26).

Anti-Yo antibodies are found in over 50% of PCDs in women with breast or ovary carcinoma (27). They are also associated with cancer of the adnexa and uterus and are rarely seen in PCDs associated with other tumours (28). Anti-Yo antibodies are absent in healthy controls and in cerebellar degeneration due to other causes (27). Occasionally anti-Yo antibodies have been found in high titres in patients with ovarian carcinoma without clinical cerebellar signs (29,30).

2. Anti-Hu syndrome

Anti-Hu antibodies, first identified in a patient with paraneoplastic sensory neuronopathy (see Chapter 8, p. 160, 161), are associated with a multifocal encephalomyelitis where lesions can be found anywhere between the cortex and sensory ganglia. The clinical expression of the paraneoplastic encephalomyelitis is determined largely by the most affected areas. When lesions predominate in the cerebellum, clinical manifestations may be similar to PCD associated with anti-Yo antibodies.

Hu antigen is a 35–40 kDa nuclear protein expressed in all CNS neurons, and also in small-cell lung carcinoma (SCLC) and neuroblastoma (31). High titres of anti-Hu are characteristic of paraneoplastic encephalomyelitis and of sensory neuronopathy. They are found in low titres in 16% of patients with SCLC without neurological paraneoplastic manifestations (32).

3. Anti-Ri syndrome

Anti-Ri antibodies are associated with opsoclonus, myoclonus, dysmetria, ataxia, and occasional encephalomyelitis. **Opsoclonus**, the cardinal sign, is characterized by involuntary chaotic, multidirectional saccadic eye movements. Not all patients with anti-Ri antibodies have opsoclonus and cerebellar signs may precede opsoclonus. **Myoclonus** is often evoked or enhanced by voluntary movements. **Ataxia** associated with anti-Ri antibodies is predominantly truncal. Anti-Ri syndrome evolves in 1 week to a few months. Its most striking clinical features are fluctuations with possible recovery. Favourable outcome may be related to the paucity of pathological lesions, including those in the midbrain.

Anti-Ri syndrome is associated almost exclusively with breast carcinoma. Ri antigens are 55 kDa and 80 kDa proteins present in all CNS neurons. Like for Yo antigens, but unlike Hu or calcium-channel antigens, Ri antigens were found in cancer tissue only in patients with specific serum or CSF antibodies.

Anti-Ri antibodies were absent in controls and in women with breast cancer without neurological signs (33), but were found in high titres (30) in 7 out of 181 women with ovarian cancer without neurological paraneoplastic syndrome, and occasionally in other non-paraneoplastic conditions (34).

Anti-Ri antibodies are not found in patients with opsoclonus associated with small-cell lung cancer or neuroblastoma (see Chapter 6, p. 108).

4. Anti-CV$_2$ syndrome

Anti-CV$_2$ antibodies have been found in 11 out of 45 patients with various paraneoplastic neurological syndromes. Cerebellar ataxia, reported in 6 of 11 patients, was the most common clinical sign. CV$_2$ antigen is a 66 kDa cytoplasmic protein present in oligodendrocytes. Serum anti-CV$_2$ antibodies were found in only two cancer patients without paraneoplastic neurological disease out of 1061 (35). A clinical response to excision of the primary tumour was reported in a patient with paraneoplastic cerebellar syndrome, optic neuritis, and CV$_2$ antibodies (36).

5. PCD associated with Hodgkin's disease (anti-Tr)

The cerebellopathy observed in patients with Hodgkin's disease resembles the syndromes described above. Unlike other paraneoplastic syndromes, the patients are predominantly males and the cerebellar disease tends to follow the diagnosis of Hodgkin's disease, although in 10 of 11 patients reported by Sanchez-Valle *et al.* (37) PCD antedated the diagnosis of Hodgkin's disease. In this study (37), all antineural antibodies showed immunoreactivity against Purkinje cells and a molecular layer of rat cerebellum, which is characteristic of Tr-antibodies. In some patients Tr-antibodies were detected only in CSF. Tr-antibody levels fell shortly after the effective treatment of Hodgkin's disease (37).

6. Anti-Ma syndromes

A pancerebellar dysfunction and symptoms of brainstem involvement have been observed in association with breast, parotid, and colon cancer by Dalmau *et al.* (38). Autopsy was performed in two patients and showed either complete absence or focal loss of Purkinje cells with Bergmann gliosis and mild inflammatory infiltration of cerebellar white matter. Antibodies reacting with Ma1 protein were found in the serum and the CSF of these patients. The Ma-antigen family contains at least five proteins. The best characterized— Ma1 (37 kDa) and Ma2 (40 kDa) seem to be restricted to neurons and spermatogenic cells of the testis.

Anti-Ma2 antibodies were found in patients with limbic (see Chapter 2, p. 37, 38) and brainstem (see Chapter 6, p. 107, 108) encephalitis associated with testicular cancer (39). Voltz *et al.* (39) reported that 3 out of 10 patients with anti-Ma2 antibodies also had cerebellar symptoms.

Significance of antibodies found in PCD

Studies of antibodies associated with PCD illustrate the remaining uncertainties concerning their significance in PCD and other paraneoplastic syndromes. A still unexplained but rare situation is the presence of specific antibodies in patients with PCD where no underlying cancer was found after a prolonged period of observation or even at autopsy. Several interpretations have been offered: the antigenic stimulus may be of non-neoplastic nature, the tumour has been missed because of its small size, or the tumour has been rejected through an immune reaction. The last interpretation fits with the observation that in patients with PCD and other neurological paraneoplasia, the underlying tumour grows slowly. The role of these antibodies in the pathogenesis of PCD is still unproven.

Typical PCD may occur in absence of specific antibodies, and high antibody titres have occasionally been observed in patients without clinical manifestations of neurological paraneoplasia. In addition, unlike the Lambert–Eaton syndrome, PCD has not been reproduced consistently in experimental models using human antibodies. Finally, the lack of efficacy of immunosuppressive therapies in most patients is another argument against the pathogenic role of these antibodies. From the clinical point of view, these antibodies strongly indicate paraneoplastic nature of the cerebellar degeneration. They are also of great help in the identification of the nature and the location of the underlying malignancy (Table 4.2).

Investigations

The first-choice examination in patients with cerebellar disorders and possible underlying malignant disease is brain MRI, which is clearly superior to CT scans in exploring the posterior fossa. A diagnostic algorithm based upon MRI scanning is shown in Fig. 4.7. MRI may reveal focal lesions, may be normal, or may show diffuse atrophy.

1. Focal lesion

The presence of a focal, frequently enhancing lesion on MRI or CT scan with mass effect is strongly suggestive of a tumour mass. In children this usually represents a primary tumour. The typical radiological appearances of dermoid tumours and haemangioblastomas are indicative of the diagnosis. In other cases, the identification of the tumour has to rely on tissue diagnosis. While in adults metastases are the most frequent cerebellar tumours, any of the primary brain tumours, particularly medulloblastoma and astrocytoma, may present in adult life.

Non-operable patients may undergo a diagnostic biopsy. The decision to perform such a biopsy relies largely upon individual judgement and the clinical situation. Even in patients known to have a systemic malignant disease, biopsy may reveal an unexpected and potentially curable pathology, such as abscess or granuloma. We feel that stereotactic biopsy is justified in the following circumstances:

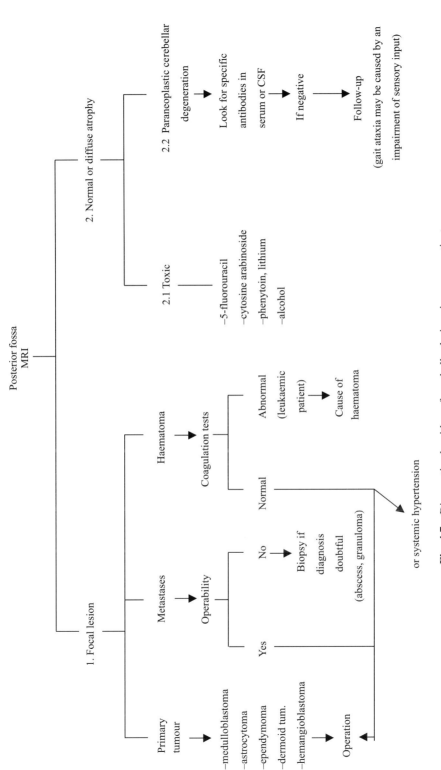

Fig. 4.7 Diagnostic algorithm of cerebellar lesions in cancer patients.

1. In the absence of known underlying malignancy or when the primary tumour is unlikely to produce brain metastases.

2. When a cerebellar haemorrhagic lesion occurs in cancer patients without coagulation disorders, and in the absence of history of systemic hypertension. In such patients, the possibility of intratumoural bleeding is high and biopsy may be advisable after the haematoma has resolved.

3. Suspected abscess not responding to an appropriate antibiotic therapy.

2. Normal or diffuse atrophy

Normal MRI or diffuse cerebellar atrophy suggests drug-induced or paraneoplastic aetiology.

2.1 Toxic aetiology   The clinical history should focus on the use of drugs toxic to the cerebellum, such as 5-fluorouracil, cytosine arabinoside, phenytoin, or lithium. Excessive alcohol consumption, which favours the development of several cancers, is also a major cause of cerebellar atrophy in adults.

2.2 Paraneoplastic cerebellar degeneration   When specific antibodies (Table 4.2) are found either in the serum or in the CSF, the diagnosis of PCD may be accepted, even in the absence of evidence of underlying malignancy. The presence of specific antibodies justifies a search for an underlying malignancy, looking particularly for treatable tumours such as Hodgkin's disease, breast cancer, or ovarian carcinoma (see Table 4.2). False-positive high titres of specific antibodies are exceptional.

In the absence of specific antibodies, the diagnosis of a paraneoplastic disease, including PCD, should be accepted with caution and only when all other diagnostic possibilities have been ruled out. A not uncommon pitfall is the diagnosis of PCD in an ataxic patient with normal brain MRI but with epidural metastases causing gait ataxia by compressing the posterior aspect of the spinal cord (40).

Therapy

The treatment of medulloblastoma and of brain metastases is considered in Chapter 12 (p. 246 to 249 and p. 255 to 261, respectively).

The management of cerebellar astrocytomas is related to the histological grade. Most pilocytic astrocytomas are composed of a tumour nodule and a cyst lined with glial membrane or tumour cells (false cyst) (Fig. 4.2.). The treatment of choice is complete resection, even though cures lasting over 20 years have been observed following partial surgical removal. The 10-year survival is 90–95% (9). The role of adjuvant radiation therapy for incompletely resected pilocytic cerebellar astrocytoma is not clear. However, it is recommended for progressive recurrent disease not amenable to complete surgical excision. Infiltrative grade 2 and high-grade cerebellar astrocytoma are usually not amenable to total resection. The benefit of adjuvant radiation and chemotherapy in the treatment of grade 2 cerebellar astrocytoma remains unproven. Adjuvant irradiation therapy is recommended after excision of high-grade tumours, but the use of adjuvant chemotherapy remains questionable.

Cerebellar deficit due to phenytoin usually subsides when serum drug concentrations fall below toxic levels. Cerebellar toxicity associated with high-dose 5-fluorouracil or cytosine arabinoside requires their discontinuation.

Most paraneoplastic cerebellar disorders are intractable. In PCD associated with Hodgkin's disease (37) and at least in one case associated with CV_2 antibodies (36), the cerebellar deficit stabilized or regressed following effective treatment of the underlying malignancy. Due to fluctuating clinical manifestations of the anti-Ri syndrome, the evaluation of treatment is difficult. Support for the hypothesis that paraneoplastic neurological disorders are caused by autoantibodies found in the serum and CSF has been demonstrated clearly in the Lambert–Eaton syndrome (41). Based on the assumption that other antibodies may be pathogenic, several studies testing immunosuppressive therapies, including plasmapheresis (42), gamma globulins, immunosuppressive drugs, or immunoabsorption (43), have been performed in patients with anti-Yo and anti-Hu syndromes. The results were generally disappointing. However, it is possible that these treatments were initiated too late, after the Purkinje cells had already been completely destroyed (see Fig. 4.6), as immunosuppressive treatment seems to be more successful when started early (44,45).

References

(1) Wessel K, Diener HE, Dichgans J *et al.* (1988). Cerebellar dysfunction in patients with bronchogenic carcinoma. *J Neurol*, **235**, 290–296.
(2) Zülch KJ. (1986). Brain tumors. Their biology and pathology, (3rd edn). Springer, Berlin.
(3) Arseni C, Cinrea AV. (1981). Statistical survey of 276 cases of medulloblastoma (1935–1978). *Acta Neurochir*, **57**, 159–162.
(4) Deutsch M, Laurent JP, Cohen ME. (1985). Myelography for staging medulloblastoma. *Cancer*, **56**, 1763–1766.
(5) Calvo FA, Hornaldo J, de la Torre A *et al.* (1983). Intracranial tumors with risk of dessimination in neuraxis. *Int J Radiat Oncol Biol Phys*, **9**, 1297–1301.
(6) Packer RJ, Schut L, Sutton LN, Bruce DA. (1989). Posterior cranial fossa brain tumors in children. In: Neurological surgery. Youmans J (ed.). Saunders, Philadelphia, pp. 3017–3040.
(7) Hayostek CJ, Shaw EG, Scheithauer B *et al.* (1993). Astrocytoma of the cerebellum. *Cancer*, **72**, 856–863.
(8) Gilles GH, Winston K, Fulchiero A, Leviton A. (1977). Histologic features and observational variation in cerebellar gliomas in children. *J Natl Cancer Inst*, **58**, 175–181.
(9) Gjerris F, Klinken L. (1978). Long-term prognosis in children with benign cerebellar astrocytoma. *J Neurosurg*, **49**, 179–184.
(10) Mamelak AN, Prados MD, Obana WG *et al.* (1994). Treatment options and prognosis for multicentric juvenile pilocytic astrocytoma. *J Neurosurg*, **81**, 24–30.
(11) Ho VB, Smirniotopoulos JG, Murphy FM *et al.* (1989). Hemangioblastoma. *AJNR*, **13**, 743–755.
(12) Richard S, Campello C, Taillandier L *et al.* (1998). Hemangioblastoma of the central nervous system in von Hippel–Lindau disease. *J Intern Med*, **243**, 547–553.
(13) Williams DW, Elster AD, Ginsberg LE *et al.* (1992). Recurrent Lhermitte–Duclos disease: report of two cases and association with Cowden's disease. *AJNR*, **13**, 287–290.

(14) Delattre JY, Krol G, Thaler HT *et al.* (1988). Distribution of brain metastases. *Arch Neurol*, **45**, 741–744.

(15) Moertel CG, Reitemeier RJ, Bolton CF, Shorter RG. (1964). Cerebellar ataxia associated with fluorinated pyrimidine therapy. *Cancer Chemother Rep*, **41**, 15–18.

(16) Riehl JL, Brown WJ. (1965). Acute cerebellar syndrome secondary to 5-fluorouracil therapy. *Neurology*, **14**, 961–967.

(17) Muggia FM, Camacho FJ, Kaplan BH *et al.* (1987). Weekly 5-fluorouracil combined with PALA: Toxic and therapeutic effects in colorectal cancer. *Cancer Treat Rep*, **71**, 253–256.

(18) Winkelman MD, Hines JD. (1989). Cerebellar degeneration caused by high dose cytosine arabinoside: a clinicopathological study. *Ann Neurol*, **14**, 520–527.

(19) Gottlieb D, Bradstock K, Koutts J *et al.* (1987). The neurotoxicity of high-dose cytosine arabinoside is age-related. *Cancer*, **60**, 1439–1441.

(20) Luton JP, Cerdas S, Billaud L *et al.* (1990). Clinical features of adrenocortical carcinoma, prognostic factors, and the effect of mitotane therapy. *N Engl J Med*, **322**, 1195–1201.

(21) Pluss JL, DiBella NJ. (1984). Reversible central nervous system dysfunction due to tamoxifen in a patient with breast cancer. *Ann Intern Med*, **101**, 652.

(22) Alpert JN. (1978). Downbeat nystagmus due to anticonvulsant toxicity. *Ann Neurol*, **4**, 471–473.

(23) Cambel WW Jr. (1980). Periodic alternating nystagmus in phenytoin intoxication. *Arch Neurol*, **37**, 178.

(24) Manto MU, Jacquy J, Hildebrand J. (1996). Cerebellar ataxia in upper limbs triggered by addition of carbamazepine to lithium treatment. *Acta Neurol Belg*, **36**, 316–317.

(25) Belli LS, De Carlis L, Romani F *et al.* (1993). Dysarthria and cerebellar ataxia: late occurrence of severe neurotoxicity in a liver transplant recipient. *Transpl Int*, **6**, 176–178.

(26) Furneaux HM, Rosenblum MK, Dalmau J *et al.* (1990). Selective expression of Purkinje-cell antigens in tumor tissue from patients with paraneoplastic cerebellar degeneration. *N Engl J Med*, **322**, 1844–1851.

(27) Jaeckle KA, Graus F, Houghton A *et al.* (1985). Autoimmune response of patients with paraneoplastic cerebellar degeneration to a Purkinje cell cytoplasmic protein antigen. *Ann Neurol*, **18**, 592–600.

(28) Greenlee JE, Dalmau J, Lyons T *et al.* (1999). Association of Anti-Yo (Type I) antibody with paraneoplastic cerebellar degeneration in the setting of transitional cell carcinoma of the bladder: detection of Yo antigen in tumor tissue and fall in antibody following tumor removal. *Ann Neurol*, **45**, 805–809.

(29) Brashear HR, Greenlee JE, Jaeckle KA, Rose JW. (1989). Anticerebellar antibodies in neurologically normal patients with ovarian neoplasms. *Neurology*, **39**, 1605–1609.

(30) Drlicek M, Bianchi G, Bogliun G *et al.* (1997). Antibodies of the anti-Yo and anti-Ri type in the absence of paraneoplastic neurological syndromes: a long-term survey of ovarian cancer patients. *J Neurol*, **244**, 85–89.

(31) Tora M, Graus F, de Bolos C, Real FX. (1997). Cell surface expression of paraneoplastic encephalomyelitis/sensory neuronopathy-associated Hu antigens in small-cell lung cancers and neuroblastomas. *Neurology*, **48**, 735–741.

(32) Dalmau J, Furneaux HM, Gralla RJ *et al.* (1990). Detection of the anti-Hu antibody in the serum of patients with small cell lung cancer—a quantitative Western blood analysis. *Ann Neurol*, **27**, 544–552.

(33) Luque FA, Furneaux HM, Ferziger R *et al.* (1991). Anti-Ri: An antibody associated with paraneoplastic opsoclonus and breast cancer. *Ann Neurol*, **29**, 241–251.

(34) Casado JL, Gil-Peralta A, Graus F *et al.* (1994). Anti-Ri antibodies associated with opsoclonus and progressive encephalomyelitis with rigidity. *Neurology*, **44**, 1521–1522.

(35) Honnorat J, Antoine JC, Derrington E *et al.* (1996). Antibodies to a subpopulation of glial cells and a 66 kDa developmental protein in patients with paraneoplastic neurological syndromes. *J Neurol Neurosurg Psychiatry*, **61**, 270–278.

(36) de la Sayette V, Bertran F, Honnorat J. (1998). Paraneoplastic cerebellar syndrome and optic neuritis with anti-CV2 antibodies. Clinical response to excision of the primary tumor. *Arch Neurol*, **55**, 405–408.

(37) Sanchez-Valle R, Dalmau J, Reñé R *et al.* (1999). Paraneoplastic cerebellar degeneration and Hodgkin's disease with anti-Tr antibodies immunological and clinical description of 11 patients. *J Neurol*, **246** (suppl. 1):1/32.

(38) Dalmau JO, Gultekin SH, Voltz R *et al.* (1999). Ma1, a novel neuronal and testis-specific protein, is recognized by the serum of patients with paraneoplastic neurologic disorders. *Brain*, **39**, 122–127.

(39) Voltz R, Gultekin SH, Rosenfeld MR *et al.* (1999). A serologic marker of paraneoplastic limbic and brain-stem encephalitis in patients with testicular cancer. *N Engl J Med*, **340**, 1788–1795.

(40) Hainline B, Tuzynski MH, Posner JB. (1992). Ataxia in epidural spinal cord compression. *Neurology*, **42**, 2193–2195.

(41) Newsom-Davis, Murray NMF. (1984). Plasma exchange and immunosuppressive drug treatment in Lambert–Eaton myasthenic syndrome. *Neurology*, **34**, 480–485.

(42) Graus F, Vega F, Delattre JY *et al.* (1992). Plasmapheresis and antineoplastic treatment in CNS paraneoplastic syndromes with antineuronal autoantibodies. *Neurology*, **42**, 536–540.

(43) Batchelor TT, Platten M, Hochberg FH. (1998). Immunoabsorption therapy for paraneoplastic syndromes. *J Neurooncol*, **40**, 131–136.

(44) Stark E, Wurster U, Patzold U *et al.* (1995). Immunological and clinical response to immunosuppressive treatment in paraneoplastic cerebellar degeneration. *Arch Neurol*, **52**, 814–818.

(45) Counsell CE, McLeod M, Grand R. (1994). Reversal of subacute paraneoplastic cerebellar syndrome with intravenous immunoglobulin. *Neurology*, **44**, 1184–1185.

5 Visual alterations

Introduction

The visual system extends all the way from the eyes to the occipital lobe. It can be affected along its long course by a number of insults. Visual disorders are very common in patients with cancer.

Clinical presentation

The type of visual abnormality is closely related to the location of the lesion, and clinical examination can identify the position of the lesion with considerable accuracy. Three lesion sites may be distinguished: prechiasmal, involving the eye and the optic nerve; chiasmal; and retrochiasmal, involving the optic tracts, optic radiations, and the occipital cortex. The principal characteristics of the three visual syndromes are summarized in Table 5.1. Visual-field abnormalities are represented schematically in Fig. 5.1.

Prechiasmal lesions cause impaired visual acuity, blurred vision, scotoma, or complete loss of vision. Patients with retinal lesions, mainly of the macula, may complain of distorted images which either appear too small or too large (metamorphia). The lesions are usually painless when the pathological process is confined to visual structures. However, some intraocular lesions, such as metastases or primary melanoma, may become painful due to secondary glaucoma. The pain associated with optic or retrobulbar neuritis is often elicited by eye movements, but this pathology is uncommon in relation to cancer. Extra-ocular lesions may cause blurred vision, often accompanied by gaze paralysis and diplopia, proptosis, and pain referred to the eye or the supraorbital region.

Chiasmal lesions cause complex alteration of visual fields. The most typical pattern is an asymmetrical, bitemporal hemianopsia. The majority of chiasmal lesions are caused by parasellar tumours. These frequently disrupt the hypothalamic–pituitary axis and cause endocrine disorders, growth abnormalities, and diabetes insipidus. Sellar and parasellar tumours may expand laterally and compress or invade the cavernous sinus. This may cause frontal pain due to involvement of the first division of the Vth cranial nerve and palpebral ptosis and diplopia due to damage of the oculomotor nerves.

Retrochiasmal lesions, involving optic tracts or radiations, cause primarily field defects (see Fig. 5.1) rather than reduced visual acuity, and may be largely unnoticed by the patient. With a right-sided lesion patients may report bumping into things on the left, or complain of loss of vision in the left eye because the temporal field is larger than the nasal field.

Bilateral cortical occipital lesions cause cortical blindness which may be denied by some patients (Anton's syndrome). Visual hallucinations due to occipital lesions usually consist of simple, possibly coloured, shapes, whereas temporal-lobe hallucinations may be much

Table 5.1 Main visual syndromes

Symptoms and signs	Prechiasmal			Chiasmal	Retrochiasmal
	Orbital	Intraocular	Optic nerve		
Visual complaints	Blurred or lost vision in one or both eyes; metamorphopsia in retinal lesions	Variable		May be unnoticed or denied; hallucinations	
Oculo-frontal pain	Frequent	If glaucoma	If optic neuritis	If associated lesion of cavernous sinus	Absent
Double vision (strabismus)	Frequent	Absent	Absent	If associated	Absent lesion of cavernous sinus
Ophthalmoscopy		Usually abnormal	Normal or optic atrophy	Normal	
Pupillary reflex		Absent or decreased		Absent or decreased	Preserved
Visual fields	Decreased acuity or loss of vision in one or both fields	Variable, typically bitemporal hemianopsia	Homonymous quadri or hemi- anopsia; cortical blindness		

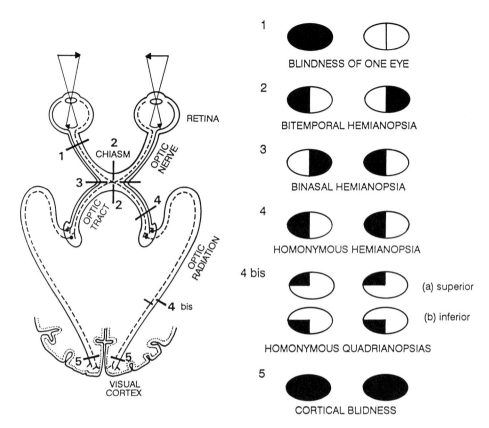

Fig. 5.1   Schematic representation of visual pathways, showing the correspondence between main visual abnormalities and lesion site.

more complex. Retrochiasmal lesions are generally painless and the pupillary reflexes are maintained.

Main aetiologies

The lesions causing visual deficits in cancer patients are summarized in Table 5.2. The direct effect of a tumour mass is the main cause of impairment of vision.

Neoplastic lesions

1. Primary tumours

In infants and children, the main primary tumours causing alteration in vision are retinoblastomas, optic gliomas, and craniopharyngiomas. In adults, primary ocular melanomas, pituitary adenomas, meningiomas, and gliomas are the most common tumours.

1.1 Retinoblastomas   Retinoblastomas, which originate from immature retinal cells, are the most common malignant ocular tumours in childhood. They account for 10–15% of all

Table 5.2 Main causes of visual alteration in cancer patients

Lesions	Causes
Neoplastic	1. Primary tumours
	1.1 Retinoblastomas
	1.2 Optic gliomas
	1.3 Craniopharyngiomas
	1.4 Primary eye melanomas
	1.5 Pituitary adenomas
	1.6 Meningiomas
	1.7 Hemispheric tumours
	2. Eye and orbit metastases
	3. Brain, pituitary, and meningeal metastases
	4. Intracranial hypertension and papilloedema
Treatment related	1. Chemotherapy
	Intracarotid
	Systemic
	2. Radiation therapy
	Eye, optic nerve lesions
	Focal radiation brain necrosis
	3. Surgery
Vascular	1. Intra-ocular haemorrhage (leukaemia)
	2. Hemispheric stroke
Paraneoplastic	Cancer associated retinopathies (rare)
	Optic neuritis (very rare)

primary ocular malignancies. Retinoblastomas are the result of mutation of the Rb tumour suppressor gene located on chromosome 13q (1). In hereditary cases, which represent about 40% of retinoblastomas, the first mutation is transmitted by germinal cells and is present in all retinal cells. The second mutation is somatic and affects the normal gene.

This 'two-hit' hypothesis fits well with the observation that in most familial cases the tumours are bilateral and multicentric whereas non-inherited retinoblastomas, which require two somatic mutations, are unilateral. In patients with family history of retinoblastoma, the diagnosis is generally made during the first year of life, and in sporadic cases usually in the second year of life. Retinoblastoma may occur in children with many other abnormalities, including mental retardation. The most common clinical manifestations of retinoblastoma are a white reflex in the pupil (cat's eye or leucocoria, Fig. 5.2) and strabismus, attributed to involvement of the macula (2,3). Ten per cent of patients develop glaucoma, causing a red, painful eye. Poor vision may be the presenting sign in slowly growing or massive tumours involving the macula. The presence of cells and debris in the vitreous may also cause impaired visual acuity. Retinoblastomas may spread intracranially and may also metastatize to the central nervous system, bones, and bone marrow (3). The risk of systemic dissemination is related to the size of the ocular tumour at diagnosis.

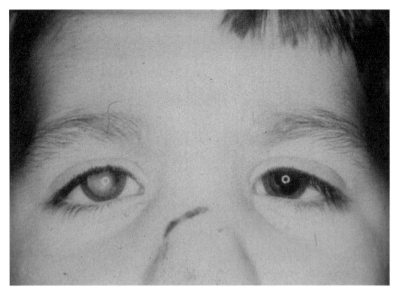

Fig. 5.2   Right-eye leucocoria in a 4-year-old boy. (Courtesy of Professor A. Zanen.)

1.2 Optic gliomas   Three-quarters of optic gliomas are diagnosed before the age of 12 years (4). They represent 5% of paediatric intracranial tumours. The majority of optic gliomas are indolent pilocytic astrocytomas. The histological characteristics of glioblastomas, which occur in fewer than 5% of cases, tend to be found in an older age group. The clinical features and prognosis of optic gliomas are related to their location and age (5).

Prechiasmal optic nerve gliomas usually occur in children. They grow very slowly or not at all, and their prognosis is particularly favourable in association with type I neurofibromatosis. They may be detected as asymptomatic lesions during investigation of type I neurofibromatosis. When symptomatic, they cause a slowly progressive visual loss. MRI or CT scans demonstrate a diffuse enlargement of optic nerve (Fig. 5.3).

Chiasmal gliomas are seen predominantly in infants or young adults. The infiltration of the chiasma causes various patterns of bilateral visual loss, most frequently an asymmetrical, bitemporal hemianopsia. MRI shows enlargement of the chiasma. Some chiasmatic glioma are exophytic (Fig. 5.4) and may cause damage to surrounding structures. Infants may develop hydrocephalus and diencephalic syndrome, characterized by emaciation and failure to gain weight despite adequate nutrition (6). Young children may present with precocious puberty and diabetes insipidus, and older children and adults with endocrinopathies (see Chapter 11, p. 206, 207).

Nearly half of optic gliomas occur in patients with **type 1 neurofibromatosis**. The diagnosis of type 1 neurofibromatosis (von Recklinghausen's disease) requires the presence of at least two of the following:

(1) six or more 'café au lait' spots;

(2) two neurofibromas or one plexiform neurofibroma;

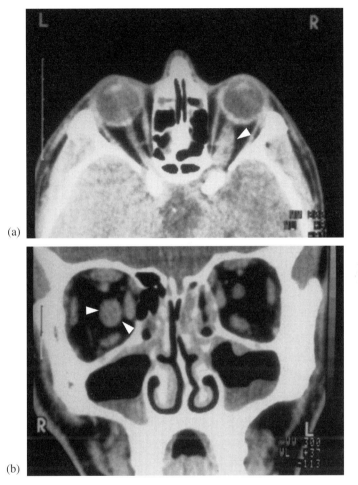

(a)

(b)

Fig. 5.3 CT scans of a fusiform enlargement (arrows) of a right optic nerve by a glioma: (a) axial and (b) cross-sectional views. (Courtesy of Professor A. Zanen.)

(3) axillary or inguinal freckling;

(4) optic glioma;

(5) sphenoid dysplasia;

(6) first-degree relative with von Recklinghausen's disease (7).

The presence of Lisch nodules (hamartoma of the iris) is a useful additional diagnostic feature. The disease is dominantly inherited, and its prevalence is 1 in 4000. The genetic abnormality is on chromosome 17q. *De novo* mutations are frequent.

1.3 Craniopharyngiomas Craniopharyngiomas are slowly growing midline tumours of the suprasellar region, accounting for 5–10% of paediatric brain tumours, with a peak incidence around the age of 10, although they can occur at any age. Over 60% of patients may present

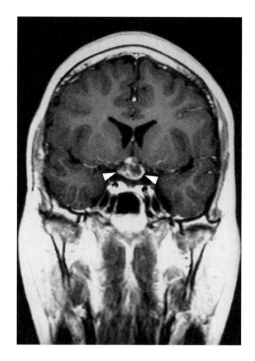

Fig. 5.4 Coronal gadolinium-enhanced T_1WI MR scan of an exophytic chiasmal glioma bulging into the hypothalamic region. The tumour appears as an heterogeneous, partially cystic mass.

with intracranial hypertension due to hydrocephalus. Half of the patients present with visual abnormalities, such as bitemporal hemianopsia, unilateral or bilateral blindness, due to chiasmal compression.

Damage to hypothalamic–pituitary axis causes growth delay, precocious puberty, or diabetes insipidus (see Chapter 11, p. 207) and in adults, amenorrhoea or impotence. Radiological features are generally diagnostic (Fig. 5.5), although epidermoid tumour of the suprasellar region and cystic pituitary adenoma may resemble craniopharyngioma. However, epidermoid tumour is more frequent in adults between the third and the fifth decade than in children, and pituitary adenomas are mainly diagnosed in adults.

1.4 Primary eye melanomas   Melanomas are the most common primary intra-ocular malignant tumours in Caucasian adults, accounting for 70% of all primary ocular malignancies (8). The diagnosis is made most frequently during the sixth decade. The tumour may arise in the iris, the ciliary body, or the choroid. Ciliary-body melanomas tend to remain asymptomatic for longer and tend to be larger at diagnosis, as they are hidden behind the iris. Anterior tumours are also more likely to compress the lens and produce astigmatism, secondary glaucoma, and invasion of the anterior chamber. Posterior uveal melanomas grow from discoid to hemispherical mass, displacing Bruch's membrane. Smaller tumours produce overlying orange pigment (Fig. 5.6). Larger tumours have a tendency to break through Bruch's membrane and to grow as pigmented, mushroom-shaped masses in the subretinal space (Fig. 5.7), with infiltration of the vitreous. The incidence of trans-scleral extension after enucleation

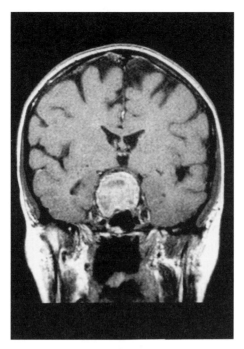

Fig. 5.5 Coronal T₁WI MR scan of a suprasellar craniopharyngioma. Gadolinium administration mostly enhances the rim of the tumour. The hypointense signals correspond to calcifications. Craniopharyngiomas are typically hypointense on T_1WI and hyperintense on T_2WI.

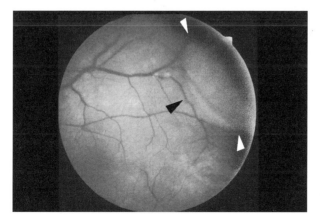

Fig. 5.6 Small intraocular melanoma. The tumour is located in the upper left periphery (arrows). It appears as a brownish choroidal lesion with some faint orange pigment raising the retina (please see plate section). (Courtesy of Professor A. Zanen.)

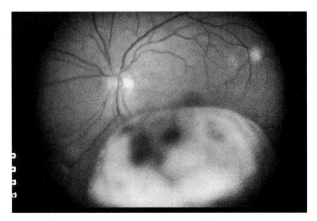

Fig. 5.7   Large intraocular melanoma. The tumour appears as a dome-shaped mass adjacent to the optic nerve. Note the dark irregular pigmentation (please see plate section). (Courtesy of Professor A. Zanen.)

ranges from 15–50% and is related to tumour size. Metastatic disease generally occurs in the first 5 years following diagnosis and therapy. The liver is the most common metastatic site, usually present when other sites of metastatic disease, including the CNS, are found.

1.5 Pituitary adenomas   Only the visual deficits caused by pituitary adenomas will be described here. Endocrine abnormalities are considered in Chapter 11 (p. 208, 209). Alteration of visual fields is caused by pituitary adenomas which extend upwards through the diaphragma sellae (Fig. 5.8). The pattern of visual-field deficit is related to the manner in which the tumour damages the optic chiasma. The classical presentation is bitemporal, often asymmetrical hemianopsia, usually starting as an upper temporal field defect. Neurological signs, including visual-field deficits, are more likely to occur as presenting features in patients with non-functional pituitary adenomas, and in patients with secreting tumours where excess hormone production remains unnoticed (9). These situations include:

(1) prolactin-secreting adenomas in men or post-menopausal women;

(2) growth hormone-secreting adenomas, particularly as acromegaly may pass unnoticed for a long time and tumours tend to be larger than in other hormonally active pituitary adenomas; and

(3) TSH-secreting adenomas in patients who have undergone prior thyroidectomy.

Conversely, visual signs are rare in ACTH-secreting pituitary adenomas (Cushing's disease).

1.6 Meningiomas   Ninety to 95% of meningiomas are benign, grade 1 tumours (10,11). They originate from the arachnoid and tend to involve the dura. Meningiomas are more common in women, with a female to male ratio of 2:1. Meningiomas generally become symptomatic in patients over 50 years of age. Several meningioma locations may injure optic pathways.

Optic nerve meningiomas usually cause painless visual deficit by compressing the nerve itself or its blood supply (Fig. 5.9). Proptosis is the second most frequent sign of optic nerve

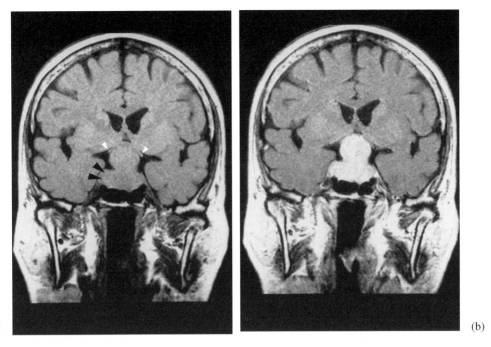

(a)   (b)

Fig. 5.8 Coronal MR scan of a voluminous pituitary macroadenoma expanding through the diaphrama sellae. The tumour displaces the optic chiasma upwards (white arrows), and extends into the right cavernous sinus (black arrows). The adenoma has typically the same signal as the cortex on T_1WI (a) and is enhanced intensely by gadolinium (b).

meningioma. Both compression and ischaemia contribute to optic nerve injury when the meningioma is located in the optic foramen.

Sphenoid ridge meningiomas compress the optic nerve from above, producing optic atrophy. They may also cause intracranial hypertension and contralateral papilloedema, giving raise to the Foster Kennedy syndrome.

In **olfactory groove meningiomas** optic atrophy may be associated with anosmia and mental changes. Meningiomas arising from the **tuberculum sellae**, the **clinoid**, or the **diaphragma sellae** tend to produce chiasmal-type visual defects or unilateral visual loss, gradually extending to the second eye. Endocrine disorders or diabetes insipidus may be associated with visual abnormalities. Foster Kennedy syndrome occurs in 5% of the patients.

1.7 Hemispheric tumours Hemispheric primary tumours may cause homonymous visual-field defects (Fig. 5.1) such as inferior quadrianopsia (parietal lesion), superior quadrianopsia (temporal lesion), or hemianopsia (occipital lesion). The most common primary tumours are intrinsic gliomas or extrinsic meningiomas.

2. *Eye and orbit metastases*

Intraocular or orbital metastases originate primarily from breast cancer (74%) in women; in men 56% of eye metastases originate from lung carcinoma (12). Nine per cent of eye and

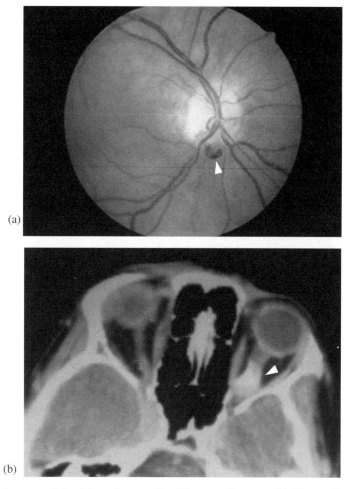

(a)

(b)

Fig. 5.9 Meningioma of the right optic nerve in a 35-year-old woman. (a) The eye fundus shows a pale optic disc with, at its inferior margin, an optociliary vessel shunt diverting the retinal venous blood from the compressed central retinal vein to the choroidal effluent vessels (arrow) (please see plate section). (b) Axial CT demonstrating an intra-orbital meningioma compressing the optic nerve (arrow) in the same patient. (Courtesy of Professor A. Zanen.)

orbit metastases are of unknown origin. A quarter of patients presenting with eye metastases have no previous history of malignant disease, and lung cancer is the most frequent underlying neoplasm. In patients with breast cancer, eye metastases usually develop in the context of previously diagnosed metastatic disease. Many other tumours may metastatize to the eye, including melanoma, gastrointestinal, renal, and prostate carcinomas, and lymphoma. About 30% of intraocular metastases are bilateral. The choroid is the most common site of eye metastases, but they may develop in other structures such as uvea, retina, or the vitreous. Intra-ocular metastases may remain asymptomatic or cause blurred vision, scotoma, and painful

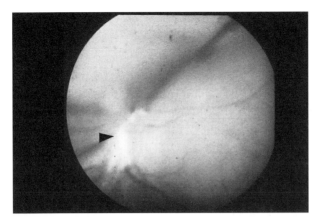

Fig. 5.10 Eye metastasis in a woman with breast carcinoma. The lesion appears as a yellowish, bilobulated ballooning, partially masking the optic disc (arrow) (please see plate section). (Courtesy of Professor A. Zanen.)

glaucoma. They appear on ophthalmoscopy as yellowish, dome-shaped lesions (Fig. 5.10). Some may cause retinal detachment.

In addition to the metastastic seedings, **orbit structures** may be invaded by adjacent tumours, including basal cell carcinomas of the eye adnexae or epithelial tumours of the anterior skull base, carcinomas of the nasal cavity, paranasal sinuses, and nasopharynx, or by anaesthesioneuroblastomas. Metastatic tumours may cause visual loss, orbital pain, proptosis, and ophthalmoplegia (Fig. 5.11).

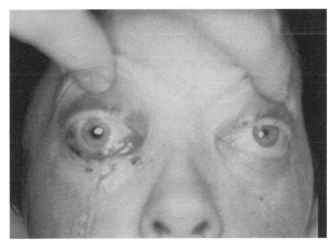

Fig. 5.11 Orbital metastasis of a lung carcinoma, causing proptosis and ophthalmoplegia of the right eye. (Courtesy of Professor A. Zanen.)

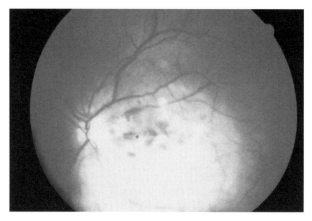

Fig. 5.12 Retinal deposit in a patient with primary non-Hodgkin's CNS lymphoma (please see plate section). (Courtesy of Dr K. Hoang-Xuan.)

Eyes are involved in up to 20% of patients with primary CNS lymphoma (PCNSL) (13,14). Lymphomatous deposits may be identified in the vitreous by slit-lamp examination, and in the choroid or retina by ophthalmoscopy (Fig. 5.12). Patients may complain of obscured or blurred vision. However, most lymphoma eye deposits are asymptomatic. Therefore, all patients with PCNSL need an ophthalmologic examination (see Chapter 12, p. 253). Conversely, at least 80% of patients presenting with ocular lymphoma eventually develop brain lesions (13). Thus any patient with ocular lymphoma should have brain MRI and lumbar puncture, and should be followed if these examinations are negative.

3. Brain, pituitary, and leptomeningeal metastases

Parenchymal **brain metastases** are multiple in about one-half of the patients and may generate various patterns of visual-field defect, including cortical blindness caused by bilateral occipital metastases.

Pituitary metastases are seen most frequently in patients with breast carcinoma (15). Visual deficits caused by metastases may mimic adenomas, but pituitary metastases differ from pituitary adenoma by an accompanying high incidence of diabetes insipidus (see Chapter 11, p. 210). They may be associated with features of cavernous sinus involvement.

Ten per cent of patients with meningeal neoplastic disease may have symptomatic infiltration of the **leptomeninges** around optic nerves and chiasma, causing visual loss (Fig. 1.4). Visual loss may be the initial symptom of the malignant disease or of its relapse (16,17). Blindness is usually progressive but vision loss may occur within 24–48 hours (18,19). The main mechanism of visual loss in patients with meningeal metastases is direct infiltration of the optic nerve by malignant cells. However, intracranial hypertension and occipital infiltration by neoplastic cells may also contribute to the visual deficits (20).

4. Intracranial hypertension and papilloedema

Papilloedema from increased intracranial pressure causes enlargement of the physiological blind spot. This is generally asymptomatic, although patients may report brief obscurations of vision. In chronic papilloedema, disc swelling subsides and the disc becomes atrophic. Optic atrophy may present with impaired colour vision and visual acuity, permanent visual-field deficit, or blindness.

Treatment-related complications

1. Chemotherapy

Visual deficits have been consistently reported after intracarotid chemotherapy for malignant hemispheric tumours, but conventional administration of anticancer drugs rarely causes impairment of vision.

Retinal toxicity ranges from impaired colour vision to decreased visual acuity and complete blindness. It has been reported after **intracarotid infusion** of nitrosoureas (BCNU (21) or HeCNU (22)), cisplatin (23) and carboplatin (24), and drug combinations (25,26). The mechanism of eye toxicity is retinal vasculitis, which appears on ophthalmoscopy as arteriolar leakage, and arterial changes ranging from narrowing to occlusion, causing macular oedema. The incidence of intracarotid chemotherapy-induced retinal toxicity is somewhat difficult to assess because it has not been recorded systematically in all trials, but the risk is approximately 10%. Factors that predispose to toxicity include: the drug dose, use of ethanol as drug solvent, and a narrow carotid artery favouring high drug concentrations. Eye toxicity is considerably diminished when the tip of the catheter is placed above the origin of ophthalmic artery (27) but this procedure may increase CNS toxicity.

Visual toxicity caused by **systemic chemotherapy** is rare. While it is occasionally reported, it is difficult to distinguish whether it is due to polychemotherapy, concomitant irradiation, infiltration of the optic pathway by neoplastic cells, or a combination of these. For example, the three patients reported by Wilson *et al.* (28) who developed a sudden and total blindness due to optic chiasma demyelination several months after treatment with oral **CCNU**, also received other anticancer drugs and whole brain irradiation to 3000–4500 cGy. The optic atrophy attributed to **vincristine** (29,30) or to intrathecal or high-dose **methotrexate** therapy (31) were reported in patients who received other treatments and may have had leptomeningeal carcinomatosis (32). Several cases of either reversible or unresolving optic neuritis reviewed by Kaplan and Wiernik (33) have been attributed to systemically administrated **cisplatin**. Prolonged administration of tamoxifen (34) and mitotane (35) has been associated with reversible ocular toxicity.

Cortical blindness due to occipital lesions has been observed within hours of the administration of cisplatin (36), vincristine (37), or polychemotherapy (38). Cortical blindness may be a manifestation of **posterior leucoencephalopathy syndrome** observed in patients treated with cyclosporin A and allogenic bone-marrow transplantation (39). This syndrome also includes raised blood pressure, headaches, seizures, and white-matter changes on CT and MRI, especially in the occipital lobes.

2. Radiation therapy

Conventional radiation therapy may cause injury to the visual system anywhere along its path.

Keratoconjunctivitis sicca results from the damage of conjunctival and corneal epithelium due to impaired tear secretion following irradiation of the lachrymal gland with doses beyond 4000–4500 cGy. This is not an invariable complication of therapy as it is prevented by early regular administration of eye lubrication with substitute tears. The conjunctival lining of the cornea is particularly sensitive to radiation injury. Corneal ulceration due to excessive dose is avoided by treating the eye open to achieve surface sparing of megavolt-age irradiation. Irradiating the cornea to 5700 cGy or more causes keratoconjunctivitis (40) within 1–2 months. Keratoconjunctivitis is characterized by severe pain and visual loss caused by ulceration, vascularization, and eventually opacification of the cornea. In addition, corneal ulceration makes the entire eye vulnerable to bacterial infections.

Post-radiation **cataract** is a common complication of eye irradiation, even when low doses are used (40).

Radiation retinopathy occurs after a delay of 1.5–6 years following doses beyond 5000 cGy at 180–200 cGy per fraction. The risk of radiation retinopathy is dose related and the delay appears longer following lower-dose irradiation. After a period of normal or nearly normal visual acuity, vision loss occurs insidiously and progresses over months, without pain unless neovascular glaucoma develops. The mechanism of radiation retinopathy is similar to the mechanism of radiation injury to the CNS, with small vessels being the primary target of injury. Progressive obliteration of small vessels causes ischaemia, oedema, microaneurysms, and retinal haemorrhages, leading to blindness. These changes are observed by ophthal-moscopy or by fluorescein angiography, which allows a detailed examination of retinal vessels including the capillary system. Cotton-wool exudes are frequently seen on ophthal-moscopic examination.

Optic atrophy can occur 1–6 years after irradiation to doses beyond 5500 cGy and the risk is related to dose per fraction. Optic atrophy is also due to ischaemia resulting from small-vessel occlusion. It causes decreased visual acuity or visual-field defect, and is detected as pallor of the optic disc on fundoscopy. In anterior lesions, pallor may be preceded by disc swelling and haemorrhage. When the injury to the optic nerve is more posterior, there is no evidence of oedema or haemorrhage on ophthalmoscopy (retrobulbar optic neuropathy).

Late-delayed **focal radiation brain necrosis** (see Chapter 2, p. 35), anywhere along the optic pathway beyond the optic chiasma, mimics brain tumour recurrence, and may produce a homonymous field defect.

3. Surgery

Visual loss occasionally follow the removal of an anterior cranial basal meningioma involv-ing sphenoid ridge, anterior clinoid, tuberculum sellae, or olfactory groove (41). The cause of visual deterioration is most likely ischaemic. Attempts of total resection of craniopharyn-giomas that are intimately associated with optic chiasma may cause permanent visual defect.

Vascular lesions

Retinal haemorrhages are seen in patients with coagulation disorders, particularly in asso-ciation with acute leukaemia (Fig. 5.13). Retinal bleeding may also occur in patients with primary or metastatic malignant intra-ocular tumours. Patients with macular haemorrhage complain of decreased visual acuity, and those with more peripheral bleeding report seeing black spots. **Optic nerve ischaemia** may result either from optic artery compression by tumours, such as optic glioma, meningioma, or metastases, or from post-radiation vascular injury.

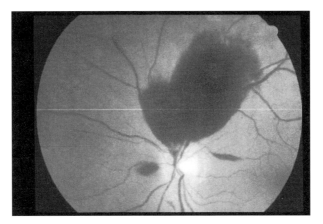

Fig. 5.13   Retinal and pre-retinal (dark red) haemorrhages in acute leukaemia (please see plate section). (Courtesy Professor A. Zanen.)

Both haemorrhagic and ischaemic stroke cause visual-field defects of retrochiasmal type, or cortical blindness. The main causes of **stroke** in cancer patients are described in Chapter 1 (p. 12, 14).

Pituitary apoplexy, due to ischaemic necrosis of the pituitary adenoma, is a rare cause of acute visual loss, often accompanied by sudden onset of headache and loss of consciousness (see Chapter 1, p. 5 and Fig. 1.3).

Paraneoplastic diseases

Visual paraneoplastic disorders are rare, and of these retinopathy is the best documented. Cancer-associated retinopathy (CAR) is characterized by a bilateral, often asymmetrical degeneration of retinal ganglion cell photoreceptors, causing a painless loss of vision which may occur suddenly but generally progress over weeks to months. The most common visual-field deficits are central scotoma and concentric constriction. In 90% of patients, CAR is associated with small-cell lung cancer and, in most cases, precedes discovery of the tumour. The auto-antibodies detected in the serum of some patients react with lung cancer antigens of approximate molecular weight 65 kDa and with a 23 kDa retinal protein (42), but antigens may differ from patient to patient. The antibodies have not been detected in sera from cancer patients without CAR, patients with retinitis pigmentosa, and normal controls.

A distinct acquired retinopathy causing progressive night blindness and 'shimmering lights' has been reported in melanoma patients (43). Fundoscopy is either normal or shows retinal vitiligo.

A few cases of pure, painless **optic neuritis**, considered as a paraneoplastic condition, have been reported in cancer patients (44,45). A case of reversible potentially immune-mediated bilateral optic neuropathy was reported in a woman with multiple myeloma (46). The visual deficit recovered after chemotherapy and the disappearance of serum paraprotein.

Investigations

The differential diagnosis of lesions affecting the visual system in cancer patients is based on the distinction between prechiasmal, chiasmal, and retrochiasmal lesions.

1. Prechiasmal lesions

Prechiasmal location is suggested by a combination of decreased visual acuity, blurred vision, scotoma, metamorphia, painful eye, unresponsive pupil, diplopia, or proptosis (Table 5.1). Direct and indirect ophthalmoscopy are usually abnormal, but the distinction between malignant and benign lesions may be difficult. For example, in children the differential diagnosis of retinoblastoma includes intraocular inflammation, infection by *Toxocara canis* (a parasite of puppies), or administration of oxygen at birth. In adults, primary ocular melanoma, lymphoma, or metastases may mimic intra-ocular inflammation. Conversely, posterior scleritis, choroid haemorrhage, or detachment may be mistaken for malignant lesions. In cancer patients many pathological processes may be bilateral. Therefore, the asymptomatic eye also needs to be examined carefully. Diseases most likely to affect both eyes are metastases, familial retinoblastoma, lesions due to chemotherapy or radiation therapy, and rare paraneoplastic syndromes. The differential diagnosis of prechiasmal lesions depends on the ability to visualize the eye by external ophthalmic examination and is based on the distinction between patients with clear or unclear eye media.

1.1 Patients with clear ocular media   In these patients the entire uvea can be examined by direct or indirect ophthalmoscopy. These examinations may reveal a large number of abnormalities, summarized in Table 5.3.

An **uveal mass** may correspond to various tumours, which can be delineated and better demonstrated by fluorescein angiography. Yellowish, dome-shaped lesions suggest metastases (Fig. 5.10), particularly in patients known to have systemic cancer, such as breast, lung, or prostate carcinoma. In doubtful cases and in patients not known to have cancer, needle biopsy should be performed. Eye involvement by non-Hodgkin's lymphoma may be demonstrated by slit-lamp examination or direct ophthalmoscopy (47). In patients with normal MRI and normal CSF, diagnostic confirmation may require aspiration of the vitreous, although lymphoma cells may be difficult to distinguish from inflammatory lymphoid cells. Small-sized primary **uveal melanomas** produce an orange pigmented lesion (Fig. 5.6) growing into a dome-shaped pigmented mass (Fig. 5.7). In experienced hands, the diagnostic accuracy of outpatient examination, including ophthalmoscopy, fluorescein angiography, and ultrasonography, is over 90% (8). Needle aspiration or incisional biopsy are rarely needed. Extrascleral extension in large tumours can be assessed by MRI. The search for distant seedings should include liver ultrasound, as the liver is the first site of metastatic spread.

In patients where **retinoblastoma** can be readily seen, the diagnosis is based on family history, direct ophthalmoscopy, slit-lamp examination, ultrasonography, or CT scan, showing calcifications. Fine-needle aspiration biopsy is not recommended and is seldom necessary.

Retinal and **anterior optic nerve infiltration**, which may cause a raised optic disc with or without **haemorrhage**, has been observed in 9% of leukaemic patients (48). It is less common in other systemic malignancies. Involvement of the optic disc and optic nerve usually heralds meningeal relapse. Intra-ocular involvement by leukaemic cells is equivalent

Table 5.3 Ophthalmoscopy abnormalities caused by cancer-related pathologies

Lesion	Investigations	Main causes
Uveal metastases	Look for systemic cancer	Breast, lung, prostate carcinoma
Primary lymphoma	Slit lamp, ophthalmoscopy	Immunodepression
	Brain MRI	
	Lumbar puncture	
	Vitreal aspiration	
Primary melanoma	Fluorescein angiography	
	Ultrasonography	
	Biopsy: rare	
Retinoblastoma	History	40% are hereditary
	Slit lamp, ultrasonography	
	CT or MRI	
Retinal infiltrate and haemorrhage	History (leukaemia)	Acute leukaemia
	Blood and bone marrow examination	Coagulation disorders
	Coagulation tests	Radiation retinopathy
Retinal vasculitis	Fluorescein angiography	Intracarotid chemotherapy
		Radiation retinitis
Retinal degeneration or retinal vitiligo	Serum antibodies (few patients)	Small-cell lung cancer
	Ophthalmoscopy	Melanoma
Papilloedema	Brain MRI or CT	Intracranial hypertension
Swollen optic disc	High-resolution MRI of retrobulbar area	Leukaemia
	Blood and bone marrow examination	Metastases of other tumours
		Primary tumours
Optic disc atrophy	MRI or CT	Papilloedema, ICHT
		Swollen disc
		Optic nerve glioma
		Meningioma
		Carcinoma
		Metastases
		Radiation therapy
		Chemotherapy
		Paraneoplasia

ICHT, intracranial hypertension.

to CNS relapse, as the eye is also a sanctuary for malignant cells, protected by the blood–retina barrier. Retinal haemorrhage may also occur in non-leukaemic patients with coagulation abnormalities or in radiation retinopathy.

Retinal **vasculitis**, which is confirmed by fluorescein angiography, may be caused by intracarotid chemotherapy or radiation therapy.

Cancer-related **retinal degeneration** is seen in CAR syndrome. Retinal vitiligo indicates a rare paraneoplastic disorder associated with melanoma. In a minority of patients with CAR, specific antibodies reacting with retinal receptors and ganglia cells are found in the serum.

Bilateral papilloedema is seen in the presence of an intracranial hypertension. Anteriorly located tumours, such as sphenoid ridge meningiomas, may cause ipsilateral optic nerve atrophy, and only later contralateral papilloedema (Foster Kennedy syndrome).

Swollen optic disc may closely resemble papilloedema but, unlike in papilloedema, visual acuity is usually altered. Swollen disc may be caused by neoplastic infiltration of optic nerve head, obstruction of the central retinal vein, or by an inflammatory reaction. Optic nerve infiltration by tumour cells may be demonstrated by high-resolution MRI.

Optic disc atrophy may be the result of either papilloedema and intracranial hypertension, neoplastic optic nerve infiltration, compression of the optic nerve, or impaired blood supply. The most common cause of optic nerve atrophy in cancer patients is pressure on the optic nerve by tumour, particularly optic glioma, meningioma, or metastases. Disc atrophy as a result of optic neuritis due to chemotherapy, radiotherapy, or to a remote effect of cancer is rare.

Visual features of prechiasmal lesion and normal fundoscopy suggest a tumour located behind the eye. High-resolution MRI and visual evoked potentials may help to identify the lesion.

1.2 Patients with unclear ocular media   In patients where fundoscopy is precluded because the ocular media is opaque due to inflammation, haemorrhage, cataract, or neoplastic infiltration, the diagnosis may be difficult. It is based on the patient's history, age, eye CT, MRI, and ultrasound examination. For example, a child under 3 years with an eye tumour showing calcium deposits on the surface on CT scan is very likely to have retinoblastoma. An adult or elderly patient with unilateral media opacity should be considered to have uveal melanoma until proven otherwise.

The differential diagnosis of prechiasmal lesions has not been based on the distinction between intrinsic and extrinsic eye lesion because the symptoms and signs often overlap. However, such a distinction may be helpful. Most tumours circumscribed to the eye globe cause painless visual impairment. They become painful only when a secondary glaucoma develops. In patients with initially extra-ocular orbital lesions, pain, diplopia, oculomotor nerve palsies, and proptosis are prominent features and visual impairment is often a late manifestation.

2. Chiasmal and retrochiasmal lesions

Normal eye examination and ophthalmoscopy point toward chiasmal or retrochiasmal lesions, although optic atrophy may be seen in the presence of chiasmal lesions. Chiasmal lesions differ from retrochiasmal injuries by the pattern of visual-field abnormalities. The differential diagnosis is summarized in Table 5.1.

2.1 Chiasmal lesions   Chiasmal lesions produce a variety of visual-field abnormalities, most typically a bitemporal quadri- or hemianopsia. **Intrinsic** chiasmatic tumours are gliomas, which are best diagnosed by high-resolution MRI (Fig. 5.4). The main **extrinsic**, suprasellar, slowly growing tumours are meningiomas, craniopharyngiomas, and pituitary adenomas. In addition to visual disorders, they may cause hydrocephalus, cavernous sinus syndrome, abnormal endocrine status, and diabetes insipidus. Although these features may help in the differential diagnosis, in practice the diagnosis is based on imaging (illustrated in Figs 5.5 and 5.8) and is generally confirmed at operation. The diagnosis of sella metastases is suggested by rapid progression of clinical signs, MRI changes, and the presence of a systemic malignancy, usually breast carcinoma (15). In patients without known systemic cancer, rapidly growing chiasma lesions should either be excised or biopsied. The suprasellar region is a typical site of spread of pineal germ-cell tumours (49). A proportion of cranial germinomas may arise in the suprasellar region.

2.2 Retrochiasmal lesions

Retrochiasmal lesions typically cause contralateral quadri- or hemianopsia. In cancer patients these lesions may be due to primary or metastatic tumours, ischaemic or haemorrhagic stroke, focal radiation necrosis, or abscess. Their differential diagnosis and investigations are discussed in Chapter 1 (p. 17 to 21). Bilateral lesions involving occipital lobes may cause cortical blindness. Cortical blindness has occasionally been attributed to chemotherapy (36–38).

Therapy

In **retinoblastomas** enucleation with resection of the optic nerve is performed in unilateral or bilateral tumours when there is no hope for restoring useful vision and the tumour completely fills the globe, disrupts the retina, or invades the anterior chamber (50). In patients with tumour extension into the orbit or optic nerve, enucleation is followed by external radiation therapy to a dose of 5000 cGy given in 5 weeks. In patients with useful residual vision, localized external irradiation to 3500–4500 cGy in a daily dose of 180–200 cGy is used, sparing the posterior surface of the lens. Laser photocoagulation is suitable for posterior-pole retinoblastomas up to 5 mm in diameter and 2.5 mm in thickness without evidence of vitreous seeding. Cryotherapy is used for tumours anterior to the eye-globe equator (51). The method is also useful in recurrent tumours following radiation therapy. Retinoblastoma is sensitive to chemotherapy. Carboplatin, vincristine, and etoposide (VP-16) are the most commonly used agents. Chemotherapy may be used to reduce tumour volume and allow more focused therapy (52) or to treat CNS, bone, or bone-marrow metastases. The use of adjuvant chemotherapy has not been established.

Optic pathway gliomas which are asymptomatic or cause minimal symptoms and have an indolent course, may be followed by surveillance alone, consisting of serial examinations of visual acuity, visual field, and imaging. This is particularly the case in optic nerve gliomas of childhood or occurring in patients with type 1 neurofibromatosis. The typical radiological features and the intrinsic nature of the tumour, involving the optic nerve and chiasma, usually preclude the need for surgery and histological confirmation of the diagnosis. Surgery is only considered in:

(1) patients with lost vision, to prevent tumour extension to chiasma or painful proptosis;

(2) rapidly growing gliomas; and

(3) exophytic tumours of the chiasma, causing mass effect or invading the hypothalamus (5).

External irradiation with 5000–5400 cGy is the treatment of choice for symptomatic and progressive chiasmal gliomas in adults and children over 5 years of age (53). Stereotactically guided fractionated irradiation provides a more localized means of radiation delivery and is especially of value in the paediatric population. To minimize intellectual, endocrine, and visual deficits due to radiation therapy, attempts have been made to use chemotherapy as the first-line treatment (54,55). These studies indicate that chemotherapy, including vincristine and carboplatin, allows treatment by irradiation to be delayed, by transient reduction or stabilization of tumour size, which may be accompanied by improvement or stabilization of visual acuity.

Treatment of **craniopharyngiomas** is considered in Chapter 11 (p. 219).

The treatment of **primary ocular melanoma** ranges from periodic observation of small, flat ($\leq$2 mm in thickness), and dormant tumours of the posterior uvea, to enucleation or large orbital exenteration of extended melanoma producing severe visual loss (56). The choice of treatment depends on:

(1) the amount of preserved vision, and intra-ocular pressure;

(2) the size, site, and growth rate of the tumour;

(3) the condition of the opposite eye; and

(4) the patient's performance status.

There is an increased tendency to use localized irradiation in the form of brachytherapy with episcleral radioactive plaques or external proton irradiation rather than resorting to enucleation. Although radiotherapy and enucleation are associated with equivalent long-term survival, irradiation carries lower immediate visual morbidity (57). Small tumours residual or recurrent after radiation therapy may be treated by photocoagulation. However, the use of this requires clear ocular media and a tumour thickness of 3 mm or less. Systemic metastases of eye melanoma may be treated with palliative intent chemotherapy, immunotherapy, and occasionally local resection or irradiation (8).

Meningiomas causing visual loss should be resected if this is feasible and the sphenoid ridge location is the most amenable to complete excision. The chances of recovery are related to the duration of visual impairment. Three-quarters of patients operated on within 2 years of the onset of symptoms have improvement in vision (58). In patients with suprasellar meningioma, vision improves in less than half of the patients. Optic nerve meningiomas can not be resected without causing blindness. Radiation therapy may control the growth of partially resected or inoperable meningiomas. The use of chemotherapy or hormone therapy in meningioma (considered in Chapter 6, p. 124) is uncertain.

The treatment of **ocular and orbital metastases** is largely palliative. Most patients should receive palliative radiotherapy with 3000–4000 cGy over 2–4 weeks. Patients with chemosensitive tumours, such as breast carcinoma may benefit from chemotherapy, and radiation therapy may be delayed or avoided. Vitreous or retinal metastases found in patients with primary non-Hodgkin's CNS lymphoma should be treated with additional irradiation following systemic chemotherapy (Chapter 12, p. 254).

Paraneoplastic retinopathies or optic nerve neuropathies do not usually respond to treatment of the underlying malignancy or to immunosuppressive drugs.

References

(1) Sparkes RS, Wilson MG, Towner JW *et al.* (1980). Regional assignment of genes for human esterase D and retinoblastoma to chromosome band 13q 14. *Science*, **208**, 1042–1044.

(2) Shields JA, Shields CL. (1992). Intraocular tumors. A text and atlas. WB Saunders, Philadelphia.

(3) Abramson DH. (1990). Retinoblastoma 1990: diagnosis, treatment and implications. *Pediatr Ann*, **19**, 387–395.

(4) Matson DD. (1969). Neurosurgery of infancy and childhood, (2nd edn). Charles C. Thomas, Springfield IL.

(5) Atler JL, Tabell NJ, Laws E Jr. (1996). Optic nerve, chiasmal and hypothalamic region tumours. In: Cancer in the nervous system. Levin VA (ed). Churchill Livingstone, New York, pp. 139–151.

(6) Pelc S. (1972). The diencephalic syndrome in infants: A review in relation to optic nerve glioma. *Eur Neurol*, **7**, 321–334.

(7) von Deimling A, Krone W. (1997). Neurofibromatosis type 1. In: Pathology and genetic. Tumours of the nervous system. Kleihues P, Cavenee WK (eds). International Agency for Research on Cancer, Lyon, pp. 172–174.

(8) Sahel JA, Steevens RA, Albert DM. (1997). Intraocular melanoma. In: Cancer principles and practice of oncology, (5th edn). De Vita VT Jr, Helleman S, Rosenberg SA (eds). Lippicott-Raven, Philadelphia, pp. 1995–2011.

(9) Thapar K, Kovacs K, Laws ER. (1997). Pituitary tumors. In: Cancer of the nervous system. Black PMcL, Loeffler JS (eds). Blackwell Science, Cambridge Mass, pp 363–403.

(10) Kepes JJ. (1982). Meningiomas: Biology, pathology and differential diagnosis. Masson, New York.

(11) Jaaskelainen J, Haltia M, Servo A. (1986). Atypical and anaplastic meningiomas: radiology, surgery, radiotherapy and outcome. *Surg Neurol*, **25**, 233–242.

(12) Shakin EP, Shields JA. (1989). The eye and ocular adnexa in systemic malignancy. In: Duane's clinical ophthalmology, Vol. 5. Tasman W, Jaeger EA (eds). JB Lippincott, Philadelphia, Chapter 34, pp. 1–7.

(13) Rockwood EJ, Zakov ZN, Bay JW. (1984). Combined malignant lymphoma of the eye and CNS (reticulum-cell sarcoma). Report of 3 cases. *J Neurosurg*, **61**, 369–374.

(14) DeAngelis LM, Yahalom J, Heinemann MH, *et al.* (1990). Primary CNS lymphoma: Combined treatment with chemotherapy and radiotherapy. *Neurology*, **40**, 80–86.

(15) Max BM, Deck MDF, Rottenberg DA. (1981). Pituitary metastasis: incidence in cancer patients and clinical differentiation from pituitary adenoma. *Neurology*, **31**, 998–1002.

(16) Olson ME, Chernik NL, Posner JB. (1974). Infiltration of the leptomeninges by systemic cancer. *Arch Neurol*, **30**, 122–137.

(17) Wasserstrom W, Glass JP, Posner JB. (1982). Diagnosis and treatment of leptomeningeal metastases from solid tumors: Experience with 90 patients. *Cancer*, **49**, 759–772.

(18) Altrocchi PH, Eckman PB. (1973). Meningeal carcinomatosis and blindness. *J Neurol Neurosurg Psychiatry*, **36**, 206–210.

(19) Fischer-Williams M, Bosanquet FD, Daniel PM. (1955). Carcinomatosis of the meninges. A report of three cases. *Brain*, **78**, 42–58.

(20) Henson RA, Urich H. (1982). Cancer and nervous system. Blackwell, Oxford, pp. 100–119.

(21) Greenberg HS, Ensminger WD, Chandler WF *et al.* (1984). Intra-arterial BCNU chemotherapy for treatment of malignant gliomas of the central nervous system. *J Neurosurg*, **61**, 423–429.

(22) Poisson M, Chiras J, Fauchon F *et al.* (1990). Treatment of malignant recurrent glioma by intra-arterial, infra-ophtalmic infusion of HeCNU 1-(2-chloroethyl)-1-nitroso-3-(2-hydroxyethyl)urea. A phase II study. *J Neurooncology*, **8**, 255–262.

(23) Newton HB, Page MA, Junck L, Greenberg HS. (1989). Intra-arterial cisplatin for the treatment of malignant gliomas. *J Neurooncology*, **7**, 39–45.

(24) Stewart DJ, Belanger JM, Grahovac Z *et al.* (1992). Phase I study of intracarotid administration of carboplatin. *Neurosurgery*, **30**, 512–517.

(25) Stewart DJ, Grahovac Z, Benoit B *et al.* (1984). Intracarotid chemotherapy with a combination of 1,3-*bis* (2-chloroethyl)-1-nitrosourea (BCNU), *cis*-diaminedichloroplatinum (Cisplatin), and 4'-*O*-demethyl-1-*O*-(4,6–0–2-thenylidene-β-D-glucopyranosyl)epipodophyllotoxin (VM-26) in the treatment of primary and metastatic brain tumors. *Neurosurgery*, **15**, 828–833.

(26) Rogers LR, Purvis JB, Lederman RJ. (1991). Alternating sequential intracarotid BCNU and cis-platin in recurrent malignant glioma. *Cancer*, **68**, 15–21.

(27) Kapp JP, Vance RB. (1985). Supraophthalmic carotid infusion for recurrent glioma. Rationale, technique and preliminary results for cisplatin and BCNU. *J Neurooncology*, **3**, 5–11.

(28) Wilson WB, Perez GM, Kleinschmidt-Demasters BK. (1987). Sudden onset of blindness in patients treated with oral CCNU and low-dose cranial irradiation. *Cancer*, **59**, 901–907.

(29) Awidi AS. (1980). Blindness and vincristine. *Ann Intern Med*, **93**, 781.

(30) Shurin SB, Rekate HL, Annable W. (1982). Optic atrophy induced by vincristine. *Pediatrics*, **70**, 288–291.

(31) Bleyer WA, Drake JC, Chabner BA. (1973). Neurotoxicity and elevated cerebrospinal fluid methotrexate concentration in meningeal leukemia. *N Engl J Med*, **289**, 770–773.

(32) Boogerd W, Moffie D, Smets LA. (1990). Early blindness and coma during intrathecal chemotherapy for meningeal carcinomatosis. *Cancer*, **65**, 452–457.

(33) Kaplan RS, Wiernik PH. (1982). Neurotoxicity of antineoplastic drugs. *Semin Oncology*, **9**, 103–130.

(34) Pavlidis NA, Petris C, Briassoulis E *et al.* (1992). Clear evidence that long-term, low-dose tamoxiphen treatment can induce ocular toxicity. A prospective study of 63 patients. *Cancer*, **69**, 2961–2964.

(35) Vizel M, Oster MW. (1982). Ocular side effects of cancer chemotherapy. *Cancer*, **49**, 1999–2002.

(36) Diamond SB, Rudolph SH, Lubicz SS *et al.* (1982). Cerebral blindness in association with cis-platinum chemotherapy for advanced carcinoma of the fallopian tube. *Obstet Gynecol*, **59**, 84S–86S.

(37) Byrd RL, Rohrbaugh TM, Raney RB, Norris DG. (1981). Transient cortical blindness second-ary to vincristine therapy in childhood malignancies. *Cancer*, **47**, 37–40.

(38) Heran F, Defer G, Brugieres P *et al.* (1990). Cortical blindness during chemotherapy: Clinical, CT, and MR correlations. *J Computer Assist Tomogr*, 14:262–266.

(39) Hinchey J, Chaves C, Appignani B *et al.* (1996). A reversible posterior leukoencephalopathy syndrome. *N Engl J Med*, **334**, 494–500.

(40) Parsons JT, Bova FJ, Fitzgerald CR *et al.* (1991). Tolerance of the visual apparatus to conventi-nal therapeutic irradiation. In: Radiation injury to the nervous system. Gutin Ph, Leibel SA, Sheline GE (eds). Raven Press, New York, pp. 283–302.

(41) DeMonte F. (1996). Surgical treatment of anterior basal meningiomas. *J Neurooncology*, **29**, 239–248.

(42) Thirkill CE, FitzGerald P, Sergott RC *et al.* (1989). Cancer-associated retinopathy (CAR syn-drome) with antibodies reacting with retinal, optic nerve and cancer cells. *N Engl J Med*, **32**, 1589–1594.

(43) Berson EL, Lessell S. (1988). Paraneoplastic night blindness with malignant melanoma. *Am J Ophthalmol*, **106**, 307–311.

(44) Tang RA, Kellaway J, Young SE. (1991). Ophthalmic complications of systemic cancer. *Oncology*, **5**, 59–71.

(45) Malik S, Furlan AJ, Sweeny PJ *et al.* (1992). Optic neuropathy: a rare paraneoplastic syndrome. *J Clin Ophthalmol*, **12**, 137–141.

(46) Lieberman FS, Odel J, Hirsh J *et al.* (1999). Bilateral optic neuropathy with IgGkappa multiple myeloma improved after myeloablative chemotherapy. *Neurology*, **52**, 414–416.

(47) Hochberg FH, Miller DC. (1988). Primary central nervous system lymphoma. *J Neurosurg*, **68**, 835–853.

(48) Ridgway EW, Jaffe N, Walton DS. (1976). Leukemic ophthalmoscopy in children. *Cancer*, **38**, 1744–1749.

(49) Fetell MR, Stein BM. (1986). Neuroendocrine aspects of pineal tumours. In: Neurologic clinics, Vol 4. Zimmerman EA, Abrams GM (eds). Saunders, Philadelphia, pp. 877–905.

(50) Shields CL, Shields JA, De Potter P. (1996). New treatment modalities for retinoblastoma. *Curr Opin Ophthalmol*, **7**, 20–26.

(51) Shields CL, Shields JA, Kiratli H, De Potter PV. (1995). Treatment of retinoblastoma with indirect ophthalmoscope laser photocoagulation. *J Pediatr Ophthalmol Strabismus*, **32**, 317–322.

(52) Murphree AL, Villablanca JG, Deegan WF *et al.* (1996). Chemotherapy plus local treatment in the management of intraocular retinoblastoma. *Arch Ophtalmol*, **114**, 1348–1356.

(53) Pierce SM, Barnes PD, Loeffler JS *et al.* (1990). Definitive radiation therapy in the management of symptomatic patients with optic glioma. Survival and long-term effects. *Cancer*, **65**, 45–52.

(54) Packer RJ, Sutton LN, Bilaniuk LT *et al.* (1988). Treatment of chiasmatic/hypothalamic gliomas of childhood with chemotherapy: an update. *Ann Neurol*, **23**, 79–85.

(55) Petronio J, Edwards MS, Prados M *et al.* (1991). Management of chiasmal/hypothalamic gliomas of infancy and childhood with chemotherapy. *J Neurosurg*, **74**, 701–708.

(56) Shields JA, Shields CL, Donoso LA. (1991). Management of posterior uveal melanoma. *Surv Ophthalmol*, **36**, 161–195.

(57) Seddon JM, Gragoudas ES, Polivogianis L *et al.* (1986). Visual outcome after proton beam irradiation of uveal melanoma. *Ophthalmology*, **93**, 666–674.

(58) Rosenstein J, Symon L. (1984). Surgical management of suprasellar meningioma. Part 2: Prognosis for visual function following craniotomy. *J Neurosurg*, **61**, 642–648.

6 Cranial nerve and brainstem lesions

Introduction

All true cranial nerves from the IIIrd to the XIIth originate in the brainstem, where their nuclei and nerve fibres are in close anatomical relation with long motor and sensory tracts. Thus the combination of cranial nerve and long-tract lesions is a hallmark of **intrinsic** brainstem injury. **Extrinsic** lesions originating from structures that surround the brainstem may either affect the nerves alone or may generate neurological deficits that combine cranial nerve and brainstem symptoms and signs. In neuro-oncological practice the distinction between intrinsic and extrinsic brainstem lesions is a common diagnostic issue. Therefore the two types of lesion have been combined and are considered in the same chapter.

Clinical presentation

Knowledge of the topographic distribution of nervous structures helps to localize the lesion. Unilateral median brainstem lesions will produce **contralateral** hemiparesis (corticospinal tract) and loss of position and vibration sense (median lemniscus). Lateral lesions will cause contralateral loss of cutaneous sensation.

   Cranial nerve abnormalities are ipsilateral and indicative of the rostro-caudal position of the lesion. However, not all cranial nerve palsies have an equal localizing value. For example, VIth nerve palsy occurring in patients with intracranial hypertension may be a false localizing sign.

   Several other important structures are located in the brainstem:

1. The **reticular formation** which is essential in maintaining normal consciousness (see Chapter 1, p. 1).
2. The **pontine gaze centre**, located near the VIth nerve nucleus. Its destruction impairs gaze towards the side of the pontine lesion.
3. The **median longitudinal fasciculus**; its lesion causes internuclear ophthalmoplegia. Unilateral lesion will impair adduction of the ipsilateral eye, and produce a nystagmus of the contralateral abducting eye.
4. The **vestibular nuclei and their connections**, their injury causes a gaze-evoked nystagmus.
5. Lesions of the **cerebellar input** and **output** pathways cause ipsilateral cerebellar symptoms and signs (Chapter 4, p. 61).

Opsoclonus (often associated with myoclonus) consists of abnormal, continuous, involuntary, chaotic, multidirectional eye movements in all directions. Opsoclonus has been putatively attributed to the lesion of pause neurons located in the paramedian pontine reticular formation. However, in view of conflicting neuropathological reports, other CNS structures, including the cerebellum, may be also involved.

Many distinct syndromes resulting from small brainstem lesions have been described, particularly in stroke patients. Most diseases involving the brainstem in cancer patients are neoplastic. They tend to be more diffuse and produce less characteristic clinical presentations. Nevertheless, the mere association of long-tract deficits with gaze-evoked nystagmus, internuclear ophthalmoplegia, cerebellar signs, or contralateral cranial nerve abnormalities points to brainstem injury.

Main aetiologies

The main causes of intra-axial and extra-axial brainstem and cranial nerve lesions are listed in Table 6.1.

Table 6.1 Main causes of intra- or extra-axial lesions involving brainstem and cranial nerve

Lesions	Intra-axial	Causes	Extra-axial
Neoplastic		Primary tumours	
	Glioma		Pineal tumours
	Ependymoma		Meningioma
			Schwannoma (neurinoma)
			Other tumours (epidermoids)
		Metastases	
	Brainstem		Leptomeningeal
			Skull base
			Head and neck
Treatment related		Chemotherapy	
			Cisplatin: VIIIth nerve
			Vinca alkaloids
		Radiation therapy	
	Brainstem necrosis (plus multiple chemotherapy)		Cranial nerves (neuromyotonia)
		Surgery	
			Cranial nerves
Infectious	Rhomboencephalitis (*Listeria monocytogenes*)		Bacterial and fungal meningitis
			Herpes zoster
Paraneoplastic	Anti-Hu, anti-Ma1, or anti-Ma2 syndromes (brainstem encephalitis)		
	Opsoclonus–myoclonus complex		

Intra-axial brainstem injuries

Neoplastic lesions

Gliomas

Two-thirds of brainstem gliomas occur before the age of 20 years, making up 10–20% of all paediatric brain tumours (1). A second small peak of incidence occurs during the fourth decade, but in adults brainstem gliomas constitute less than 2% of all brain tumours. Brainstem glioma occupy three distinct sites, which differ in their clinical manifestations, pathological features, and prognosis.

   Approximately 70% of brainstem gliomas infiltrate the pons (Fig. 6.1) and present with progressive:

(1) cranial nerve palsies, mainly of the VIth and VIIth nerves, which are often the initial signs;

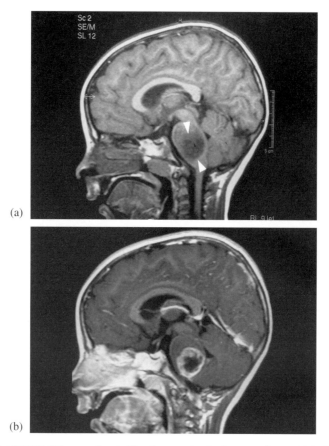

(a)

(b)

Fig. 6.1   Sagittal T_1WI MRI scan of an infiltrating pontine brainstem glioma, (a) before and (b) after gadolinium administration.

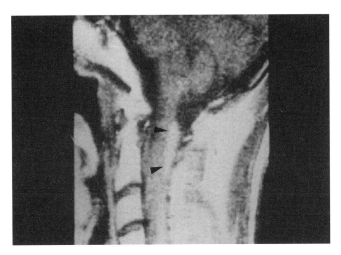

Fig. 6.2 Sagittal gadolinium-enhanced T_1WI MR scan of a partially exophytic glioma located at the cervicomedullary junction (arrows). (Courtesy of Professor J. Brotchi.)

(2) long-tract deficits, causing limb weakness, gait difficulty, and sensory ataxia; and

(3) cerebellar signs, including gait ataxia and nystagmus.

Some children may display personality changes or cognitive disorders, such as a decline in school performance. These abnormalities have been observed even in the absence of hydrocephalus, and their pathogenesis is not fully understood.

Up to 20% of brainstem gliomas are located at the cervicomedullary junction. They often present an exophytic growth (Fig. 6.2) which can fill the fourth ventricle. The tumours are frequently more benign than pontine gliomas and can be pilocytic astrocytomas. Cervicomedullary gliomas commonly present with headaches, projectile vomiting, dysphagia, and dysarthria.

About 10–15% of brainstem gliomas are located in the midbrain. They also present with headaches, vomiting, and papilloedema related to obstructive hydrocephalus. Tectal midbrain gliomas may cause Parinaud's syndrome (see p. 108).

MRI allows an accurate and early diagnosis of all brainstem gliomas. In children with infiltrating gliomas, characteristic radiological features (Fig. 6.1) preclude the need for a diagnostic biopsy (2).

Ependymomas

In children, ependymomas represent 10–20% of posterior fossa tumours before the age of 15 years, surpassed in frequency only by medulloblastomas and gliomas. In children, two-thirds of ependymomas arise infratentorially, typically from the floor of the fourth ventricle. The majority of ependymomas occurring in adults are supratentorial (3). Ependymomas have a relatively indolent natural history and clinical manifestations usually precede the diagnosis by few months. The most common presentation is intracranial hypertension caused by filling of the fourth ventricle and occlusion of CSF outflow (Fig. 6.3). The complaint is headache

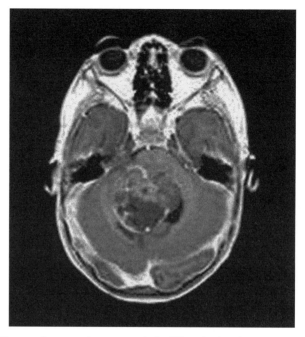

Fig. 6.3 Axial MR scan of an ependymoma entirely filling the fourth ventricle. On this T$_1$WI scan the tumour is heterogeneously enhanced by gadolinium.

and vomiting, with frequent papilloedema. Ependymomas infiltrating the brainstem may mimic pontine glioma by causing multiple cranial nerve lesions, limb weakness, and sensory ataxia. Tumours extending into the cerebellopontine angle cause cerebellar signs resembling medulloblastoma (Fig. 6.4).

Ependymomas that infiltrate the upper portion of the spinal cord produce neck stiffness and head tilt. Craniospinal dissemination occurs in 3–15% of patients (4,5). It is more common in posterior fossa lesions and in anaplastic tumours. There are several pathological classifications of ependymomas. Although the prognostic value of histological grading remains controversial (5,6), as it has not been consistently proven that the survival of patients with 'malignant', 'undifferentiated', or 'high-grade' lesions was shorter, a separation into grades 2 and 3 is proposed in the current WHO classification. The issue is further confounded by inclusion of ependymoblastomas. They occur before the age of 5 years, have poor prognosis, and are regarded as PNETs (primitive neuroectodermal tumours) or embryonal tumours (7). It is possible that the poor prognosis of young children with ependymoma observed in several studies is, at least partially, due to the inclusion of children with ependymoblastoma.

Metastases

As the distribution of metastases in the brain is roughly random and in proportion to the brain mass of a specific region, the presence of metastases in the brainstem is relatively rare,

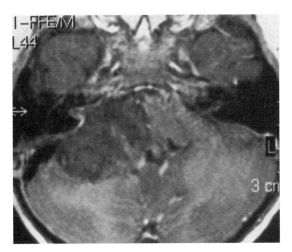

Fig. 6.4 Axial gadolinium-enhanced T_1W1 MR scan showing fourth ventricule ependymoma extending to the cerebellopontine angle.

although not exceptional (8,9) (Fig. 1.7). Unlike primary intrinsic brainstem tumours, metastases occur predominantly in adults. They often cause gaze and cranial nerve palsy, and gait ataxia, progressing over weeks. They tend to be small and MRI may be necessary to visualize them.

Treatment-related lesions

Intrinsic brainstem lesions caused by anticancer treatments are rare. Multifocal pontine lesions characterized by loss of myelin, loss and swelling of axons, have been observed in patients treated with multiple chemotherapy regimens and radiation therapy. Their pathogenesis is unclear but is probably due to direct damage by combined anticancer therapy (10).

Infections

Infections limited to brainstem are rare. *Listeria monocytogenes*, which infects immunosuppressed individuals preferentially, particularly patients with leukaemia or lymphoma, has a tendency to involve the brainstem and may cause focal brainstem deficits (11).

Paraneoplasia

Paraneoplastic brainstem encephalitis

Paraneoplastic brainstem encephalitis may occur as a predominant location or as part of a more diffuse anti-Hu syndrome which includes limbic encephalitis (Chapter 2, p. 37, 38), cerebellar degeneration (Chapter 4, p. 68 to 72), and sensory neuronopathy (Chapter 8, p. 160, 161) and lower motor neuron lesion (Chapter 7, p. 144). Clinical features of brainstem involvement include ophthalmoplegia, diplopia, nystagmus, dysarthria, and dysphagia.

More recently brainstem encephalitis has been associated with two other antibodies. Voltz *et al.* (12) reported 13 patients with testicular cancer and paraneoplastic limbic and brainstem encephalitis associated with Ma2 antibodies. Three of four patients with Ma1 antibodies and a variety of malignancies also had brainstem and cerebellar dysfunction, and one patient had dysphagia and weakness (13).

Paraneoplastic opsoclonus–myoclonus

In infants and children paraneoplastic opsoclonus is associated with neuroblastoma (14) and in up to 50% of these patients opsoclonus precedes tumour diagnosis. In adults, paraneoplastic opsoclonus–myoclonus is less frequent than in children. The likelihood of detecting an underlying tumour, particularly lung cancer, is about 20% (15). Paraneoplastic opsoclonus may remit spontaneously, and in many patients neuropathological abnormalities were not found, even in the brainstem. Opsoclonus–myoclonus, clinically similar to that found in cancer patients, may also be caused by infectious, toxic, or metabolic diseases. The paraneoplastic nature of the syndrome is based on the allegedly high incidence of association with malignancies, as no specific antibody markers have been found, unlike opsoclonus–myoclonus seen in anti-Ri syndrome, where it is associated with cerebellar dysfunction (Chapter 4, p. 70, 71).

Extra-axial brainstem injuries

Extrinsic lesions causing damage to the brainstem and the cranial nerves are predominantly neoplastic in cancer patients.

Neoplastic lesions

Pineal tumours

Pineal tumours are rare, accounting for about 0.5% of intracranial malignancies in Europe and North America. They affect adolescents and young adults, with a peak incidence in the second and the third decades. **Germ-cell tumours** account for about 40% of pineal tumours (16). Two-thirds are germinomas and others are non-germinomatous germ-cell tumours.

Non-germinomatous tumours containing yolk-sac elements may produce α-fetoprotein, and those containing choriocarcinoma elements produce human β-chorionic gonadotrophin. Human β-chorionic gonadotrophin may be also produced by syncytiotrophoblasts in otherwise pure germinoma. Measurement of human β-chorionic gonadotrophin and α-fetoprotein in serum and CSF is useful in diagnosis and treatment monitoring. Elevated α-fetoprotein is diagnostic of non-germinomatous tumours, as are high levels of human β-chorionic gonadotrophin. A moderate rise in human β-chorionic gonadotrophin may be seen in germinomas and non-germinomatous germ cell tumours.

Neoplasms arising from pinealocytes account for about 20% of all pineal tumours. They may be either **pineocytomas** or highly malignant **pineoblastomas**, which predominate in children and are considered to be PNETs. **Glial tumours** of the pineal region are mainly astrocytomas, of various malignancy grades.

Tectal compression due to pineal tumours (Fig. 6.5) is characterized by Parinaud's syndrome. It consists of impaired upward gaze and poor pupillary response to light, with preserved response to accommodation. Further tectal compression may cause unequal pupil size, impaired convergence, and retractory nystagmus. Pineal tumours frequently compress

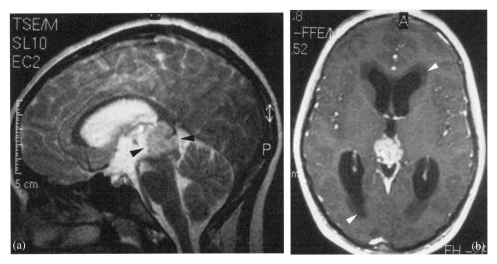

Fig. 6.5 MR scan of a pineocytoma in a 12-year-old boy. (a) Sagittal T_2WI shows tectal and peri-aqueductal depression by the tumoral mass (arrows). (b) Axial enhanced T_1WI shows hydrocephalus with CSF extrusion into the periventricular white matter (arrows).

the aqueduct causing hydrocephalus and intracranial hypertension (Fig. 6.5). Extension of tumour to superior cerebellar peduncles may cause cerebellar signs, and extension to the cavernous sinus produces hypoaesthesia, pain in the territory of the ophthalmic branch of the Vth nerve, and diplopia. Diabetes insipidus and endocrine disorders associated with tumours of the pineal region are considered in Chapter 11 (p. 208).

Meningiomas

Meningiomas are classified according to the site of attachment (17). However, tumours with a similar base may extend in different directions and the cranial nerve lesions may only tentatively indicate primary meningioma location (Table 6.2).

Table 6.2 Cranial nerve lesions caused by meningiomas

Location (attachment)	Most common cranial nerve lesion	Other early or frequent symptoms and signs
Sphenoid ridge (inner part)	VI, III, IV, V_1	Progressive visual loss
		Optic atrophy
Olfactory groove	I (anosmia), II (visual loss)	Mental changes, seizures
Cavernous sinus	V_1, (V_2), III, IV, VI	
Cerebellopontine angle	VIII, VII, V, IX–X	Cerebellar, brainstem signs
Clivus:		
Middle and rostral	III, V, VIII, VII, VI	
Posterior	XI, IX–X, XII	
Cerebellar convexity	Late vision abnormalities (optic atrophy)	Intracranial hypertension, hydrocephalus, cerebellar signs
Foramen magnum	Lower cranial nerves (V and VII, rare)	Cervical and upper-limb pain, sensory loss, and weakness

Schwannomas

The VIIIth nerve is the most common site of intracranial schwannomas (18). Vestibular schwannomas constitute 80% of cerebellopontine angle tumours, with meningiomas (10%), epidermoid tumours, and metastases occurring infrequently. Bilateral vestibular schwannomas are found in about 5% of all cases and are diagnostic of **type 2 neurofibromatosis**, which is a dominantly inherited disease. Other features of type 2 neurofibromatosis include intracranial schwannomas of other intracranial nerves, meningiomas and gliomas, posterior lens opacities, cerebral calcifications, and rare cutaneous schwannomas. Sporadic vestibular schwannomas are generally diagnosed during the fifth or sixth decade, but tumours occurring in patients with type 2 neurofibromatosis are usually discovered during the first or second decade of life.

All patients with a vestibular schwannoma present with features of nerve involvement. The initial complaint is tinnitus and impaired hearing, particularly high-frequency hearing loss, and this is followed by facial paresis. MRI is particularly useful at detecting an enhancing cerebellopontine angle mass, and MRI can usually distinguish vestibular schwannoma from meningioma (Figs 6.6 and 6.7). Evoked brainstem potentials may contribute to early diagnosis (Fig. 6.8).

If there is poor access to modern imaging, the tumour may remain undiagnosed and continue to grow, causing damage to other cranial nerves, including the Vth, IX–Xth, and VIth nerves, and may lead to cerebellar and brainstem compression. Eventually intracranial hypertension may develop.

Schwannomas may arise from other cranial nerves listed in Table 6.3. The initial symptoms and signs allow for accurate localization of tumours, with the exception of differential diagnosis between VIIth and VIIIth nerve schwannoma, as both tumours cause hearing loss and facial weakness. Large intracranial schwannomas late in the course of disease may damage several cranial nerves and compress the brainstem, making precise clinical localization difficult. The occurrence of multiple intracranial schwannomas suggest the diagnosis of type 2 neurofibromatosis.

Epidermoid tumours

Between 40 and 50% of cranial epidermoid tumours are found in the cerebellopontine angle and constitute the third most common mass in this location after schwannoma and meningioma. About 15% are suprasellar or midline posterior fossa tumours. Intracranial epidermoid tumours are congenital, but their diagnosis is made mostly around the fourth decade. Cerebellopontine epidermoids cause irritation of the Vth nerve and may present with a 'tic douloureux'. Epidermoids are cystic tumours with MRI signal characteristics similar to those of CSF (Fig. 6.9).

Leptomeningeal metastases

Cranial nerve palsies are a cardinal feature of leptomeningeal metastases (19). They are often associated with other signs of meningeal carcinomatosis, such as encephalopathy, hydrocephalus, meningeal irritation, and spinal root deficits. Diplopia and ocular paresis followed by facial weakness, hearing and visual loss are the most common manifestations, but any cranial nerve may be involved. Untreated disease progresses rapidly, usually over a few

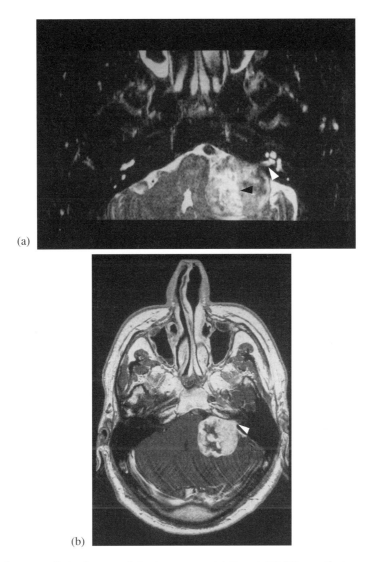

(a)

(b)

Fig. 6.6 Large vestibular (or acoustic) schwannoma. (a) On axial T$_2$WI scan the tumour is heterogeneous and slightly hyperintense to the cerebral tissue. (b) Axial post-contrast T$_1$WI MR scan shows
a strong, heterogeneous enhancement. Note the foci of cystic degeneration (black arrows) and the
intracanalicular segment of the tumour (white arrows) shown on T$_1$ and T$_2$ images.

weeks, and cranial nerve abnormalities develop during the course of the disease in up to 70%
of the patients. The primary tumours causing leptomeningeal metastases are listed in Table
1.4. Damage to cranial nerves occurs more frequently in meningeal involvement by solid
tumours than in leukaemic meningitis (20). The diagnosis is confirmed by detecting neoplastic cells in the CSF (see Chapter 1, p. 17). MRI changes suggestive of leptomeningeal
spread of malignancy (see Fig. 1.4) are found in about 70% of patients and contribute to the
diagnosis.

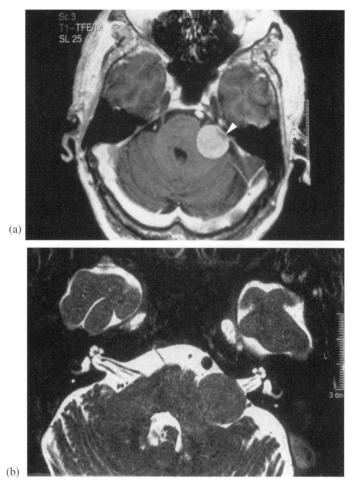

(a)

(b)

Fig. 6.7 Axial MR scan of a cerebellopontine angle meningioma. (a) T_1WI shows a strong enhancement by gadolinium. (b) On T_2WI the tumour is isointense with cerebral tissue. Compared with vestibular schwannoma (Fig. 6.6), note the dural tail (arrow), the absence of cystic degeneration, and no intracanalicular tumour location.

Metastases of the base of the skull

Cranial nerve lesions caused by skull metastases are very common. They may indicate widespread bone metastases or they may be the initial manifestation of a malignant disease. The latter is exemplified by patients with numb chin syndrome reported by Massey *et al.* (21). Of 19 cancer patients presenting with this syndrome, 16 died of cancer within 17 months.

The location of skull metastases may be indicated by a specific combination of cranial nerve lesions (22). They are grouped into individual syndromes in Table 6.4. However, in practice, these syndromes are either incomplete or overlap, and most are unilateral.

Bony metastases may be visualized by plain X-rays but are best demonstrated by CT scan. MRI reveals not only bone lesions, it also demonstrates their intra- and extra-cranial extent (Fig. 6.10). Isotopic bone scan, using technetium, is a sensitive screening examin-

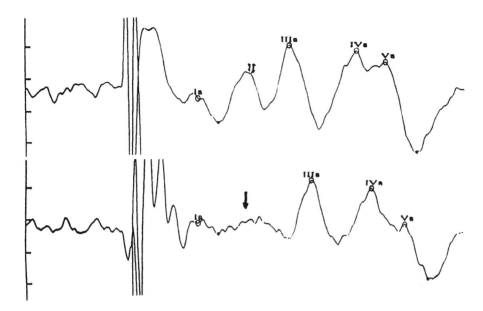

Fig. 6.8 Brainstem auditory evoked potentials (BAEP) in a patient with acoustic schwannoma. Compared to the normal side (upper trace) the abnormal BAEP (lower trace) shows the absence of wave II (arrow) and a delay in waves III to V. (Courtesy of Dr Ph. Voordecker.)

Table 6.3 Clinical presentation of cranial nerve schwannomas

Location (nerve)	First symptoms and signs	Other (later) features
III–IV–VI	Diplopia, strabismus	Brainstem compression
V	Facial numbness, dysaesthesia, neuralgia	Diplopia
VII	Unilateral hearing loss, facial dysaesthesia and facial weakness	
VIII (most common)	Tinnitus, unilateral hearing loss	Vth, IX–Xth, VIth nerve lesion, signs of cerebellar and brainstem compression
	Facial weakness	
IX–X–XI	Hoarseness, dysphagia, shoulder weakness (trapezius and sternocleidomastoid)	
XII (very rare)	Hemiatrophy and weakness of the tongue	

ation (Fig. 6.11). However, it is important to stress that radiological lesions do not always match clinical manifestations.

Head and neck primary tumours and metastases

Cranial nerves are frequently affected by malignant tumours arising from the head and neck region bordering the skull base and cervical spine. Tumours can either invade through the nerve foramina, directly through skull invasion, or by microscopic extension along cranial

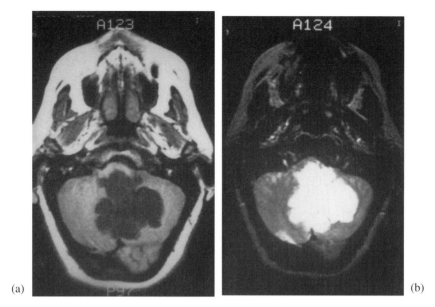

(a)   (b)

Fig. 6.9 Axial view of a midline posterior fossa epidermoid tumour. The tumour is lobulated and shows a slightly hyperintense, thin rim. The signal of the central cystic material is similar to CSF on (a) T_1W1 and (b) T_2W1 MR scan. (Courtesy of Professor J. Brotchi.)

nerves, such as that seen with adenoid cystic carcinoma. The risk of cranial nerve damage relates to the tumour invasiveness and the proximity to neural structures.

The most common head and neck tumour associated with cranial nerve damage is **nasopharyngeal carcinoma**. This tumour originates from the fossa of Rosenmüller and tends to enter the cranial cavity through the foramen lacerum. Neurological complications of nasopharynx carcinoma have been analysed by Turgman *et al.* (23) in a nationwide Israeli survey. Seventy-four of 150 patients seen during 9-year period developed neurological complications, of which 92% were limited to cranial nerve dysfunction. In 23 patients (34%) the initial presentation was a neurological deficit. The most frequently involved cranial nerves were VIth (68%) and Vth (65%), although potentially every cranial nerve can be affected.

Other tumours, such as paranasal sinus carcinomas involving the ethmoid sinuses and parotid tumours, can cause damage of cranial nerves in their proximity.

Upper cervical tumours causing cranial nerve lesions include thyroid, laryngeal, and tongue carcinomas, sarcomas, lymphomas, and cervical lymph node metastases. Neurological signs are often unilateral and involve the IX–Xth, XIth and XIIth cranial nerves. Episodes of hypotension and bradycardia occasionally causing syncope may be a manifestation of IX–Xth nerve involvement by metastatic tumours. This has been attributed to stimulation of brainstem nuclei inhibiting the sympathetic tone (24). These patients may also report paroxysmal neck pain.

Lower cervical and mediastinal tumours may injure the recurrent laryngeal nerve (causing hoarseness), the phrenic nerve, and the cervical sympathetic ganglion.

Table 6.4 Main cranial nerve syndromes caused by skull metastases

Symptoms	Signs	Nerves involved	Most probable metastatic location
Frontal eye pain		II	Orbit
Diplopia	Oculomotor paresis	III–IV–VI	Sphenoidal
	Frontal hypoaesthesia	V_1	
Frontal eye pain	Proptosis, decreased visual acuity	III–IV–VI	
Diplopia	Oculomotor paresis	V_1	Parasellar (cavernous sinus)
	Frontal hypoaesthesia But vision less often affected and vein turgescence instead of proptosis		
Facial numbness or pain	Facial hypoaesthesia	V_2 and V_3	Middle fossa
Diplopia	Paresis of eye abduction	VI	
Facial paresis	Facial paresis	VII	
Hearing loss, tinnitus	Decreased auditive acuity	VIII	Pontocerebellar angle
Facial pain	Facial hypoaesthesia	V_2 and V_3	
Dysphagia – hoarseness	Unilateral palate, vocal cord	IX–X	
Pharynx pain	Weakness and decreased gag reflex		Jugular foramen
Drooping shoulder	Weakness and atrophy of sternocle idomastoid and trapezius muscles	XI	
Occipital pain	Neck stiffness	XII	Occipital condyle
Dysarthria	Tongue atrophy and weakness		
Numb chin	Mental hypoaesthesia	Partial V_3 (mental nerve)	Anterior mandible

Combinations of these lesions lead to three syndromes which are useful in the diagnosis of lung carcinoma. The syndrome combining a lesion of the left recurrent laryngeal nerve, which loops around the arch of the aorta, with a paralysis of the left phrenic nerve points to a metastatic enlargement of the lymph nodes around the carina. The combination of the right recurrent laryngeal nerve, which loops around the subclavian artery, with right phrenic nerve dysfunction, indicates a lesion at the apex of the right lung. Horner's syndrome indicates a lesion of sympathetic innervation.

Treatment-related lesions

Cranial nerve lesions may occur as a consequence of chemotherapy, irradiation, or surgery.

Chemotherapy

The most common cranial nerve lesion due to chemotherapy is VIIIth nerve toxicity caused by cisplatin. **Cisplatin** toxicity causes tinnitus and loss of hearing (25,26). Tinnitus is not dose related. It does not accompany loss of hearing and the onset is not predictive of imminent changes in hearing. Hearing loss is bilateral but not always symmetrical. It is due to a

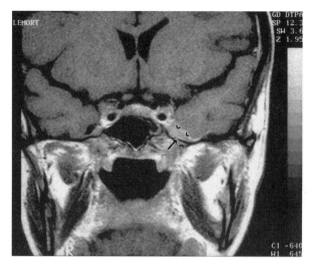

Fig. 6.10   Gadolinium-enhanced T_1WI MR scan of a skull base metastasis in a patient with breast carcinoma. Note the destruction of the greater sphenoid wing (arrow), the intracranial extent of the malignant tissue (arrowheads), and the contrast enhancement of the dura. The gasserian ganglion was also involved in this patient, causing facial pain. (Courtesy of Dr M. Lemort.)

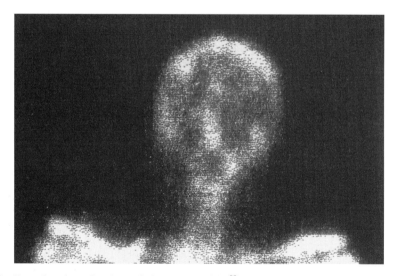

Fig. 6.11   Posterior view of an isotopic bone scan with [^{99}Tc^m]MDP, showing multiple skull metastases in a man with prostate carcinoma. (Courtesy of Professor A. Schoutens.)
MDP: methyldiphosphanate

lesion of hair cells in the organ of Corti and is generally irreversible. The deficit predominantly affects high frequencies above the speech range. Audiometric changes are therefore more frequent than symptomatic deafness. The reported incidence of cisplatin ototoxicity varies from 4 to 91%. The wide variation is largely due to methods and intensity of assessment, and the criteria by which ototoxicity is defined, as well as due to treatment-related factors. Cisplatin ototoxicity is enhanced by several factors, including the cumulative dose of cisplatin, magnitude of the individual dose, hydration, frequency of drug administration and perhaps even the rate of infusion, and the patient's age (older adults and possibly very young children (27) show greater sensitivity). Concomitant administration of other ototoxic drugs such as aminoglycoside antibiotics, actinomycin, or bleomycin, concomitant renal toxicity, pre-existing hearing loss, and concomitant radiation therapy may also enhance cisplatin ototoxicity. Because of these individual variations in drug sensitivity, severe ototoxicity is difficult to predict, and monitoring of high frequencies (around 8000 Hz) is recommended, especially in high-risk patients, young children, and all patients committed to longer cisplatin therapy. Bilateral symptomatic hearing loss has been reported following intracarotid cisplatin administration combined with intravenous BCNU (28). Vestibular toxicity heralded by dizziness and vertigo, and corroborated by electronystagmography, is rare (29) following cisplatin.

Several neurotoxic vinca alkaloids are used in cancer chemotherapy. During **vincristine** administration recurrent laryngeal (30), oculomotor (31), and facial nerve palsies have been observed (31). However, it would be unwise to attribute unilateral cranial nerve deficit occurring in the absence of clear signs of peripheral neuropathy to chemotherapy alone, and metastatic nerve lesions are a much more likely cause.

Radiation therapy

Cranial nerve lesions due to irradiation correspond to different pathogenic processes (32). The effect of irradiations on rapidly dividing receptor cells of the olfactory bulb accounts for the acute anosmia reported during radiation therapy. A similar acute and reversible damage of the cochlea may cause transient tinnitus and hearing loss. However, the principal cause of hearing loss following radiation therapy is radiation-induced otitis media without cranial nerve damage. Rare single cases of late anosmia and damage to the organ of Corti have also been attributed to irradiation.

Most delayed post-radiation cranial nerve lesions are due to a combination of vascular and axonal damage and to perineural fibrosis. Berger and Bataini (33) reported 35 cranial nerve palsies observed in 25 patients irradiated for head and neck tumours and the palsies were assumed to be due to radiation injury. The XIIth nerve was involved in 19 of 25 patients, the recurrent laryngeal in 9, the XIth in 5, and the Vth in only one. Several other authors have reported post-radiation hypoglossal or recurrent nerve palsies (32). Most post-irradiation cranial nerve lesions occur after a delay of several years following doses of 6000 cGy or more. The reason why lower cranial nerves are more often involved is not clear. It is more likely to be due to their location within areas treated with high radiation doses as used for head and neck tumours, rather than due to higher intrinsic sensitivity to irradiation.

Neuromyotonia is a rare clinical manifestation due to a delayed muscle relaxation after voluntary contraction. Neuromyotonia has been reported after irradiation of the motor branch of the trigeminal nerve (34) and oculomotor nerves (35).

Although, in cancer patients, cranial nerve palsies may be due to irradiation, they are outnumbered by cranial nerve damage due to metastatic lesions. In a study of 37 women with breast cancer and vocal cord paralysis, the neurological lesion was caused by metastases in 32, and by radiation fibrosis in only two (36).

Surgery

Cranial nerve lesions are common after extensive resection of head and neck tumours. The most frequently involved nerves are the XIth nerve, causing drooping of the shoulder; the mandibular branch of the VIIth nerve; and the XIIth nerve causing tongue hemiatrophy. Lesions of the sympathetic innervation cause ipsilateral Horner's syndrome. IXth, Xth and phrenic nerve damage is less frequent (37).

Posterior fossa surgery, usually for resection of meningioma, is also a common cause of cranial nerve lesions. Cranial nerves are often wrapped in the meningeal tumours and their dissection can be difficult, even with the operating microscope. The frequency of postoperative cranial nerve injuries is related to tumour size and location.

Resection of anterior tentorial meningiomas leads to spontaneously resolving lesions of cranial nerves (38) . Cranial nerve lesions, mostly of the Vth nerve, may follow the operation of cavernous sinus meningioma. All cranial nerves from the IIIrd to the XIIth are at risk during resection of petroclival meningiomas (39) and removal of foramen magnum meningiomas may be followed by IX–Xth, XIth, and XIIth nerve lesions. In cerebellopontine angle meningiomas, the facio-acoustic complex is at risk, but is usually less frequently injured than following surgery for vestibular schwannoma, where facial nerve palsy may occur in up to one-third of operated patients, especially in large tumours.

Infections

Herpes zoster is the most frequent infection of the nervous system in cancer patients and is seen especially in Hodgkin's disease, non-Hodgkin's lymphoma, and leukaemia. It may affect cranial nerves, particularly the ophthalmic division of the Vth nerve and the VIIth nerve (geniculate herpes zoster). In immunosuppressed patients disseminated infection may follow localized disease.

Cranial nerves can be damaged in bacterial and tuberculous meningitis. Hearing loss occurs in up to 15% of patients with pneumococcus meningitis, although during the acute phase hearing loss may be overshadowed by other clinical manifestations.

Investigations

In patients presenting with brainstem and cranial nerve lesions, brain MRI is the most useful first examination. If it is normal, a CT scan may help to demonstrate bone lesions. The diagnostic algorithm shown in Fig. 6.12. is based on MRI or CT scan features.

1. Normal MRI and CT scans

In cancer patients where both MRI and CT scan (and isotope bone scan of the skull) are normal, lumbar puncture is performed to exclude leptomeningeal metastases, as MRI is normal in about 30% of patients with this disease. The identification of neoplastic cells in the CSF is diagnostic of leptomeningeal disease, but it may require repeated examinations. Repeated lumbar punctures are justified when CSF protein levels are high and the glucose is low. Inflammatory CSF changes may be caused by infectious diseases such as herpes zoster, brainstem listeriosis, or by paraneoplastic brainstem encephalitis, which may be confirmed by high titres of anti-Hu, anti-Ma1 or Ma2 antibodies in the serum or CSF. Children with

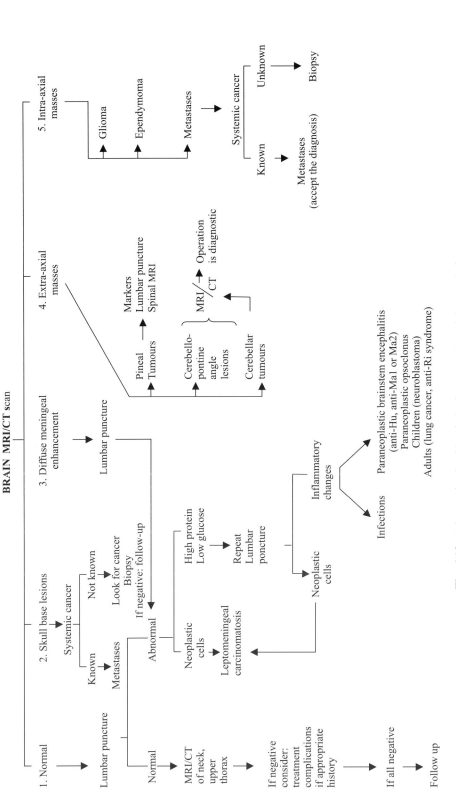

BRAIN MRI/CT scan

1. Normal

Lumbar puncture

Normal

MRI/CT of neck, upper thorax

If negative consider: treatment complications if appropriate history

If all negative

Follow up

2. Skull base lesions

Systemic cancer

Known → Metastases

Not known → Look for cancer
Biopsy
If negative: follow-up

3. Diffuse meningeal enhancement

Lumbar puncture

Abnormal

Neoplastic cells → Leptomeningeal carcinomatosis

High protein
Low glucose → Repeat Lumbar poncture

Neoplastic cells

Inflammatory changes

Infections

Paraneoplastic brainstem encephalitis (anti-Hu, anti-Ma1 or Ma2)
Paraneoplastic opsoclonus
Children (neuroblastoma)
Adults (lung cancer, anti-Ri syndrome)

4. Extra-axial masses

Pineal Tumours → Markers
Lumbar puncture
Spinal MRI

Cerebello-pontine angle lesions

Cerebellar tumours

} MRI/CT → Operation is diagnostic

5. Intra-axial masses

Glioma

Ependymoma

Metastases →

Systemic cancer

Known → Metastases (accept the diagnosis)

Unknown → Biopsy

Fig. 6.12 Diagnostic algorithm in brainstem and cranial nerve lesions.

opsoclonus (with or without inflammatory CSF changes) should have a work-up for neurob-lastoma including chest X-ray, abdominal CT, and determination of 24-hour urine vanillyl-mandelic acid and metanephrine. In adults with opsoclonus, chest X-rays or CT should be performed. Determination of anti-Ri antibodies may be useful in women, especially if there is associated cerebellar dysfunction.

In cancer patients with **lower cranial nerve** (IX–XIIth) lesions, normal cranial imaging and CSF examination point to involvement by tumours of the neck or the upper thoracic region. If MRI or CT scan of the neck and thorax are normal, cranial nerve or brainstem lesions may be due to treatment-related complications, providing this ties in with an appro-priate history of exposure to drugs or radiation. Patients without clear diagnosis need careful follow-up, as small malignant lesions may be missed on initial MRI.

2. Skull-base lesions

When MRI or CT scans in a patient with systemic cancer demonstrate lesions of the skull base, the diagnosis of bone metastases causing cranial nerve injury may be accepted. Lumbar puncture in patients with extradural cranial metastases is not recommended as, in our expe-rience, neoplastic cells are rarely found.

In patients not known to have malignant disease, an extensive search of an underlying neo-plasia is justified as cranial nerve lesions may be the first manifestation of distant malignancy arising from breast, lung, or prostate. Accessible lesions should be biopsied.

3. Diffuse meningeal enhancement

In patients with known malignancy, the combination of meningeal enhancement on MRI with cranial nerve lesions, suggests leptomeningeal carcinomatosis. Although positive CSF cytology is an important component of the diagnostic process, the diagnosis of lep-tomeningeal carcinomatosis in patients with negative CSF cytology can be based on clinical and typical radiological features alone (40).

4. Extra-axial masses

The differential diagnosis of extra-axial masses causing brainstem and cranial nerve lesions is based on radiological features, and factors such as tumour location, age, gender, and the rate of progression of neurological deficit.

Pineal region tumours are diagnosed primarily in the second and third decades. Unless high serum or CSF levels of α-fetoprotein or β-chorionic gonadotrophin (which are markers of non-germinomatous germ-cell tumours) are found, the diagnosis needs to be based on the pathological examination of surgically removed material. The approach to obtaining tissue includes stereotactic biopsy, endoscopic biopsy, open biopsy under direct vision, or attempted tumour removal. The choice depends on the presumed diagnosis. Open surgery should be undertaken by an experienced surgeon, and complete resection should be attempted in benign tumours. Therapeutic trial of low-dose radiation therapy of pineal region tumours is no longer appropriate or acceptable, as the response to irradia-tion is not specific and tissue diagnosis is essential. Patients with malignant germ-cell tumours should have CSF examination and contrast-enhanced MRI to search for cranial and spinal metastases.

Schwannomas represent 80% of **cerebellopontine angle tumours**. Bilateral vestibular schwannomas are diagnostic of type 2 neurofibromatosis.

Meningiomas are the second most common tumours of the cerebellopontine angle and represent about 10% of cases. The differential diagnosis between schwannoma and meningioma is based on the radiological features illustrated in Figs 6.6 and 6.7. In meningiomas hearing is more often spared. The cerebellopontine angle is also the most common location of epidermoid tumours, but they rarely cause hearing loss. Epidermoid tumours, in contrast to meningiomas and schwannomas, do not generally enhance on CT or MRI and their signal is almost isointense with CSF.

The diagnosis of **metastases** should be considered in adults with systemic cancer. In patients with cerebellopontine angle metastases the progression of symptoms is more rapid than in most primary tumours.

Primary cerebellar tumours, such as medulloblastomas or astrocytomas (described in Chapter 4, p. 63) may compress the brainstem and cause cranial nerve lesions.

The distinction between medulloblastoma, astrocytoma, other glioma, or ependymoma may be difficult on imaging criteria, and pathological confirmation of the diagnosis is essential.

5. *Intra-axial masses*

Primary intra-axial brainstem tumours are seen predominantly in children and young adults. The typical radiological features of **intrinsic brainstem glioma** are usually sufficient for diagnosis and biopsy, particularly in children, is not considered necessary (41). In adults, stereotactic biopsy is appropriate as 30% of patients may have other tumours, including metastasis, ependymoma, or lymphoma (42).

The radiological features of brain glioma infiltrating the pons (Fig. 6.1) can be diagnostic and easily distinguished from ependymomas which tends to arise from the floor of the fourth ventricle and fill the fourth ventricle (Figs 6.3 and 6.4). The presence of spinal dissemination favours the diagnosis of ependymomas but is uncommon at diagnosis. Exophytic gliomas of the cervicomedullary junction, ependymomas, and medulloblastomas invading the fourth ventricle may be radiologically indistinguishable and require tissue diagnosis.

In adults with systemic malignancy, enhancing intracranial lesions suggest **brainstem metastases**. Brainstem metastases are inoperable and the decision to perform a diagnostic biopsy is largely based on clinical judgement. Diagnostic biopsy is justified in patients with controlled primary tumour, without other metastases, and in malignancies seldom associated with brain metastases. Biopsy should also be performed in patients at high risk of CNS infection, and is mandatory in patients without a previous history of cancer.

Therapy

Posterior fossa tumours frequently present with signs of hydrocephalus and intracranial hypertension. CSF diversion may be performed trough ventriculostomy (fenestration of the floor of the third ventricle) or by ventriculoperitoneal shunt. In patients with malignant tumours, shunting may carry a potential risk of peritoneal and systemic dissemination of neoplastic cells, although this remains a rare event. However, in current practice CSF diversion is best avoided if tumour resection or subsequent antitumour therapy are likely to restore CSF flow.

Brainstem gliomas

Surgery has no role in the treatment of diffuse intrinsic brainstem glioma. Even the use of diagnostic stereotactic biopsy is not necessary in children (2,41). Exophytic, partly cystic, tumours of the cervicomedullary junction should be resected and, if histology shows pilocytic astrocytoma, further therapy is not required.

Radiation therapy (5000–5500 cGy given in 180–200 cGy daily fractions) is the treatment of choice for infiltrating intrinsic brainstem glioma. Hyperfractionated schedules (43), using 100–125 cGy twice a day to doses of 7200 cGy or higher are not associated with improved survival while they carry higher toxicity.

Recurrent brainstem gliomas occasionally respond to chemotherapy with etoposide (VP16) or nitrosourea-containing regimens. Of 12 patients treated with VP16 by Chamberlain, one had a complete and three a partial response (44). The use of adjuvant chemotherapy remains unproven (45).

Not all brainstem gliomas require immediate therapy. Patients with indolent, often well-circumscribed tumours may be offered initial observation alone with radiotherapy reserved

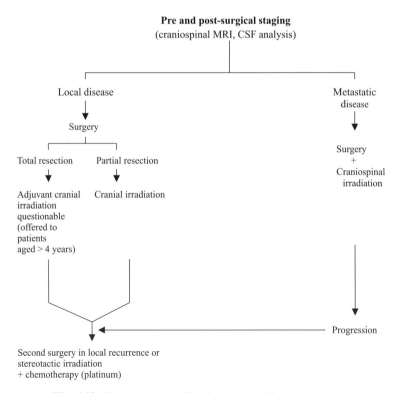

Fig. 6.13   Treatment algorithm in subtentorial ependymomas.

for progressive symptomatic diseases. The median survival of children with brainstem glioma is only 9–12 months. Unlike many other tumour types, adults with brainstem glioma tend to have a more favourable outcome with longer survival than children (46).

Posterior fossa ependymomas

Staging with pre- and post-operative brain and spinal MRI, and CSF examination identifies three groups of patients:

(1) patients with macroscopically total tumour resection;

(2) those with partial tumour removal; and

(3) a small group with disseminated disease at diagnosis.

The treatment algorithm shown in Fig. 6.13 is based on this distinction.

Radical surgical excision is the treatment of choice in patients with non-disseminated ependymomas. The extent of resection is an independent prognostic factor for survival (47), probably much more important than histology; however, histological grading of ependymoma is a predictor of outcome in some studies (48). Following macroscopically total resection, 5-year survival is 60–80%, as compared to 30% following incomplete resection. The value of radiation therapy following total tumour resection remains undefined, although it is generally offered to all patients over 4–5 years of age. After subtotal tumour removal, radiotherapy using 180–200 cGy daily doses to a total dose of 5000–5500 cGy is recommended, as retrospective studies (49,50) suggest improved disease control. The superiority of hyperfractionated irradiation over the conventional schedule has not been established. Prophylactic craniospinal irradiation in patients without demonstrable seeding is not appropriate (51).

Patients with metastatic disease are treated with surgery and craniospinal irradiation, with radiation boost to the sites of macroscopic disease. Occasional patients with one or two sites of dissemination may be considered for radical excision.

Most ependymomas recur locally and may be treated with second surgery and radiation therapy if considered save, particularly with the use of stereotactic techniques. Recurrent ependymomas not amenable to local therapeutic measures may be treated with palliative chemotherapy containing cisplatin (52,53).

Pineal tumours

Open surgical resection is curative in patients with lipomas, benign teratomas, epidermoid tumours, benign cysts, meningiomas, and well circumscribed pineocytomas. In other patients, tissue material obtained by biopsy is sufficient for subsequent treatment with radiation and chemotherapy. Tumours with elevated serum or CSF β-chorionic gonadotrophin and α-fetoprotein do not need pathological confirmation, except in the situation of slight elevation of β-chorionic gonadotrophin, which cannot distinguish between germinoma and nongerminomatous tumours.

CNS germinoma are cured by irradiation, with 90–100% 5-year survival (54–56). A local dose of 4000 cGy given in 20 fractions is usually sufficient (57) and the role of prophylactic craniospinal irradiation is debated. Germinomas are chemosensitive tumours (see ref. 58,

Table 3, p. 252), with a reported response rate of 84% following a combination regimen of carboplatin, etoposide (VP16), bleomycin, and cyclophosphamide (59). However, the recurrence rate following chemotherapy is high and the regimen is toxic. Primary chemotherapy is not an appropriate treatment for germinoma, although it has been used in conjunction with radiation therapy to allow for a reduction in radiation dose and as a potential substitute for prophylactic craniospinal irradiation.

Non-germinomatous germ-cell CNS tumours are rarely cured by radiation alone, with a 5-year survival in the region of 20% (55,57,60). Non-germinomatous tumours such as testicular teratomas are chemosensitive (see ref. 58, Tables 4a and 4b, pp. 254 and 256, respectively) to drug combinations including platinum derivatives, VP16, and bleomycin (61,62) as well as high-dose cyclophosphamide (63). The appropriate treatment of patients with non-germinomatous germ-cell tumours is primary chemotherapy followed by craniospinal irradiation and a localized irradiation boost. Surgery is considered for patients with resectable residual tumours.

Pineoblastomas are highly malignant tumours with a peak incidence in the first decade of life. They resemble PNETs and are treated like medulloblastomas (see Chapter 12). Neoadjuvant chemotherapy is used to delay craniospinal irradiation in children under 3 years of age.

Meningiomas

Total surgical resection is the mainstay therapy in meningiomas. However, posterior fossa meningiomas frequently involve cranial nerves and tumour resection is sometimes deliberately incomplete. Adjuvant radiation therapy is therefore more frequently considered and this can be delivered with stereotactic techniques, particularly for small tumours. Adjuvant radiation is considered a standard treatment in patients with atypical (grade 2) or anaplastic (grade 3) meningiomas, although its value has not been demonstrated in prospective trials.

There is no proven benefit of hormone and chemotherapy in the treatment of meningiomas. Meningiomas were treated with anti-oestrogens because they are twice as common in women, because their growth seems more rapid during pregnancy, and because they occur in association with breast carcinoma. However, meningiomas do not express significant amounts of oestrogen receptors, and anti-oestrogen treatment failed to produce tumour regression. Also, the administration of progesterone receptor antagonists has been tried with little success, although meningiomas express these receptors abundantly. A small number of patients have been treated with prolonged administration of hydroxyurea (64), with some success, but these results need to be confirmed.

Intracranial schwannomas

Several factors contribute to therapeutic decision:

(1) the rate of tumour growth, which ranges from less than 1 mm to 1 cm in diameter per year;
(2) patient's condition, and life expectancy;
(3) the severity of the neurological deficit; and
(4) uni- versus bilateral location.

Treatment of vestibular schwannoma therefore varies from expectant follow-up in elderly patients with quiescent tumours causing mild disability, to urgent removal of a large neurinoma causing gait instability or intracranial hypertension. Microsurgical resection allows complete tumour removal in 91–100% of cases (18) with less than 1% mortality. Single-fraction or fractionated stereotactic radiation therapy (radiosurgery) is considered as a safe alternative to microsurgery, and appears particularly successful in smaller tumours less than 3 cm in diameter. However, there has been no formal comparison of the two methods with objective evaluation of toxicity and efficacy.

The suggestion is that radiosurgery is more likely to preserve hearing and facial nerve function than surgery (65) and the risk of cranial nerve damage may be less with fractionated techniques.

Miscellaneous lesions

Epidermoid and **dermoid tumours** are treated by surgical removal only. The management of **leptomeningeal metastases** is reviewed in Chapter 12 (p. 261–268) . Conventional irradiation with 3000–4500 cGy is appropriate for **metastases of the base of the skull** causing cranial nerve lesions. The results are inversely correlated with the duration and the severity of symptoms and signs. As skull base metastases are not protected by the blood–brain barrier, the response to chemotherapy is similar to that of other bone locations. When cranial nerve lesions are **attributed to chemotherapy**, the drug should be discontinued. However, peripheral nerve deficits may progress for up to 2 months after discontinuation of vincristine or cisplatin. Treatment of **opportunistic infections** is summarized in Table 1.7.

The opsoclonus–myoclonus complex occurring in infants and children may respond to the treatment of underlying neuroblastoma or to ACTH or glucocorticosteroids. The management of paraneoplastic brainstem encephalitis remains disappointing.

References

(1) Albright A, Price RA, Guthkelch AN. (1983). Brain-stem gliomas of children. A clinicopathological study. *Cancer*, **52**, 2313–2319.
(2) Albright AL, Packer RJ, Zimmerman R *et al.* (1993). Magnetic resonance scans should replace biopsies for the diagnosis of diffuse brain stem gliomas: a report from the children's cancer group. *Neurosurgery*, **33**, 1026–1029.
(3) Polednak AP, Flannery JT. (1994). Histology of cancer incidence ad prognosis. SEER Population based data, 1973–1987. Brain, other central nervous system and eye cancer. *Cancer*, **75**, 330–337.
(4) Pollack IF. Brain tumors in children. *N Engl J Med*, **331**, 1500–1507.
(5) Shaw EG, Evans RG, Scheithauer BW *et al.* (1987). Postoperative radiotherapy of intracranial ependymoma in pediatric and adult patients. *Int J Radiat Oncol Biol Phys*, **13**, 1457–1462.
(6) Chiu J, Woo SY, Ater J *et al.* (1992). Intracranial ependymoma in children: analysis of prognostic factors. *J Neurooncol*, **13**, 283–290.
(7) Schiffer D. (1997). In: Brain Tumours, (2nd edn). Springer, Berlin, pp. 252–253.
(8) Derby BM, Guiang RL. (1975). Spectrum of symptomatic brain-stem metastasis. *J Neurol Neurosurg Psychiatry*, **38**, 888–895.

(9) Hunter KMF, Rewcastle NB. (1968). Metastatic neoplasm of the brainstem. *Can Med Assoc J*, **98**, 1–7.

(10) Breuer AC, Blank NK, Schoene WC. (1978). Multifocal pontine lesions in cancer patients treated with chemotherapy and CNS radiotherapy. *Cancer*, **41**, 2112–2120.

(11) Bach MC, Davis KM. (1987). Listeria rhombencephalitis mimicking tuberculous meningitis. *Rev Infect Dis*, **9**, 130–133.

(12) Voltz R, Gultekin SH, Rosenfeld MR *et al.* (1999). A serologic marker of paraneoplastic limbic and brain-stem encephalitis in patients with testicular cancer. *N Engl J Med*, **340**, 1788–1795.

(13) Dalmau J, Gultekin SH, Voltz R *et al.* (1999). Mal, a novel neuro- and testis-specific protein, is recognized by the serum of patients with paraneoplastic neurological disorders. *Brain*, **122**, 27–39.

(14) Solomon GE, Chutorian AM. (1968). Opsoclonus and occult neuroblastoma. *N Engl J Med*, **279**, 475–477.

(15) Digre KB. (1986). Opsoclonus in adults. Report of three cases and review of literature. *Arch Neurol*, **43**, 1165–1175.

(16) Allen JC, Bruce J, Kun LE, Langford LA. (1996). Pineal Region Tumors. In: Cancer in the nervous system. Levin VA (ed.). Churchill Livingstone, Edinburgh, pp. 171–185.

(17) Mefty AL (ed). (1991). Meningiomas. Raven Press, New York.

(18) Flickinger JC, Kondziolka D, Lundsford LD. (1997). Vestibular schwannomas. In: Cancer of the nervous system. Black PMcL, Loeffler JL (eds). Blackwell Science, pp. 404–413.

(19) Grisold W, Drlicek M, Setinek U. (1998). LC Clinical syndrome in different primaries. *J Neurooncol*, **38**, 103–110.

(20) Hildebrand J. (1978). In: Lesions of the nervous system in cancer patients. Raven Press, New York, Table 3.2 p. 36.

(21) Massey EW, Moore J, Schold SC Jr. (1981). Mental neuropathy from systemic cancer. *Neurology*, **31**, 1277–1281.

(22) Greenberg HS, Deck MD, Vikram B *et al.* (1981). Metastasis to the base of the skull : Clinical findings in 43 patients. *Neurology*, **31**, 530–537.

(23) Turgman J, Braham J, Modan B, Goldhammer Y. (1978). Neurological complications in patients with malignant tumors of the nasopharynx. *Europ Neurol*, **17**, 149–154.

(24) Onrot J, Wiley RG, Fogo A *et al.* (1987). Neck tumour with syncope due to paroxysmal sympathetic withdrawal. *J Neurol Neurosurg Psychiatry*, **50**, 1063–1066.

(25) Melamed LB, Selim MA, Schuchman D. (1985). Cisplatin ototoxicity in gynecologic cancer patients. A preliminary report. *Cancer*, **55**, 41–43.

(26) Schaefer SD, Post JD, Cose LG, Wright CG. (1985). Ototoxicity of low- and moderate-dose cisplatin. *Cancer*, **56**, 1934–1939.

(27) McHaney VA, Thibadoux G, Hayes FA, Green AA. (1983). Hearing loss in children receiving cisplatin chemotherapy. *J Pediatrics*, **102**, 314–317.

(28) Recht L, Fram RJ, Strauss G *et al.* (1990). Preirradiation chemotherapy of supratentorial malignant primary brain tumors with intracarotid cisplatinum and IV BCNU. *Am J Clin Oncol*, **13**, 125–131.

(29) Schaefer SD, Wright CG, Post JD, Frenkel EP. (1981). Cis-platinum vestibular toxicity. *Cancer*, **47**, 857–859.

(30) Whittaker JA, Griffith IP. (1977). Recurrent laryngeal nerve paralysis in patients receiving vincristine and vinblastine. *Br Med J*, **1**, 1251–1252.

(31) Sandler SG, Tobin W, Henderson ES. (1969). Vincristine-induced neuropathy. A clinical study of fifty leukemic patients. *Neurology*, **19**, 367–374.

(32) Giese WL, Kinsella TJ. (1991). Radiation injury to peripheral and cranial nerves. In: Radiation injury to nervous system. Gutin Ph, Leibel SA, Sheline GE (eds). Raven Press, New York, pp. 383–403.

(33) Berger PS, Bataini JP. (1977). Radiation-induced cranial nerve palsy. *Cancer*, **40**, 152–155.

(34) Diaz JM, Urban ES, Schiffman JS, Peterson AC. (1992). Post-irradiation neuromyotonia affecting trigenimal nerve distribution: An unusual presentation. *Neurology*, **42**, 1102–1104.

(35) Lessell S, Lessell IM, Rizzo JF. (1986). Ocular neuromyotonia after radiation therapy. *Am J Ophthalmol*, **102**, 766–770.

(36) Westbrook KC, Ballantyne AJ, Eckles NE, Brown GR. (1974). Breast cancer and vocal cord paralysis. *South Med J*, **67**, 805–807.

(37) Swift TR. (1970). Involvement of peripheral nerves in radical neck dissection. *Am J Surg*, **119**, 694–698.

(38) Cantore G, Ciappetta P. (1991). Tentorial meningiomas. In: Meningiomas and their surgical treatment. Schmidek HH (ed.). Sanders, Philadelphia, pp. 390–395.

(39) Samii M, Ammirati M, Mahran A *et al.* (1989). Surgery of petroclival meningiomas: report of 24 cases. *Neurosurgery*, **24**, 12–17.

(40) Straathof CS, de Bruin HG, Dippel DWJ, Vecht CJ. (1999). The diagnostic accuracy of magnetic resonance imaging and cerebrospinal cytology in leptomeningeal metastasis. *J Neurol*, **246**, 810–814.

(41) Levivier M, Massager N, Brotchi J. (1998). Management of mass lesions of the brainstem. *Crit Rev Neurosurg*, **8**, 338–345.

(42) Franzini A, Allegranza A, Melcarne A *et al.* (1988). Serial stereotactic biopsy of brainstem expanding lesions: considerations on 45 consecutive cases. *Acta Neurochir (Wien)*, Suppl. **42**, 170–176.

(43) Packer RJ, Boyett JM, Zimmerman RA *et al.* (1993). Hyperfractionated radiation therapy (72 Gy) for children with brainstem glioma. A children cancer group phase I/II trial. *Cancer*, **72**, 1414–1421.

(44) Chamberlain MC. (1993). Recurrent brainstem gliomas treated with oral VP-16. *J Neurooncol*, **15**, 133–139.

(45) Jenkin RD, Boesel C, Ertel I *et al.* (1987). Brain-stem tumors in childhood a prospective randomized trial of irradiation with and without adjuvant CCNU, VCR and prednisone. *J Neurosurg*, **66**, 227–233.

(46) Landolfi JC, Thaler HT, DeAngelis LM. (1998). Adult brainstem gliomas. *Neurology*, **51**, 1136–1139.

(47) Healey EA, Barnes PD, Kupsky WJ *et al.* (1991). The prognostic significance of post-operative residual tumour in ependymoma. *Neurosurgery*, **28**, 666–672.

(48) Vanuytsel LJ, Bessell EM, Ashley SE *et al.* (1992). Intracranial ependymoma: long term results of a policy of surgery and radiotherapy. *Int J Radiat Oncol Biol Phys*, **23**, 313–319.

(49) Rousseau P, Habrand JL, Sarrazin D *et al.* (1994). Treatment of intracranial ependymomas of children. *Int J Radiat Oncol Biol Phys*, **28**, 381–386.

(50) Donahue B, Steinfeld A. (1998). Intracranial ependymoma in the adult patient: successful treatment with surgery and radiation therapy. *J Neurooncol*, **37**, 131–133.

(51) Vanuytsel L, Brada M. (1991). The role of prophylactic spinal irradiation in localised intracranial ependymoma. *Int J Radiat Oncol Biol Phys*, **21**, 825–830.

(52) Bertolone SJ, Baum ES, Krivit W and Hammond GD. (1989). A phase II study of cisplatin therapy in childhood tumours. *J Neurooncol*, **7**, 5–11.

(53) Sexauer CL, Khan A, Burger PC *et al.* (1985). Cisplatin in recurrent pediatric brain tumours. A POG phase II study. *Cancer*, **56**, 1497–1501.

(54) Haddock MG, Schild SE, Scheithauer BW, Schomberg PJ. (1997). Radiation therapy for histologically confirmed primary central nervous system germinoma. *Int J Radiat Oncol Biol Phys*, **38**, 915–923.

(55) Matsutani M, Sano K, Takakura K *et al.* (1997). Primary intracranial germ cell tumors: a clinical analysis of 153 histologically verified cases. *J Neurosurg*, **86**, 446–455.

(56) Shirato H, Nishio M, Sawamura Y *et al.* (1997). Analysis of long-term treatment of intracranial germinoma. *Int J Radiat Oncol Biol Phys*, **37**, 511–515.

(57) Shirato H. (1998). Radiotherapy for CNS GCTs in intracranial germ cell tumours. Sawamura Y, Shirato H, de Tribolet N (eds). Springer, New York, pp. 283–315.

(58) Balmaceda C, Modak S, Finlay J. (1998). Chemotherapy for CNS GCTs. In: Intracranial germ cell tumours. Sawamura Y, Shirato H, de Tribolet N (eds). Springer, New York, pp. 244–281.

(59) Balmaceda C, Heller G, Rosenblaum M *et al.* (1996). Chemotherapy without irradiation – a novel approach for newly diagnosed central nervous system germ cell tumors: results of an international cooperative trial. *J Clin Oncol*, **14**, 2908–2915.

(60) Dearnaley DP, A'Hern RP, Whittaker S, Bloom HJG. (1990). Pineal and CNS germ cell tumors. Royal Marsden experience 1962–1987. *Int J Radiat Oncol Biol Phys*, **18**, 773–781.

(61) Patel SR, Buckner JC, Smithson WA *et al.* (1992). Cisplatin-based chemotherapy in primary central nervous system germ cell tumors. *J Neurooncol*, **12**, 47–52.

(62) Sebag-Montefiore D, Douek E, Kingston J, Plowman P. (1992). Intracranial germ cell tumors: I. Experience with platinum based chemotherapy and implications for curative chemoradiotherapy. *Clin Oncol*, **4**, 345–350.

(63) Allen JC, Kim JH, Packer RJ. (1987). Neoadjuvant chemotherapy for newly diagnosed germ-cell tumors of the central nervous system. *J Neurosurg*, **67**, 65–70.

(64) Schrell UM, Rittig MG, Anders M *et al.* (1997). Hydroxyurea for treatment of unresectable meningiomas. Decrease in the size of meningiomas in patients treated by hydroxyurea. *J Neurosurg*, **86**, 840–844.

(65) Pollock BE, Lunsford LD, Kondziolka D *et al.* (1995). Outcome analysis of acoustic neuroma management: a comparison of microsurgery and stereotactic radiosurgery. *Neurosurgery*, **36**, 215–225.

7 Spinal cord lesions

Introduction

Spinal cord diseases included in this chapter cause neurological deficits of a central type. Lesions of lower motor neurons, spinal roots, or cauda equina are considered in Chapters 8 and 9, which deal with peripheral neurological deficits. This separation is convenient for distinguishing peripheral from central nervous lesions. However, in clinical practice, this distinction is somewhat artificial as many patients combine both types of neurological deficits. This is illustrated by extramedullary spinal tumours that initially produce predominantly radicular symptoms but, if untreated, will cause spinal cord compression; or by amyotrophic lateral sclerosis, which usually combines upper and lower neuron lesions.

Anatomical structures and clinical presentation

Spinal cord lesions produce motor deficit, sensory impairment, and autonomic nervous system lesions, including sphincter disorders.

The **corticospinal tract**, the major descending motor pathway, is located in the lateral columns of the spinal cord. Lesions of the cortical spinal tract cause spastic weakness with brisk tendon reflexes, clonus, and extensor plantar reflex (Babinski's sign). Muscle atrophy is only slight and occurs late. The integrity of the corticospinal tract can be tested by motor evoked potentials.

There are three **ascending sensory** tracts:

1. The **posterior medial lemniscal** system carries sensation of discriminative touch, vibration, and joint position from the ipsilateral side of the body. The integrity of the lemniscal system may be explored by sensory evoked potentials (Fig. 7.1).

2. The **lateral spinothalamic** tracts convey crude touch, pain, and temperature sensation from the opposite side of the body.

3. The **lateral spinocerebellar** tracts provide information about the position of body segments in space and relative to each other. This sensory modality is often affected in hereditary degenerative disorders.

The autonomic nervous system has two major, predominantly efferent components. The sympathetic component originates entirely from the thoracolumbar spinal cord. The parasympathetic system outflows from the brainstem and sacral spinal cord. The main clinical features of spinal autonomic nervous system damage are sphincter disturbances, postural hypotension, and Horner's syndrome.

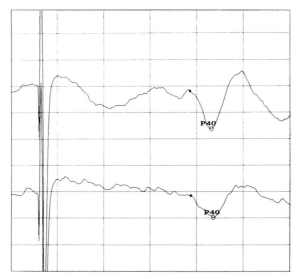

Fig. 7.1 Somatosensory evoked potential in a patient with thoracic (T4–T5) medullary astrocytoma, complaining only of back pain. The P40 wave is delayed bilaterally; 55.4 ms on the right (upper trace) and 54.8 ms on the left (lower trace) for an upper normal value of 44.5 ms. There is a significant asymmetry (>33 percent) of P40 amplitude between the right (1.8 μV) and the left (0.7 μV) sides. (Courtesy of Dr Ph. Voordecker.)

Bladder and bowel function are largely controlled by autonomic nervous system. In patients with spinal cord diseases, bladder disorders occur earlier and are more common and more troublesome than bowel abnormalities. The spinal cord contains neuronal pathways by which the **pontine micturition centre** controls urine storage, bladder emptying, and detrusor–sphincter synergia. Continence is ensured by signals descending from suprapontine structures and the pontine centre, which inhibits the parasympathetic innervation of the detrusor muscle, and by contraction of striatal pelvic floor muscles and uretheral sphincter. The latter is controlled by the tonic activity of motor neurons of **Onuf's nucleus** (S2–S4). Normal voiding requires co-ordination between the relaxation of striatal uretheral sphincter and contraction of the detrusor muscle.

Spinal lesions located above sacral segments leave intact sacral segmental reflex but interrupt ascending and descending connections to the pontine micturition and higher centres. Spinal shock usually causes urinary retention due to bladder areflexia. With time, reflex contraction of the detrusor in response to bladder stretch is usually regained. Although this reflex can be useful for micturition, it may also result in urgency and incontinence. Hypertonicity of the bladder may reduce its capacity and compliance, with raised pressure within the bladder that may cause ureteric reflux, hydronephrosis, pyelonephritis, and eventually renal failure. The external urethral sphincter may be capable of reflex contraction and may be more or less spastic, resulting in detrusor–sphincter dyssynergia and incomplete voiding, which predisposes to urinary infection and stone formation. Patients will complain of frequent voiding and urgency when detrusor hyperreflexia predominates, of dysuria or retention when urethral spasticity prevails.

Sacral cord lesions may destroy the parasympathetic neurons and the anterior horn cells supplying the pelvic floor and external sphincter. This leads to flaccid bladder and sphincters, with retention and/or incontinence.

In summary, similar urinary symptoms may be caused by different functional bladder–sphincter disorders. Urodynamic studies may be necessary to elucidate the pathogenic mechanism and define appropriate management.

Orthostatic hypotension occurs in severe cervical and upper thoracic spinal cord lesions and is due to a lack of control of vascular reflexes. The syndrome is observed mainly in acute lesions of the spinal cord. We have seen two patients with severe upper thoracic compression by epidural metastases who repeatedly lost consciousness, even in the seated position, due to postural hypotension.

Horner's syndrome is due to ipsilateral sympathetic denervation. It is characterized by myosis, ptosis, and facial anhydrosis. The lesion may be either central and involve lateral brainstem or cervical spinal cord, or peripheral and cause damage to pre- or post-ganglionic structures.

Clinical syndromes

In **complete transection** of the spinal cord, deficits are located below the lesion and combine spastic paraplegia or tetraplegia, brisk tendon reflexes and Babinski's sign, loss of all sensory modalities, and loss of bladder and bowel control. In acute spinal injury, this presentation may be preceded by a transient spinal shock phase, characterized by hypotonia, areflexia, and urinary retention.

Partial spinal cord lesions give rise to more complex clinical presentations. Two of them are common in neuro-oncologic practice:

1. **Unilateral spinal cord lesion** causes ipsilateral weakness, hyperreflexia, spasticity, loss of position and vibration sense, and contralateral loss of pain and temperature sensation. This clinical presentation is called **Brown–Séquard syndrome**. It is common in spinal cord lesions seen in cancer patients but does not usually occur in its pure form.

2. **Central spinal cord lesions** that occur in the cancer population are caused by tumours or, rarely, by radiation therapy. They produce a **syringomyelia-like syndrome**, characterized usually by bilateral segmental deficit combining impaired pain and temperature sensation (favouring painless burns and wounds), distal atrophy, and weakness. Large central lesions may interrupt the descending and ascending tracts below the lesion.

Gait disorders

In humans, gait is a remarkable skill that requires the ability to maintain an upright position and balance, and to initiate and maintain rhythmic stepping. Gait abnormality is a very common neurological sign. It may be caused by lesions involving various parts of central or peripheral nervous system. Gait disorders are very frequent in spinal cord lesions, where both equilibrium (ascending tracts) and locomotion (descending tracts) may be disturbed. It is particularly important to elicit subtle gait changes which are often the presenting sign of a slowly progressive intramedullary lesion.

Main aetiologies

The causes of spinal cord injury seen in cancer patients are summarized in Table 7.1.

Neoplastic lesions

The neoplastic lesions described in this chapter are restricted to the spinal cord. Tumours such as ependymomas of the cauda equina or filum terminale, which cause neurological deficits of mainly peripheral type, are considered in Chapter 9.

Primary intramedullary tumours

Most intrinsic spinal cord tumours occur in children and young adults. The most common pathologies are ependymomas and astrocytomas; each pathology accounts for 25–30% (1,2) of all intramedullary tumours. Gangliogliomas made up to 14% of intramedullary tumours in the series of Constantini and Epstein (2), but only 2.9% in that of Fischer and Brotchi (1). Other less-frequent pathologies are haemangioblastomas, epidermoid and dermoid tumours, lipomas, primary melanomas, and lymphomas.

Table 7.1   Main causes of spinal cord lesions in cancer patients

Lesions	Causes
Neoplastic	Primary tumours
	Intramedullary
	Ependymoma
	Astrocytoma
	Other
	Intradural, extramedullary
	Schwannoma
	Neurofibroma
	Meningioma
	Metastatic tumours
	Epidural
	Meningeal
	Intramedullary
Treatment induced	Intrathecal chemotherapy
	Radiation therapy
	Early delayed myelopathy
	Late-delayed myelopathy
	Epidural lipoma induced by glucocorticoids
Infectious	Epidural abscess (on catheter)
Vascular	Epidural haematoma (thrombocytopenia)
Paraneoplastic	Necrotizing myelopathy
	Amyotrophic lateral sclerosis
	Stiff-person syndrome

Ependymomas and astrocytomas

While primary spinal cord tumours occur at any age, most astrocytomas are diagnosed before the age of 20 years, and ependymomas are mostly seen in adults before the age of 50 years. Astrocytomas are more frequently thoracic (42%) (1), whereas approximately two-thirds of ependymomas are cervical or cervicothoracic.

Most ependymomas and astrocytomas are slowly growing, grade 1 or grade 2 tumours. They produce similar clinical manifestations. The most frequent presenting symptom is local neck or back pain, which predominates in vertebral segments located over the tumour. Pain may be exacerbated in recumbent position and at night, but this feature was found in only a minority of patients reported by Fischer and Brotchi (1). Cervical tumours may cause torticolis. Low cervical tumours produce dysaesthesia, radicular pain, weakness, and muscle atrophy in the upper limbs. A thoracic location tends to cause lower-limb weakness and progressive gait disorders. Sphincter abnormalities are rarely the presenting feature. In patients with low-grade astrocytoma or ependymoma, several years may elapse between the first symptoms and diagnosis, but intra-tumoral bleeding may occur even in non-malignant ependymomas. In such patients, the neurological deficit evolves over a few days or weeks, and may be indistinguishable from the clinical course of malignant tumours. Malignant forms, especially high-grade astrocytoma, follow a rapid course, often existing only a few weeks (3) before the diagnosis is made.

MRI has replaced invasive diagnostic studies and is the investigation of first choice in patients with suspected intramedullary tumour (4). T_1-weighted images with and without gadolinium allow us to delineate the solid and the cystic components of the tumour. T_2-weighted images provide a 'myelographic' picture of the tumour. Although radiological features help to distinguish astrocytoma and ependymoma (Figs 7.2 and 7.3), MRI can not be considered a surrogate for pathological examination to differentiate the two tumour types. Typical MRI appearances characterize lipoma (Fig. 7.4), haemangioblastoma (Fig. 7.5), dermoid, and epidermoid tumours (Fig. 7.6). The tumour location helps further in the differential diagnosis: lipomas, dermoids, and epidermoids occur preferentially in the lumbar spinal cord and in the region of the conus terminalis or cauda equina.

Primary intradural extramedullary tumours

The most common intradural extramedullary neoplasms are nerve sheath tumours and meningiomas (see also Chapter 9, p. 170, 171). There are two pathological types of **nerve sheath tumours: schwannomas** and **neurofibromas**. They usually arise from dorsal sensory roots. In 15% of cases nerve sheath tumours may have an extradural extension, giving rise to the characteristic 'dumb-bell' shape (Fig. 7.7) (5). Rarely, nerve sheath tumours may grow into the cord (6) or be only intramedullary (7). Sporadic schwannomas and neurofibromas are mostly diagnosed in adults (around the fourth decade of life), with men and women being equally affected. In patients with type 1 (NF1) or type 2 neurofibromatosis (NF2) their diagnosis is usually made before the age of 20 years. Neurofibromas occurring in NF1 have a greater propensity for malignant degeneration than sporadic cases. Multiple schwannomas are characteristic of NF2 (Fig. 7.8).

Spinal meningiomas are the second most common intradural extramedullary tumours. They present most frequently in elderly women, usually as solitary lesions. Meningiomas may be firmly attached to the dura (Fig. 7.9) and sometimes to the nerve roots.

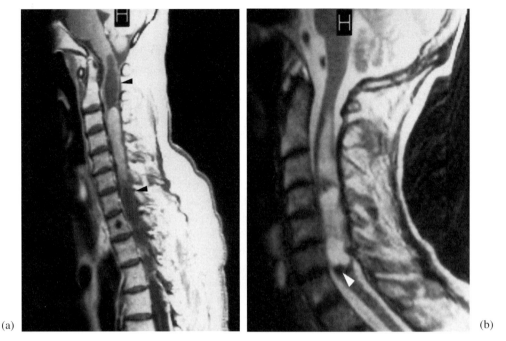

(a)   (b)

Fig. 7.2 Sagittal MR scan of cervical intramedullary ependymomas in two different patients.
(a) On the precontrast T_1W1 scan the tumour appears almost isointense with normal spinal cord, and
is delineated by polar cysts (arrows). The solid part of the tumour was strongly enhanced by
gadolinium (not shown). (b) On the T_2W1 scan the tumour is hyperintense. Note the 'cap' sign
(arrow) which corresponds to the deposit of haemosiderin due to chronic haemorrhage.

   Both nerve sheath tumours and spinal meningiomas first cause radicular symptoms and
signs, described in Chapter 9 (p. 169). However, if the diagnosis is not made at an early stage,
enlarging tumours will cause symptoms and signs of spinal cord compression.

Metastatic tumours

The epidural space is the most common site of metastases which cause injury to the spinal
cord. Leptomeningeal metastases are also frequent, but they rarely present with isolated signs
of spinal cord lesion. Intramedullary metastases are rare.

Epidural spinal metastases

Epidural metastases are found at autopsy in approximately 5% of patients who die of
cancer (8), but not all are symptomatic (9). In our series, signs of spinal cord compression
developed in 1.3% of hospitalized cancer patients (10). The most common mechanism of
invasion of the epidural space is direct extension from the vertebral bodies. Therefore,
the main primary tumours associated with epidural spinal metastases are 'osteotropic'.
Brihaye *et al.* (11) reviewed almost 1500 patients with epidural metastases and found

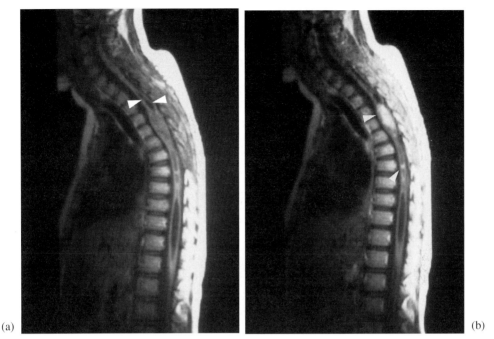

(a)   (b)

Fig. 7.3 Sagittal MR scan of upper thoracic intramedullary grade 2 astrocytoma. (a) On pre-contrast T$_1$WI the tumour is isointense to the spinal cord with hypointense cysts (arrows). (b) The post-contrast enhancement is multifocal (arrows) and heterogeneous. Note the syringomyelic cavity below the tumour.

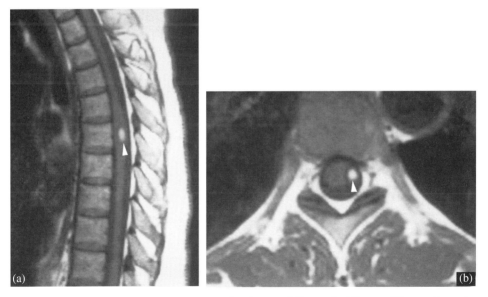

Fig. 7.4 Sagittal (a) and axial (b) T$_1$WI scan of an intramedullary spinal lipoma. The unenhanced MR scan shows a typical high-intensity fat signal (arrow).

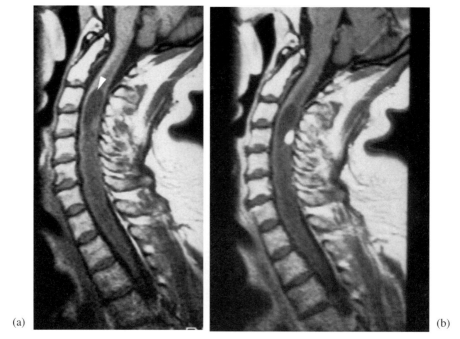

(a)   (b)

Fig. 7.5 Typical MR scan of a cervical spinal haemangioblastoma. The tumour is formed by a cyst (arrow) and a solid nodule which is isointense to the cord on T_1WI (a) and is intensely enhanced by gadolinium (b).

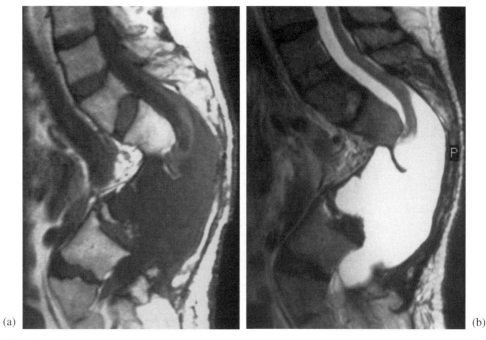

(a)   (b)

Fig. 7.6 Sagittal MR scan of an extensive recurrent epidermoid tumour of thoracolumbar region. The signal characteristics are close to the CSF on T_1WI (a) and T_2WI (b).

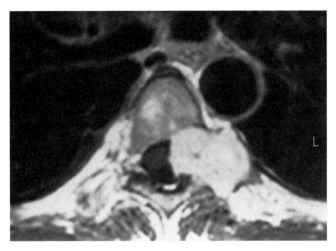

Fig. 7.7   Axial post-contrast T$_1$WI MR scan of a thoracic intradural schwannoma with extradural extension (dumb-bell shape).

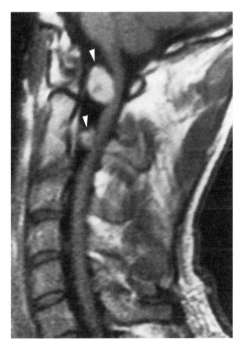

Fig. 7.8   Sagittal post-contrast T$_1$WI MR scan showing multiple spinal schwannomas (arrows) in a patient with type 2 neurofibromatosis.

that 16.5% originated from breast, 15.6% from lung, 9.2% from prostate, 6.5% from kidney, and 4.6% from gastrointestinal carcinoma. The miscellaneous group included myelomas and lymphomas. Lymphomas usually originate from paravertebral adenopathies and reach the epidural space through vertebral foramina without necessarily causing bony destruction (12).

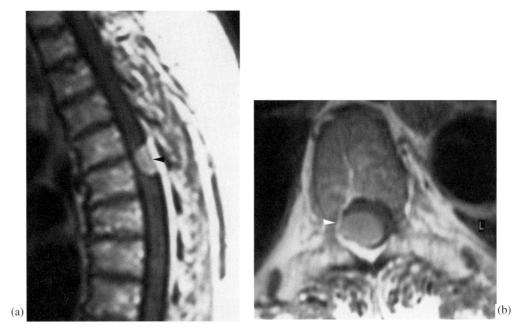

(a)   (b)

Fig. 7.9 Post-contrast T₁WI MR scan of an intradural, extramedullary thoracic meningioma. Sagittal view (a) and axial view (b), showing the attachment of the tumour to the inner aspect of the dura (arrow).

Symptoms and signs of epidural metastases are stereotyped and unrelated to the nature of the primary tumour. Pain is the prominent presenting symptom in at least 90% of adults, although it is less frequent in children (13). Midline backache, at the level of epidural metastases, precedes radicular pain, but is usually less severe.

Radicular pain may be either unilateral or bilateral. It may be elicited or exacerbated by vertebral compression and movement, especially flexion or Valsalva manoeuvre, and is not alleviated—and can even be enhanced—by recumbency. Lhermitte's sign (described on p. 142) has occasionally been reported in patients with epidural cervical metastases. However, it is much more common in demyelinating diseases or following radiation therapy (14). At the stage of radicular pain, depression of tendon reflexes, weakness, and sensory changes may be found in the territory corresponding to the roots injured by epidural seeds. Radicular signs are more conspicuous in the limbs than at thoracic or abdominal level. The symptoms and signs of spinal cord dysfunction, such as paraparesis, sensory disturbances, and bowel and bladder disorders, typically follow the pain. In patients with thoracic epidural metastases, which is the most common site, weakness usually involves the lower limbs, causing gait disorders. Gait difficulties may also be caused by sensory ataxia due to posterior compression of the spinal cord and may be wrongly attributed to cerebellar metastases, drug toxicity, or paraneoplastic manifestation (15). Sensory deficit is characterized by an upper limit which may follow an ascending course, and cause an incorrect tumour location in the early stages of spinal cord compression. Sphincter disturbances are rarely the presenting complaint, except when the metastatic lesion involves the conus (16). In approximately 20% of cases, progression to paralysis evolves over a few hours. Such a rapid progression can not be explained simply by an increase in tumour size and is most likely related to vascular changes such as thrombosis, ischaemia, or oedema. Slowly progressive paraplegia is attributed to gradual compression of the spinal cord by the tumour mass.

The diagnosis of epidural metastases is usually confirmed by radiological studies. Plain X-rays demonstrate vertebral abnormalities in over 80% of cases. The most common findings are loss of definition of vertebral pedicles, 'winking owl' sign, vertebral collapse, and bone dislocation (Fig. 7.10). The disc space, unlike in infectious diseases, tends to be preserved. Isotope bone scan is more sensitive than plain X-ray in detecting bony metastases and can confirm vertebral involvement and identify patients at risk (Fig. 7.11).

Conventional and CT-scan myelography have been progressively replaced by MRI but may be employed if MRI is not readily available. MRI offers several advantages over conventional CT or CT myelography (Fig. 7.12). It is more sensitive, shows the extraspinal extent of the tumour, the upper and lower limit of epidural metastasis, and may demonstrate multiple epidural lesions in about 16% of cases (17,18).

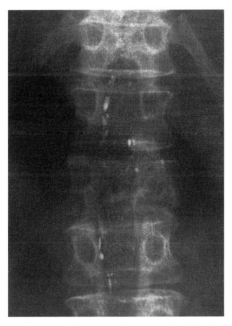

Fig. 7.10   Spinal X-ray in a patient with breast carcinoma and epidural metastasis. The second lumbar vertebra is collapsed and the definition of the left pedicle is lost (winking owl sign). (Courtesy of Dr M. Lemort.)

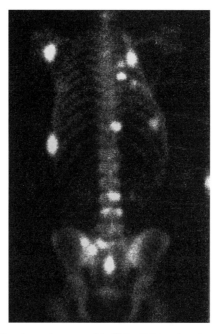

Fig. 7.11   Posterior view of an isotopic scan with [^{99}Tc^m]MDP, showing multiple bone metastases including vertebrae T10, L3, and L4 in a 30-year-old patient with a carcinoid tumour and no sign of spinal cord compression. (Courtesy of Professor A. Schoutens.)
MDP: methyldiphosphanate

Lumbar puncture is not recommended unless it is performed during myelography. It is potentially hazardous because of the coning phenomenon, and its diagnostic value is limited as neoplastic cells are seldom found in patients with epidural metastases.

Leptomeningeal metastases
The main spinal symptoms and signs caused by leptomeningeal metastases are deficits of peripheral type caused by root and cauda equina lesions. They manifest as pain, weakness, and sphincter disorders. Although bulky spinal leptomeningeal lesions are frequently seen on MRI or at autopsy, in our experience, signs of spinal cord compression in leptomeningeal carcinomatosis are rare.

Intramedullary spinal metastases
Intramedullary metastases are rare. Only 4% 1117 intramedullary tumours reviewed by la Société de Neurochirurgie de Langue Française were metastatic (19). The distribution of primary tumours is similar to that of brain metastases (see Table 1.3). Lung carcinoma, especially small-cell lung cancer is the leading primary malignancy, followed by breast cancer and melanoma (20,21). In 41 out of 112 patients with intramedullary metastases reviewed by Jacquet *et al.* (21), spinal cord symptoms and signs were the first manifestation of disseminated malignant disease.

The clinical picture may mimic the features of epidural metastases. Pseudo-radicular pain is present in most patients and is the initial symptom in about half. Lower-limb weakness and

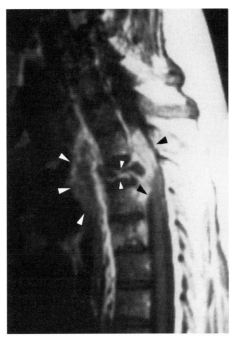

Fig. 7.12   Post-contrast sagittal T$_1$WI MR scan of breast carcinoma epidural metastasis showing: a pre-spinal neoplastic mass (three large, white arrows), vertebral collapse (two small white arrows), and the epidural mass compressing the spinal cord (two black arrows).

sphincter disorders are more frequent and occur earlier than in epidural metastases. Most patients are paraplegic within 2 months. Dissociated sensory loss, considered typical of intramedullary lesions, is frequent.

MRI is the investigation of choice and can demonstrate intramedullary metastases clearly (Fig. 7.13). It is far superior to CT scan or CT myelography.

Treatment-related lesions

Myelopathies associated with intrathecal chemotherapy
Acute or subacute paraparesis or quadriparesis may occur after intrathecal administration of various agents, including anaesthetics, analgesics, and contrast media. In cancer patients, these disorders have been observed after intrathecal administration of methotrexate, cytosine arabinoside, or thiotepa. Myelopathy due to intrathecal chemotherapy can be clinically separated into three groups (22) based on the time of onset following drug administration and the extent of deficit.

Groups 1 and 2 present acutely within 48 hours of intrathecal therapy. In the third group the symptoms are delayed and slowly progressive. The clinical presentation in groups 1 and 2 is characterized by severe radicular pain in the legs, followed by an ascending paraplegia or quadriplegia. The distinguishing feature of the first group is encephalopathy with a rapid progression to stupor, coma, and respiratory distress. In the second group, the neurological

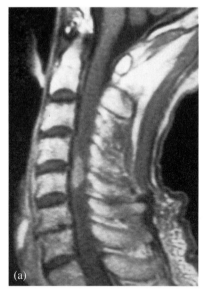
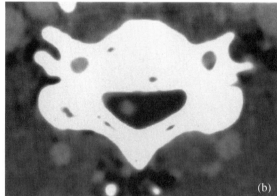

Fig. 7.13 Intramedullary spinal metastasis of an epidermoid carcinoma of unknown origin: (a) sagittal and (b) axial post-contrast T_1WI MR scan.

signs are restricted to spinal cord or spinal roots. Some patients have a clear sensory level. In Graus's review (22) spontaneous partial or total recovery occurred within hours to few days in the two groups, but three patients of the first group died of acute pulmonary oedema.

Scanty pathological data indicate that, in acute myelopathy, lesions may affect spinal cord structures, spinal roots, and cauda equina (23,24), but the precise pathogenesis is not clear. Putative pathogenic mechanisms include high drug concentrations, neurotoxicity of drug preservatives (methylhydroxybenzoate, propylhydroxybenzoate, benzylalcohol), and a hypersensitivity reaction.

In the third group, paraparesis or quadriparesis with tendon hyperreflexia and Babinski's sign developed progressively weeks to months after the last intrathecal treatment (25–27). Some patients had sensory level and sphincter dysfunction. The clinical features and the pathological examination indicated that in patients of the third group nervous lesions were restricted to the spinal cord. This subacute myelopathy is probably caused by direct drug toxicity, mainly of cytosine arabinoside.

Radiation therapy

Radiation therapy may cause two main types of spinal cord lesion.

Early delayed radiation myelopathy

Lhermitte's sign characterizes early delayed myelopathy. It consists of a sensation like an electric shock, elicited by neck flexion. Lhermitte's sign occurs in about 15% of patients 2–4 months after irradiation of the cervical spinal cord (28). Early delayed radiation myelopathy is usually self-limiting, although occasionally it may persist longer. Lhermitte's sign does not predict the occurrence of late-delayed myelopathy. Early-delayed radiation myelopathy, by analogy with multiple sclerosis where Lhermitte's sign is common, is attributed to reversible demyelination of posterior spinal columns.

Late-delayed radiation myelopathy

Chronic progressive myelopathy occurs several months to several years following irradiation. In a review of 83 patients with late radiation myelopathy reported in seven studies, the delay from irradiation ranged from 3 to 50 months (mean 13 months and median 12 months) (29). The incidence of myelopathy varies from 0.15% (30) to 2.9% (31) of irradiated patients and is related to the dose per fraction and the total dose. The overlapping of adjacent irradiation fields may cause localized radiation overdose and consequent radiation myelopathy.

Initial clinical features are numbness or painful, burning paraesthesia without precise radicular distribution. They usually start in the lower limbs, and follow an ascending course up to the level of the segment damaged by irradiation. Patients may also complain of inability to perceive pain or temperature. Brown–Séquard syndrome is observed in 25–30% of patients (32,33) but usually represents a transient stage. Weakness is rarely a presenting feature. Weakness also follows an ascending course, leading progressively to paraplegia or quadriplegia, depending on the site of the lesion, with sphincter abnormalities. Late-delayed myelopathy is generally irreversible, although it may stabilize at a particular level of deficit.

Histologically, radiation myelopathy is characterized by demyelination, axonal degeneration, and small-vessel occlusion. More severe forms may lead to frank coagulative or haemorrhagic necrosis, which predominates in the lateral and posterior spinal tracts. Occasionally, these lesions may be demonstrated by MRI. In advanced stages, conventional or CT-scan myelography may show spinal cord atrophy, which may be preceded by spinal cord enlargement (34).

Supportive treatments

Epidural lipoma

Epidural lipoma is a rare manifestation of fat redistribution caused by chronic administration of glucocorticosteroids. It can cause progressive symptomatic spinal cord compression (35). Lipomas tend to diminish in size when glucocorticosteroids are discontinued, although occasionally surgical decompression may be required. The typical fat density on CT or MRI scan makes the diagnosis easy.

Infection

Epidural abscess

Epidural abscess is an occasional complication of intrathecal or epidural catheter used for administration of opiates for pain control (36). In a series of 11 patients reported by Smitt *et al.* (37) pain at the catheter site exacerbated by drug injection was the typical symptom suggestive of an abscess. The abscess was in the posterior epidural space and was clearly demonstrated by MRI. The pathogen was usually of skin origin and included *Staphylococcus epidermidis* in eight, and *Staphylococcus aureus* in three, patients.

Vascular lesions

Epidural haematomas are a rare complication of thrombocytopenia, and may be favoured by even mild trauma. They usually produce an acute spinal cord compression. The characteristic high signal intensity of blood on MRI and CT scans and the absence of vertebral lesions distinguish haematomas from epidural metastases in most patients.

Paraneopastic diseases

Necrotizing myelopathy

This very rare disorder was first reported by Mancall and Rosales in seven patients with lung carcinoma (38). Since that time the disease has been observed in patients with a variety of tumours, particularly lymphomas (39). Myelopathy usually affects the thoracic spinal cord. It presents with a radicular pain followed by acute or subacute flaccid paraplegia, sensory loss below the level of the lesion, and loss of bladder and bowel control. MRI is usually normal, but it may show spinal cord swelling or focal contrast enhancement. CSF proteins are usually increased. Pathological lesions are restricted to the spinal cord, which may be swollen in a fusiform fashion. Diffuse necrosis affects both the grey and white matter. There is no inflammatory or glial reaction.

Motor neuron disease (MND)

Amyotrophic lateral sclerosis (ALS) is a progressive disease of unknown cause which combines degeneration of upper and lower motor neurons; a less common variant of MND is limited to lower motor neuron degeneration. The overwhelming majority of patients with ALS MND do not have cancer. Epidemiological studies do not support an association between cancer and ALS (40). In addition, ALS seen in cancer patients is clinically and histologically indistinguishable from the disease found in the general population. Some observations, however, suggest that in certain circumstances ALS may be a paraneoplastic disease. There seems to be a disproportionate incidence of ALS in patients with lymphoproliferative disorders with or without monoclonal paraproteinaemia (41). In a few cases, ALS is associated with anti-Hu-antibodies, and lower motor neuron lesions are prominent in up to 20% of patients with paraneoplastic encephalomyelitis (42). However, patients with anti-Hu antibodies almost always present signs of involvement of other areas of the nervous system. In a recently reported woman with lower motor neuron syndrome and breast cancer, serum antibodies directed against an antigen concentrated at axonal proximal segments and nodes of Ranvier were found (43). Finally, in rare reports ALS signs have regressed after successful treatment of the associated tumour, suggesting a relationship between the two diseases.

Stiff-person syndrome

Stiff-person syndrome is a rare disorder characterized by progressive but fluctuating muscle stiffness and painful spasms. Typically, an early involvement of axial muscles may lead to spinal deformity. The disease slowly spreads to involve proximal limb musculature and impairs gait. Spasm is precipitated by sudden auditory (startle) or tactile stimuli. Stiff-person syndrome may be associated with insulin-dependent diabetes and other autoimmune disorders, such as pernicious anaemia or thyroiditis. Electromyography (EMG) shows continuous motor unit activity in agonist and antagonist muscles (44) despite attempted muscle relaxation. Stiff-person syndrome is heterogeneous and the pathogenesis, particularly of the neoplastic form, is not fully elucidated (45). About 60% of patients present antibodies against glutamic acid decarboxylase in serum and CSF (46). Only a minority of stiff-person syndromes are paraneoplastic and are associated with a variety of tumours. Antibodies directed against amphiphysine, a synaptic protein, have been found in patients with breast carcinoma and stiff-person syndrome (47). But they have also been detected in an atypical case of stiff-person syndrome without evidence of malignancy (48).

Investigations

MRI is the principal diagnostic examination in cancer patients with spinal cord pathology. The degree of urgency with which MRI should be performed is inversely related to the rate of symptom progression. However, the rate of progression is not always predictable. Therefore MRI should be performed urgently in all patients with early symptoms suggestive of cord involvement, such as radicular pain or persistent backache accompanied by early neurological signs. If urgent MRI is not available, plain X-rays, CT scan, and conventional or CT myelography may demonstrate spinal lesions. However, they are considerably less sensitive in exploring intramedullary structure, and negative findings should not be taken as evidence of the absence of a spinal cord lesion.

MRI helps to differentiate between epidural, intradural extramedullary, and intramedullary lesions, and the diagnostic algorithm shown in Fig. 7.14 is based on this distinction.

1. Epidural lesion

Metastases are the most common epidural lesions found in cancer patients. Patients with lesions suggestive of epidural metastases without known underlying malignancy should have histological confirmation of the diagnosis either as part of a decompressive procedure or just for diagnostic purposes. It may be appropriate to obtain tissue material from a more easily accessible site, particularly if anticancer therapy is likely to produce shrinkage of tumour at the metastatic site without the need for decompressive surgery. This is particularly true for chemo- and radiosensitive tumours. In the presence of easily identifiable diagnostic features, such as multiple skeletal lesions and the presence of protein in myeloma or skeletal metastases, prostatic mass and elevated PSA (prostate specific autigen) in prostatic carcinoma, the need for histological confirmation depends on the need for decompressive surgery. In patients where the primary tumour is unknown, histology may contribute to the identification of the primary tumour, and occasionally it may reveal a non-neoplastic and potentially curable lesion such as epidural abscess or granuloma.

2. Intradural, extramedullary lesion

Intradural extramedullary lesions are usually slowly growing **nerve-sheath tumours** (schwannomas or neurofibromas) or **meningiomas**. The differential diagnosis may be difficult on MRI alone unless a dumbbell-shaped image typical of nerve-sheath tumours is found. In most of these patients the diagnosis is made by tumour resection. In patients with

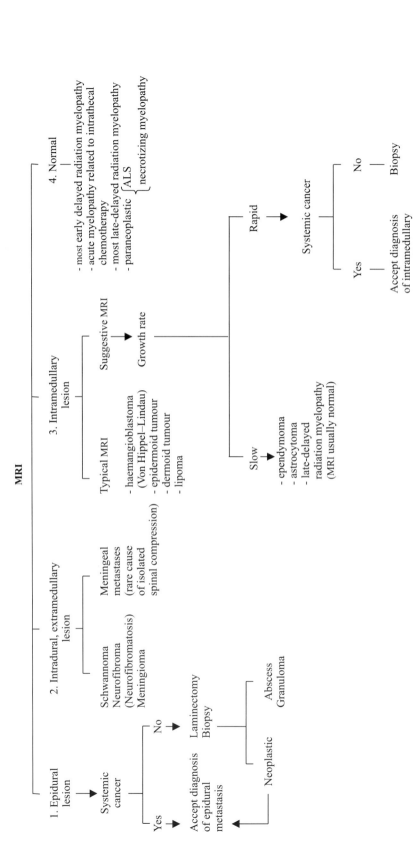

Fig. 7.14 Diagnostic algorithm in spinal lesions

type 1 or 2 neurofibromatosis, the probability of neurofibroma or schwannoma is very high and only symptomatic lesions are operated on.

Leptomeningeal metastases are usually associated with widespread neurological deficits, and they seldom produce isolated, clinically symptomatic, spinal cord compression.

3. Intramedullary lesion

The MRI aspect of certain intramedullary tumours such as **haemangioblastoma** (as a possible manifestation of von Hippel–Lindau disease), **epidermoid**, and **dermoid** tumours or **lipomas** can be diagnostic. In the majority of patients with an intramedullary lesion, the diagnosis can not rely on MRI alone, even though the radiological images may be suggestive of the diagnosis of ependymoma or astrocytoma (Figs 7.2 and 7.3), which are the most common, primary, slowly growing, intramedullary tumours. The majority of patients require histological confirmation and occasionally unexpected infectious or granulomatous lesions are discovered (49). In **late-delayed radiation myelopathy** MRI is usually normal but occasionally it may demonstrate a hypointense gadolinium-enhanced focal lesion on T_1-weighted images (50). Its diagnosis is largely based upon a history of prior irradiation.

The rate of progression may also help in the diagnosis. Rapidly growing intramedullary lesions include **malignant gliomas, primary melanomas, lymphomas**, or **metastases**. In patients known to have cancer, particularly lung, breast carcinoma, or melanoma, the diagnosis of metastatic seeding is usually accepted without biopsy. Diagnostic biopsy is recommended in other cases.

4. Normal MRI

MRI remains normal or non-contributive in **early delayed radiation myelopathy** (Lhermitte's sign) and in **acute radiculomyelitis** caused by intrathecal chemotherapy. The diagnosis is based on clinical features and a treatment history with negative MRI. In cancer patients, Lhermitte's sign may also be caused by **cisplatin** administration without irradiation (51). The diagnosis of **late-delayed myelopathy** is also based primarily upon clinical history, and MRI is usually normal. MRI is also normal in most patients with paraneoplastic necrotizing myelopathy and amyotrophic lateral sclerosis.

It is important to remember that a medullary lesion may be missed by scanning the wrong spinal cord segment. This may occur because a neurological deficit caused by cervical or upper thoracic lesions may begin in the lower limbs and subsequently follow an ascendant course.

Therapy

Intramedullary tumours

Total surgical removal is the mainstay therapy in most **primary** intramedullary tumours. The use of cavitron ultrasound aspiration (CUSA) has greatly increased the number of patients in whom this goal can be achieved. Occasionally surgery will be performed even in paraplegic patients to prevent cervical extension of thoracic spinal tumours located above the level of T4. Not all medullary neoplasms are equally amenable to macroscopically total resection.

Ependymomas present a clear cleavage plane between the dark purple or brownish tumour tissue and the surrounding white matter. These characteristics contribute to macroscopically total removal of the tumour, which was achieved in 86 out of 93 patients operated on by Brotchi and Fischer (52). Extensive ependymomas may require more than one operation. In low-grade myelopapillary ependymomas, adjuvant radiation therapy is not recommended, even after incomplete tumour removal (52). In adults with incompletely resected, undifferentiated (malignant) ependymomas, spinal irradiation with 5000 cGy has been advocated, but its benefit is unproven.

Intramedullary astrocytomas are infiltrating tumours, which are difficult to resect completely. Nevertheless, macroscopically total removal was achieved by Fischer and Brotchi in 15 (37%) of 41 patients (1). The relatively firm consistency of the tumour and its greyish coloration may guide the resection. Occasionally cleavage plane or satellite cysts may facilitate tumour removal. In low-grade astrocytomas in children, adjuvant radiation therapy is generally not recommended (53). Even in histologically malignant forms, the role of adjuvant irradiation remains unproven, although it is generally used by analogy with malignant cerebral gliomas. The treatment of **gangliogliomas** is comparable to that of astrocytomas.

Surgery is the appropriate primary therapy for benign spinal cord tumours of non-glial origin. **Haemangioblastoma**, which are visible on the posterior or posterolateral aspect of the spinal cord, may be removed without opening the medullary cord. Piecemeal removal should be avoided in operating on intramedullary haemangioblastoma, and this may occasionally require pre-operative embolization (54). In patients with von Hippel–Lindau disease, asymptomatic spinal haemangioblastoma may be observed initially (55). Intramedullary **lipomas** which present on the surface of the spinal cord are recognizable by their yellow colour and fibrous texture. They are adherent to the nervous tissue and removal is usually partial, even with the use of CUSA. Resection of the capsule which surrounds epidermoid and dermoid tumours may also be difficult, with residual tissue causing delayed tumour recurrence (1).

Primary intramedullary lymphomas are treated as primary non-Hodgkin's CNS lymphomas, with a combination of glucocortisteroids, chemotherapy, and radiation therapy (see Chapter 12, p. 249, 253 & 254). The prognosis of **primary intramedullary melanomas** is less gloomy than that of metastatic melanoma (56). Treatment consists of surgical removal followed by radiation therapy. **Intramedullary metastases** which develop during the course of widespread cancer and are not associated with leptomeningeal seedings are irradiated.

Isolated intramedullary metastases which are the presenting sign of a systemic cancer (21) are usually biopsied or resected. Subsequent treatment depends on tumour histology and generally consists of local irradiation.

Primary intradural extramedullary tumours

The primary aim in the treatment of **spinal nerve-sheath tumours** is complete resection, which is curative. Dumb-bell tumours may require a combined intradural and extradural approach. In large schwannomas and neurofibromas, the involved nerve root is often sacrificed and this generally causes minimal neurological deficit. In patients with neurofibromatosis, tumours may be multiple, and only symptomatic lesions should be removed. **Neurofibrosarcomas** are highly malignant tumours, usually associated with distant metastases and poor prognosis (57).

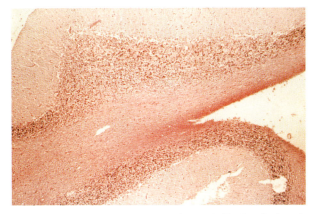

Plate 1 Complete disappearance of Purkinje cells in the cerebellar hemisphere in subacute paraneoplastic cerebellar degeneration diagnosed in a woman with carcinoma of the ovary. (Courtesy of Professor J.J. Vanderhaeghen.)

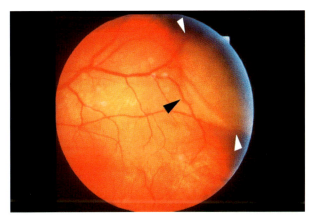

Plate 2 Small intraocular melanoma. The tumour is located in the upper left periphery (arrows). It appears as a brownish choroidal lesion with some faint orange pigment raising the retina. (Courtesy of Professor A. Zanen.)

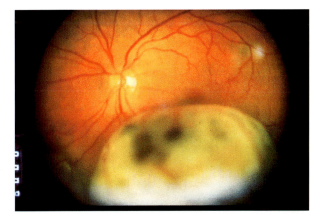

Plate 3 Large intraocular melanoma. The tumour appears as a dome-shaped mass adjacent to the optic nerve. Note the dark irregular pigmentation. (Courtesy of Professor A. Zanen.)

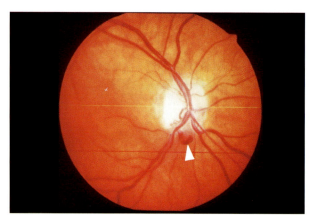

Plate 4   Meningioma of the right optic nerve in a 35-year-old woman. The eye fundus shows a pale optic disc with, at its inferior margin, an optociliary vessel shunt diverting the retinal venous blood from the compressed central retinal vein to the choroidal effluent vessels (arrow). (Courtesy of Professor A. Zanen.)

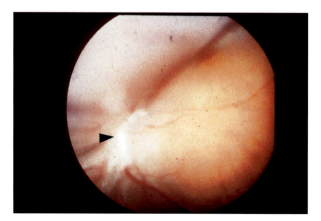

Plate 5   Eye metastasis in a woman with breast carcinoma. The lesion appears as a yellowish, bilobulated ballooning, partially masking the optic disc (arrow). (Courtesy of Professor A. Zanen.)

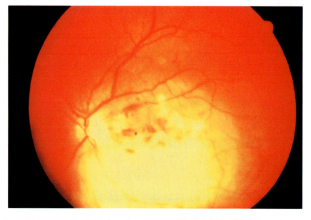

Plate 6   Retinal deposit in a patient with primary non-Hodgkin's CNS lymphoma. (Courtesy of Dr K. Hoang-Xuan.)

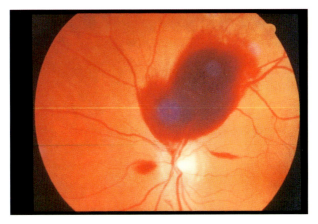

Plate 7   Retinal and pre-retinal (dark red) haemorrhages in acute leukaemia. (Courtesy Professor A. Zanen.)

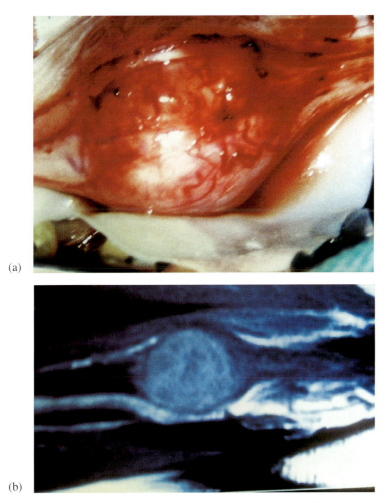

(a)

(b)

Plate 8   (a) T_1WI MR scan of a schwannoma of tibialis posterior nerve; (b) same tumour viewed at operation. (Courtesy of Professor J. Noterman.)

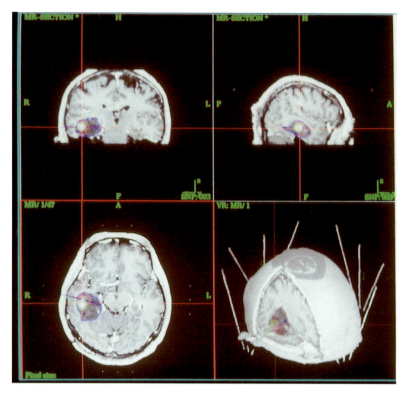

Plate 9 Neurosurgical planning for resection of a right temporal anaplastic astrocytoma. The multiplanar view of T_1WI MR scan performed in stereotactic condition delineates the tumour (blue contour), the contrast-enhanced area (green contour), and the hypermetabolic area of [18]FDG-PET scan (red contour). (Courtesy of Professor M. Levivier.)

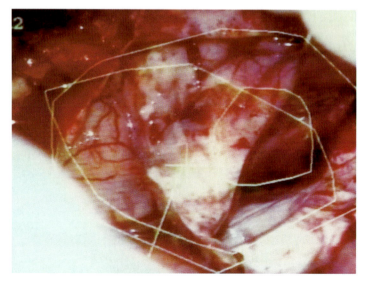

Plate 10 The three contours defined in Fig. 12.1 are projected on the operation field during tumour removal. (Courtesy of Professor M. Levivier.)

Surgery is the cornerstone therapy of spinal **meningiomas**. In a series of 174 patients Solero *et al.* (58) reported a post-surgical recurrence rate of 6% after complete, and 17% after partial tumour resection. If second operation can not be performed, radiation therapy may be used to improve local control tumour control.

Epidural lesions

The management of **epidural metastases** is considered in Chapter 12 (p. 268–272). Symptomatic **epidural lipoma**, induced by glucocorticosteroids, may require surgical removal.

Treatment of spinal **epidural abscess** is by antibiotic chemotherapy and surgical drainage (59,60). Intravenous administration of appropriate antibiotics should start immediately and be maintained for 4–6 weeks. It is followed by prolonged oral antibiotics when osteomyelitis is present. A posteriorly located abscess requires urgent laminectomy and drainage whenever the patient's general condition permits.

References

(1) Fischer G, Brotchi J. (1996). Intramedullary spinal cord tumors. Thième, Stuttgart.
(2) Constantini S, Epstein FJ. (1996). Primary spinal tumors. In: Cancer and the nervous system. Levin VA (ed). Churchill Livingstone, New York, pp. 127–137.
(3) Cohen AR, Wisoff JH, Allen JC, Epstein F. (1989). Malignant astrocytomas of the spinal cord. *J Neurosurg*, **70**, 50–54.
(4) Brotchi J, Dewitte O, Levivier M *et al.* (1991). A survey of 65 tumors within the spinal cord: surgical results and the importance of preoperative magnetic resonance imaging. *Neurosurg*, **29**(5), 651–657.
(5) Li MH, Holtas S, Larsson E-M. (1992). MR imaging of intradural–extramedullary tumors. *Acta Radiol*, **33**, 207–212.
(6) Gorman Ph, Rigamonti D, Joslyn JN. (1889). Intramedullary schwannoma of cervical spinal cord: case report. *Surg Neurol*, **32**, 459–462.
(7) Ross DA, Edwards MSB, Wilson CB. (1986). Intramedullary neurilemomas of the spinal cord: report of two cases and review of the literature. *Neurosurgery*, **19**, 458–464.
(8) Barron KD, Hirano A, Araski S *et al.* (1959). Experiences with metastatic neoplasm involving the spinal cord. *Neurology*, **9**, 91–106.
(9) Longeval E, Hildebrand J, Vollont GH. (1975). Early diagnosis of metastases in the epidural space. *Acta Neurochir (Wien)*, **31**, 177–184.
(10) Hildebrand J. (1978). Metastases of extradural space and spinal cord. In: Lesions of the nervous system in cancer patients. Raven Press, New York, pp. 19–30.
(11) Brihaye J, Ectors P, Lemort M, Van Houtte P. (1988). The management of spinal epidural metastases. *Adv Tech Stand Neurosurg*, **16**, 121–176.
(12) Perry JR, Deodhare SS, Bilbao JM *et al.* (1993). The significance of spinal cord compression as the initial manifestation of lymphoma. *Neurosurgery*, **32**, 157–162.
(13) Raffel C, Neave VC, Lavine S, McComb JG. (1991). Treatment of spinal cord compression by epidural malignancy in childhood. *Neurosurgery*, **28**, 349–352.
(14) Ventafridda V, Caraceni A, Martini C *et al.* (1991). On the significance of Lhermitte's sign in oncology. *J Neurooncol*, **10**, 133–137.

(15) Hainline B, Tuszynski MH, Posner JB. (1992). Ataxia in epidural spinal cord compression. *Neurology*, **42**, 2193–2195.

(16) Constans JP, de Divitiis E, Donzelli R *et al.* (1983). Spinal metastases with neurologic manifestations. A review of 600 cases. *J Neurosurg*, **59**, 111–118.

(17) Kaminski HJ, Diwan VG, Ruff RL. (1991). Second occurrence of spinal epidural metastases. *Neurology*, **41**, 744–746.

(18) van der Sande JJ, Kroger R, Boogerd W. (1990). Multiple spinal epidural metastases: an unexpectedly frequent finding. *J Neurol Neurosurg Psychiatr*, **53**, 1001–1003.

(19) Fischer G, Brotchi J. (1994). Les tumeurs intramedullaires. *Neurochirurgie*, **40**, (Suppl 1):1–110.

(20) Costigan DA, Winkelman MD. (1985). Intramedullary spinal cord metastasis. A clinicopathological study of 13 cases. *J Neurosurg*, **62**, 227–233.

(21) Jacquet G, Godart J, Katranji H. *et al.* (1993). Metastases intramedullaires des cancers viscéraux, à propos de trois cas opérés et revue de la littérature. *Rachis*, **5**, 35–48.

(22) Graus F. (1990). Acute meningospinal syndromes: Acute myelopathy and radiculopathy. In: Neurological adverse reactions to anticancer drugs. Hildebrand J (ed.). Springer-Verlag, Berlin, pp. 87–92.

(23) Saiki JH, Thompson S, Smith F, Atkinson R. (1972). Paraplegia following intrathecal chemotherapy. *Cancer*, **29**, 370–374.

(24) Mena H, Garcia JH, Velandia F. (1981). Central and peripheral myelinopathy associated with systemic neoplasia and chemotherapy. *Cancer*, **48**, 1724–1737.

(25) Breuer AC, Pitman SW, Dawson DM, Schoene WC. (1977). Paraparesis following intrathecal cytosine arabinoside. A case report with neuropathologic findings. *Cancer*, **40**, 2817–2822.

(26) Clark AW, Cohen SR, Nissenblatt MJ, Wilson SK. (1982). Paraplegia following intrathecal chemotherapy: neuropathologic findings and elevation of myelin basic protein. *Cancer*, **50**, 42–47.

(27) Dunton SF, Nitschke R, Spruce WE *et al.* (1986). Progressive ascending paralysis following administration of intrathecal and intravenous cytosine arabinoside. A pediatric oncology group study. *Cancer*, **57**, 1083–1088.

(28) Word JA, Kalokhe UP, Aron BS *et al.* (1980). Transient radiation myelopathy (Lhermitte's sign) in patients with Hodgkin's disease treated by mantle irradiation. *Int J Oncol Biol Phys*, **6**, 1731–1733.

(29) Hildebrand J. (1978). Neurotoxicity of radiation therapy. In: Lesions of the nervous system in cancer patients. Raven Press, New York, pp. 71–88.

(30) Kaplan HS. (1972). Hodgkin's disease. Harvard University Press, Cambridge, Mass.

(31) Palmer JJ. (1972). Radiation myelopathy. *Brain*, **95**, 109–122.

(32) Jellinger K, Sturm KW. (1971). Delayed radiation myelopathy in man. Report of twelve necropsy cases. *J Neurol Sci*, **14**, 389–408.

(33) Combes PF, Daly N, Schlienger M and Humeau F. (1974). Les myélopathies radiques tardives progressives. *J Radiol*, **56**, 815–825.

(34) Tugendhaft P, Baleriaux D, Gerard JM, Hildebrand J. (1984). Sequential CT scanning in radiation myelopathy. *J Neurooncology*, **2**, 249–252.

(35) Haddad SF, Hitchon PW, Godersky JC. (1991). Idiopathic and glucorticoid-induced spinal epidural lipomatosis. *J Neurosurg*, **74**, 38–42.

(36) Du Pen SL, Peterson DG, Williams A, Bogosian AJ. (1990). Infection during chronic epidural catheterization: diagnosis and treatment. *Anesthesiology*, **73**, 905–909.

(37) Sillevis-Smitt P, Tsafka A, van den Bent *et al.* (1999) Spinal epidural abscess complicating chronic epidural analgesia in 11 cancer patients: clinical findings and MR-imaging. J Neurology **246**, 815–820.

(38) Mancall EL, Rosales RK. (1964). Necrotizing myelopathy associated with visceral carcinoma. *Brain*, **87**, 639–656.

(39) Richter RB, Moore RY. (1968). Non-invasive central nervous system disease associated with lymphoid tumors. *Johns Hopkins Med J*, **122**, 271–283.

(40) Rosenfeld MR and Posner JB. (1991). Paraneoplastic motor neuron disease. In: Advances in neurology Vol 56, Amyotrophic lateral sclerosis and other motor neuron diseases. Rowland LP (ed.). Raven Press, New York, pp. 445–459.

(41) Gordon PH, Rowland LP, Younger DS *et al.* (1997). Lymphoproliferative disorders and motor neuron disease: An update. *Neurology*, **48**, 1671–1678.

(42) Dalmau J, Graus F, Rosenblum MK, Poner JB. (1992). Anti-Hu–associated paraneoplastic encephalomyelitis/sensory neuronopathy. A clinical study of 71 patients. *Medicine*, **71**, 59–72.

(43) Ferracci F, Fassetta G, Butler MH *et al.* (1999). A novel antineural antibody in a motor neuron syndrome associated with breast cancer. *Neurology*, **53**, 852–855.

(44) Meinck HM, Ricker R, Hulser PJ, Solimena M. (1995). Stiff-man syndrome: neurophysiological findings in eight patients. *J Neurol*, **242**, 134–142.

(45) Kissel JT, Elble RJ. (1998). Stiff-person syndrome. Stiff opposition to a simple explanation. *Neurology*, **51**, 11–14.

(46) Solimena M, Folli F, Denis-Donini S *et al.* (1988). Autoantibodies to glutamic and decarboxylase in patients with stiff-man syndrome, epilepsy, and type I diabetes mellitus. *N Engl J Med*, **318**, 1012–1020.

(47) Folli F, Solimena M, Cofiell *et al.* (1993). Autoantibodies to a 128-kd synaptic protein in three women with stiff-man syndrome and breast cancer. *N Engl J Med*, **328**, 546–551.

(48) Schmierer K, Valdueza JM, Bender A *et al.* (1998). Atypical stiff-person syndrome with spinal MRI findings, amphiphysin autoantibodies and immunosuppression. *Neurology*, **51**, 250–252.

(49) Levivier M, Brotchi J, Baleriaux D *et al.* (1991). Sarcoidosis presenting as an isolated intramedullary tumor. *Neurosurgery*, **29**, 271–276.

(50) Michikawa M, Wada Y, Sano M *et al.* (1992). Radiation myelopathy: significance of gadolinium-DPTA enhancement in the diagnosis. *Neuroradiology*, **33**, 286–289.

(51) Ecles R, Talt DM, Peckham MJ. (1986). Lhermitte's sign as a complication of cisplatin containing chemotherapy of testicular cancer. *Cancer Treat Rep*, **70**, 905–907.

(52) Brotchi J, Fischer G. (1998). Spinal cord ependymomas. *Neurosurgery Focus*, **4**, 1–5.

(53) Brotchi J. (1997). Intramedullary spinal cord astrocytomas: diagnosis and treatment. *Crit Rev Neurosurg*, **7**, 83–88.

(54) Tampieri D, Leblanc R, TerBrugge K. (1993). Preoperative embolization of brain and spinal hemangioblastoma. *Neurosurgery*, **33**, 502–505.

(55) Resche F, Moisan JP, Mantoura J *et al.* (1993). Haemangioblastoma, haemangioblastomatosis and von Hippel–Lindau disease. In: Advances and technical standards in neurosurgery, Vol. 20. Symon L (ed.). Springer, Vienna, pp. 197–304.

(56) Larson TC, Houser OW, Onofrio BM, Piepgras DG. (1987). Primary spinal melanoma. *J Neurosurg*, **66**, 47–49.

(57) Storm FK, Eilber FR, Mirra J, Morton DL. (1980). Neurofibrosarcoma. *Cancer*, **45**, 126–129.

(58) Solero CL, Fornari M, Giombini S *et al.* (1989). Spinal meningiomas: Review of 174 operated cases. *Neurosurgery*, **25**, 153–160.

(59) Hlavin ML, Kaminski HJ, Ross JS, Ganz E. (1990). Spinal epidural abscess: A ten-year perspective. *Neurosurgery*, **27**, 177–184.

(60) Darouiche RO, Hamill RJ, Greenberg SB *et al.* (1992). Bacterial spinal epidural abscess. Review of 43 cases and literature survey. *Medicine*, **71**, 369–385.

8 Diffuse lesions of the peripheral nervous system

Introduction

The diseases considered in this chapter are caused by diffuse, generally symmetric lesions of the peripheral nervous system (PNS). The structures involved are peripheral nerves and spinal roots, sensory neurons located in spinal ganglia, and lower motor neurons.

Clinical presentation

Clinical examination and neurophysiological tests allow us to make a distinction between four separate clinical syndromes, summarized in Table 8.1:

(1) sensory-motor dying back polyneuropathy;

(2) polyradiculoneuritis;

(3) sensory neuronopathy; and

(4) lower motor neuron disease.

The distinction of these syndromes helps in localization of the pathogenic process, and may indicate its nature.

Sensory-motor dying back polyneuropathy is the most common type of peripheral neuropathy in the general population and cancer patients. The clinical manifestations are symmetrical, begin in the distal part of the largest and longest nerve fibres, and progress proximally. Feet and legs are affected first and more severely than hands and forearms. In milder forms the upper limbs may be spared. The most prominent symptoms and signs are spontaneous paraesthesia (tingling, electric sensations), unpleasant cutaneous dysaesthesia, early depression of tendon reflexes, progressive muscle atrophy, weakness, and decreased sensation. Vibratory sense is usually affected before position and tactile senses. Troublesome autonomic disorders such as paralytic ileus or postural hypotension are fairly common in peripheral neuropathies seen in cancer patients.

Peripheral polyneuropathies caused by chemotherapeutic drugs are primary due to axonal lesion. In axonal neuropathies, the earliest neurophysiological abnormality is a decreased amplitude of compound muscle action potential (CMAP). Changes of nerve conduction velocity occur later and are not appropriate for monitoring axonal dying back neuropathy. Demyelinating neuropathies are less common in cancer patients and are often associated with an abnormal serum paraprotein.

Table 8.1 Characteristics of peripheral nerve syndromes

Syndrome	Structure involved	Main features	
		Clinical	Neurophysiologic
Sensory-motor dying back polyneuropathy	Peripheral nerves	Distal symmetric, proximally progressing deficits	╱ CMAP amplitude
		Lower limbs are predominantly involved	╱ Sensory and motor conduction velocity
			Neurogenic pattern of motor unit potentials
Polyradiculoneuritis	Spinal roots, peripheral nerves	Motor and sensory symptoms may be predominantly proximal or distal	Conduction blocks in demyelinating forms
			Delayed or absent F response
Sensory neuronopathy	Spinal ganglia, posterior spinal tracts	Purely sensory changes	╱ Amplitude of sensory nerve action potentials and sensory nerve velocity
		May predominate in lower or upper limbs, in proximal or distal segments	CMAP and motor conduction velocity are normal
Lower motor neuron disease (motor neuronopathy)	Lower motor neurons	Purely motor changes	Fibrillations
		Predominantly distal	Neurogenic pattern of motor unit potentials
		Bilateral, often asymmetric	╱ CMAP amplitude
			Normal sensory examinations

Abbreviations: CMAP, compound muscle action potential; ╱, decreased.

In **polyradiculoneuritis** the lesions involve both the spinal roots and the peripheral nerves. Unlike in dying back neuropathy, clinical manifestations do not necessarily start or predominate in distal segments. In some patients both motor and sensory deficits are predominantly proximal. The early electrophysiological abnormality of demyelinating polyradiculoneuritis, such as paraneoplastic Guillain–Barré syndrome, are conduction blocks (Fig. 8.1). A delayed F response indicates proximal peripheral nerve or nerve root lesion (Fig. 8.2) (1).

Sensory neuronopathy results from lesions of sensory neurons located in spinal ganglia, and spreading to spinal posterior tracts. Sensory neuronopathy is less common than dying back neuropathy. However, it occurs more frequently in cancer patients than in the general population because some of its causes, including cisplatin or Taxol® toxicity or paraneoplastic neuronopathy, are related to cancer. Clinical features consist of paraesthesia, pain, decrease or loss of tendon reflexes, and sensory changes mainly of vibratory and position

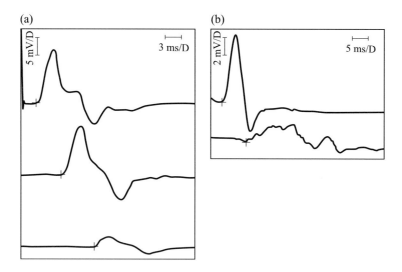

Fig. 8.1 Electrophysiological abnormalities in acute demyelinating polyradiculoneuritis. (a) A proximal conduction block. The amplitude of the compound muscle action potential (CAMP) of adductor digiti minimi shows a 75% decrease between axillar (midline) and supraclavicular (Erb-point, lower line) stimulation of the ulnar nerve. (b) A marked temporal dispersion of the CAMP of abductor pollicis brevis is shown when the median nerve is stimulated at the elbow (lower line) as compared to normal CAMP when the stimulation is at the wrist. (Courtesy of Professor P. Van den Bergh.)

sense. The deficits may predominate in the upper or the lower limbs, begin proximally and involve the trunk and the face. Sensory deafferentation frequently causes gait ataxia. There is no weakness and no muscle atrophy. Electrophysiological changes are characterized by an early decrease of amplitude of sensory nerve action potentials, and sensory nerve conduction velocity. The testing of the motor function is normal.

   Lower motor neuron lesions, or motor neuronopathy, presents with clinical and electrophysiological features opposite to sensory neuronopathy. Patients complain of weakness, which usually predominates, as does muscle atrophy, in distal segments of the limbs. Tendon reflexes are depressed or lost. Pain and cramps may be present, but there are no sensory changes. Electrophysiological features of low motor neuron lesions include fibrillations, neurogenic pattern of motor unit potentials (Fig. 8.3), and reduced CMAP amplitude. Motor nerve conduction velocity is usually normal unless the loss of motor fibres is severe. Sensory function is normal.

Main aetiologies

The main causes of diffuse PNS lesions in cancer patients are summarized in Table 8.2.

Neoplastic lesions

Widespread tumoral lesions of the PNS may be caused by metastatic infiltrations. They involve most commonly the spinal roots, as part of leptomeningeal carcinomatosis.

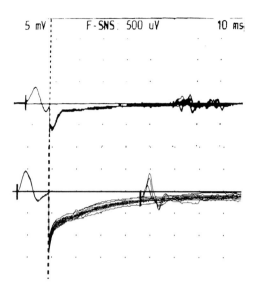

Fig. 8.2 F response in the peroneal nerve in a patient with proximal demyelinating neuropathy. The response is delayed (69.9 ms, upper trace) as compared with a matched control (55.8 ms, lower trace). (Courtesy of Dr J.M. Caroyer.)

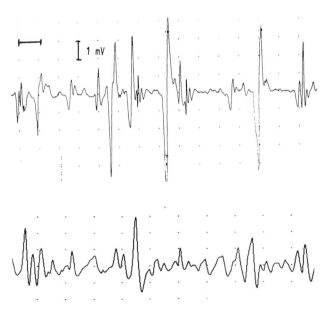

Fig. 8.3 Electromyographic recording in the first dorsal interosseous muscle. The upper trace shows a neurogenic pattern characterized by high amplitude (>6 mV) and polyphasic motor unit potentials in a patient with lower motor neuron disease. The lower trace shows the same recording in a matched control.(Courtesy of Dr J.M. Caroyer.)

Table 8.2   Main causes of peripheral neuropathy in cancer patients

Lesions	Causes
Neoplastic	Leptomeningeal metastases (spinal roots)
	Peripheral nerve infiltration (leukaemia, lymphoma)
Treatment related	Chemotherapy
	Supportive treatments
Paraneoplastic	Subacute sensory neuronopathy (anti-Hu syndrome)
	Associated with monoclonal paraproteinaemia (myeloma, Waldenström disease)
	Associated with carcinoma or lymphoma (with or without paraproteinaemia)
	Due to paraneoplastic vasculitis

Neoplastic infiltration limited to peripheral nerves is uncommon, and mainly occurs in patients with haematological malignancies.

Spinal root lesions are present in about 70% of patients with leptomeningeal carcinomatosis (2). Primary malignancies causing leptomeningeal metastases are acute leukaemias, lymphomas, and solid tumours (summarized in Table 1.4). The main spinal root symptoms and signs are radicular pain, weakness, and loss of tendon reflexes. Their distribution is random and usually asymmetrical. Leptomeningeal carcinomatosis is a multifocal disease, also causing encephalopathy, intracranial hypertension, meningeal irritation, and cranial nerve lesions. However, purely spinal forms have been reported (3,4). We have observed two patients with lung cancer and predominantly spinal leptomeningeal carcinomatosis, in both patients the initial diagnosis was paraneoplastic Guillain–Barré syndrome.

Widespread metastatic involvement of **peripheral nerves** causing symptomatic neuropathy is very rare. Polyneuropathy has been documented in leukaemia (5,6) and non-Hodgkin's lymphoma (6–8), particularly T-cell lymphoma (9), where a distal sensory-motor polyneuropathy with normal CSF and pathologically proven nerve infiltration has been documented (10).

Treatment-related complications

Chemotherapy

In the general population the main causes of peripheral neuropathy are toxic or metabolic. Not surprisingly, in cancer patients, chemotherapy is the leading cause of peripheral neuropathy. A barrier, similar to the blood–brain barrier, also surrounds the peripheral nerves (11). However, the blood–nerve barrier does not protect the proximal and distal extremities of peripheral nerves against many neurotoxic drugs (listed in Table 8.3). PNS toxicity is a major dose-limiting factor for drugs such as vincristine, cisplatin, or Taxol®. For other drugs it may only be a mild side-effect (Table 8.3). Not all peripheral neuropathies due to chemotherapy have the same clinical presentation. Distal dying back neuropathy is the most frequent presentation. Sensory neuronopathy is caused by cisplatin and sometimes Taxol®. Suramin and cytosine arabinoside produce Guillain–Barré-like polyradiculoneuritis (Table 8.3).

Table 8.3 Chemotherapy-induced peripheral neuropathies

Drugs	Severity of neuropathy	Clinical presentation
Vincristine	+++	Predominantly motor dying back neuropathy
Vindesine	++	
Vinorelbine	++	
Vinblastine	+	
Taxol®, Taxotere®	+++	Most common: sensory neuronopathy involving all modalities
		Less common: sensor-motor dying back neuropathy
VP-16 (etoposide)	+	Sensory-motor dying back neuropathy
Cisplatin	+++	Sensory neuronopathy
Procarbazine	+	Predominantly sensory dying back neuropathy
Mizonidazole, mitronidazole	++	Sensory-motor dying back neuropathy
Suramin	++	Guillain–Barré-like syndrome
Cytosine arabinoside	+ (rare)	
Hexamethylmelamine	+	Ataxia, weakness, muscle tenderness
5-Azacytidine	+	
Mitotane	+	

+++, Severe; ++, moderate; +, mild.

Neurotoxicity of drugs interacting with tubulin   Several **vinca alkaloids** are used in the treatment of cancer: vincristine, vinblastine, vindesine, and, more recently, vinorelbine. The clinical features of the dying back neuropathy produced by these drugs are similar, but their severity varies considerably. Vincristine is the most neurotoxic, vinblastine is only mildly neurotoxic, vindesine and vinorelbine have an intermediate neurotoxicity (12–15). Axonal peripheral neuropathy is found almost invariably in patients treated with vincristine. The reported percentage of affected patients depends largely on the scrutiny and methods used for its detection. The examination of neuromuscular biopsies has shown that a variable degree of peripheral neuropathy is present in all patients treated with vincristine (13). The usual earliest manifestations are tingling, burning, and pricking sensations, or numbness in feet, hands, and the perioral area. Ankle jerks disappear during the early stages of vincristine administration, and are followed by the depression of patellar and upper-limb tendon reflexes. Distal and symmetrical weakness, starting in the lower limbs, appears gradually, usually for a cumulated dose above 15 mg. Early signs of weakness, such as difficulty of walking on the heels, justifies a delay or discontinuation of the treatment. Motor deficit due to vincristine is very slowly reversible and may progress for weeks after treatment discontinuation. The persistence of neurological signs is possibly related to the lack of collateral regeneration of terminal axons, demonstrated in muscle biopsy study (13). Contrasting with motor signs and sensory symptoms, sensory signs are mild and present only in about 5% of clinically tested patients. The features of vincristine neuropathy are symmetrical, and, in our opinion, marked asymmetry of the neurological deficit is seldom consistent with the diagnosis of vincristine toxicity only. Although vincristine neuropathy is dose related, higher total doses of vincristine may be administered by increasing the interval between courses. Conversely, the sensitivity of the peripheral nervous system to vincristine may be enhanced by several factors, such as:

(1) age: adults are at least three times more sensitive than children (16);

(2) pre-existing neuromuscular lesions, such as sensory-motor hereditary neuropathy (17), or myotonia dystrophica (18);

(3) associated diseases, such as diabetes or liver dysfunction;

(4) co-administration of potentially neurotoxic drugs, such as isoniazid (19), procarbazine (20), or other vinca alcaloids (21).

The nature of the primary tumour is not considered as a factor influencing the severity of the peripheral neuropathy. However, at least in one study, vincristine-induced neurotoxicity was abnormally severe in lymphoma patients (22).

The major site of autonomic nervous system damage is the alimentary tract. Colicky abdominal pain and constipation occur in about one-third of patients and may be an early manifestation of vincristine toxicity. Urinary retention, atonic bladder, impotence, and postural hypotension (23) are less frequent. However, the incidence of postural hypotension is often underestimated, as it is not systematically investigated. Signs of cardiovascular autonomic neuropathy, such as abnormal variation in blood pressure on standing, or in heart rate during deep breathing or standing, are more common in patients treated with vincristine than control cancer patients (24), but in most patients these changes are clinically asymptomatic.

Taxol® (paclitaxel) and Taxotere® (docetaxel) are plant alkaloids that promote and stabilize microtubular assembly. Taxol® neurotoxicity was first recognized in a trial where half of the patients who received 250 or 275 mg/m^2 developed, usually within few days, a predominantly sensory peripheral neuropathy (25). Even a single administration of high-dose Taxol® is able to produce a reversible peripheral neuropathy (26). Early symptoms include paraesthesia, dysaesthesia, numbness or shooting pain beginning in the hands or simultaneously in the upper and lower limbs. Sensory changes involve all the modalities: proprioception, vibration, temperature, pinprick, and touch. Loss of tendon reflexes is an early and common sign. Limb weakness may be predominantly proximal or distal. Features of autonomic system damage are unusual when Taxol® is used alone, but have been observed in patients with pre-existing neurotoxic factors such as alcoholism, diabetes, or treatment with cisplatin or vinca alcaloids. Clinical and physiological features indicate that, in the majority of patients, Taxol® causes a sensory neuronopathy involving both thick and thin sensory fibres. However, in some patients distal sensory-motor neuropathy resembling dying back polyneuropathy is seen. Peripheral neuropathy caused by Taxotere® is similar to that due to Taxol® and has been observed after a cumulative dose of 600 mg (27).

The neurotoxicity of podophyllum resin is attributed to **podophyllotoxin**, one of its chemical constituents. Two podophyllotoxin derivatives, VP-16 (etoposide) and VM-26 (teniposide), are used in cancer treatment and have been reported to be toxic for both the central and the peripheral nervous system (28,29). However, in our opinion, their toxicity toward peripheral nerves is uncertain. Merwe *et al.* (29) have observed a mild, reversible, and dose-related 'peripheral neuritis' in 6 out of 65 patients treated with VP-16, 300–400 mg/day, with a 9-day rest period between each course. However, in other studies with VP-16, no peripheral nerve toxicity was reported, even with higher doses, despite the presence of central nervous system toxicity (30). The lack of enhancement of vincristine neurotoxicity by VP-16 (31) also indicates that VP-16 toxicity for peripheral nerves is minimal, if at all present.

We are not aware of peripheral neurotoxicity imputable to VM-26 (teniposide). For instance, in patients treated by the EORTC Brain Tumour Group with the combination of VM-26 (60 mg/m^2 every 6 weeks) plus CCNU, and followed until tumour recurrence or death, no sign of peripheral neuropathy has been found (32).

Cisplatin, which accumulates in spinal ganglia, invariably produces a dose-related sensory neuronopathy (33,34). The earliest manifestations develop around a cumulative dose of 300–350 mg/m^2 and, by 600 mg/m^2, almost all patients have neurological symptoms and signs, starting with tingling or numbness in the fingers and the toes. Clinical presentation is very characteristic. Vibratory sense is most severely and most frequently affected, and precedes changes in joint position, touch, and pinprick sensation. Sensory ataxia eventually leads to impaired walking; going down a staircase may become arduous. Lhermitte's sign, which points to a lesion of posterior columns (see Chapter 7, p. 142, 143), has been reported in patients treated with cisplatin, who did not receive spinal radiation therapy (35). This sign developed in parallel to a peripheral neuronopathy, but lasted for a shorter time. Muscle strength remains normal, unless other neurotoxic agents are given concomitantly, but tendon reflexes are decreased or abolished. Features of cisplatin neuronopathy may progress for weeks to months after the treatment has been stopped and persist as long as 2 years after its discontinuation. Autonomic neuropathy is exceptional (36).

Paraesthesia and depression of tendon reflexes have been observed in 10% of patients treated with oral **procarbazine** by Brunner and Young (37) and in 17% of those treated by Samuels *et al.* (38). The peripheral neuropathy caused by procarbazine is reversible and mild. It is very seldom a limiting factor when procarbazine is administered orally, unless it is used in combination with other neurotoxic agents (39).

Mizonidazole and its analogue **mitronidazole** have been used as radiosensitizers of anoxic cells in the treatment of various cancers. However, the initially encouraging results were not confirmed in subsequent randomized trials (see Chapter 12, p. 234, 235), and the use of these agents in cancer management may be historical. At a cumulative dose of about 12 g/m^2, mizonidazole produces a predominantly distal sensory-motor peripheral neuropathy characterized by dysaesthesia in feet and hands, impaired vibratory, touch, and pinprick sensations, and depression of tendon reflexes. Weakness is mild and rare. In the EORTC Brain Tumour Group trial, 10% of patients who received a mean total dose of 11.7 g/m^2 in 3 weeks developed reversible and mild symptoms of peripheral neuropathy (40).

Suramin has an antitumour activity in adrenal, renal, and prostate carcinomas. For blood levels of 350 µg/l or more, suramin produces a Guillain–Barré-like syndrome, starting as distal extremity numbness, areflexia and weakness, which may progress to paraplegia within weeks. Severe autonomic failure and diminished vital capacity may occur. Nerve conduction studies reveal conduction blocks and signs of severe demyelination, confirmed on biopsy. CSF protein levels are increased. The syndrome is reversible and dose-related (41,42).

Peripheral neuropathy is very rare in patients treated with **cytosine arabinoside**. Occasionally a Guillain–Barré-like syndrome has been reported in high-dose treatment (43).

Symptoms and signs suggesting neuromuscular lesions have been observed during treatment with **hexamethylmelamine, 5-azacytidine**, and **mitotane**. However, the occurrence of a peripheral neuropathy has not been established unequivocally for these drugs, because the symptoms are mild, non-specific, and inconstant. Only a small percentage of patients treated with hexamethylmelamine complain of paraesthesia and show hyporeflexia and loss of vibratory and proprioceptive sense. These symptoms and signs suggest peripheral neuropathy (44). There is also evidence that hexamethylmelamine enhances cisplatin neurotoxicity (45). Eight of 17 adult leukaemic patients treated with intravenous 5-azacytidine 200–250 mg/m^2/day for 5 days, experienced muscle weakness and tenderness in addition to CNS side-effects (46). Weakness interpreted as a sign of peripheral neuropathy (neuritis) has been reported in one-fifth of 115 patients treated with mitotane for adrenal cortical carcinoma (47).

Supportive treatments

Several drugs frequently used in cancer patients, such as phenytoin (48), and probably other anti-epileptics including carbamazepine (49), tricyclic antidepressants (50), or cyclosporin (51), may cause peripheral neuropathy. When these drugs are used alone the neurotoxicity is mild and often limited to paraesthesia, but they may potentiate neurotoxic effects of the anti-cancer drugs listed in Table 8.3.

Paraneoplastic diseases

Peripheral neuropathies seen in cancer patients illustrate the difficulty of defining the concept of neurological paraneoplastic diseases. Not all so-called paraneoplastic peripheral neuropathies are equally suggestive of a remote effect of cancer. In his monograph, Posner rightly makes a distinction between 'classic' paraneoplasias, which are highly evocative of an underlying cancer, as opposed to syndromes sometimes associated with cancer but more often seen in patients without malignancy. During the past decade the diagnosis of many classic paraneoplasias has been made easier by the identification, in the serum and the CSF, of specific antibodies directed towards antigenic epitopes shared by the tumour and the nervous tissues (52). These antibodies are not only helpful in diagnosis of neurological paraneoplasia but are also reliable markers of the underlying cancer (see Table 4.2) Four groups of paraneoplastic peripheral nerve diseases have been described:

(1) subacute sensory neuronopathy, which corresponds to the definition of classic paraneoplasia;

(2) peripheral neuropathies associated with paraproteinaemia;

(3) sensory-motor neuropathies in patients with carcinoma or lymphoma—their paraneoplastic nature is uncertain and based on the allegedly increased frequency of association with cancer;

(4) peripheral neuropathies caused by paraneoplastic vasculitis.

1. Subacute sensory neuronopathy

Subacute sensory neuronopathy was first identified by Denny-Brown in two patients with bronchogenic carcinoma. The syndrome may also occur in otherwise healthy individuals or in association with autoimmune diseases. However, its occurrence justifies the search for an underlying cancer, as in about 50% of patients a malignant tumour, mostly small-cell lung carcinoma (80%), will eventually be found. In about half of the cases paraneoplastic sensory neuronopathy is part of a more widely spread encephalomyelitis, and occurs in association with limbic encephalitis (see Chapter 2, p. 36, 37), cerebellar degeneration (see Chapter 4, p. 70), brainstem, or lower motor neuron lesions (see Chapter 6, p. 107). Paraneoplastic encephalomyelitis is often associated with high titres of Hu antibody, which are found in the serum in 20% of patients with isolated sensory neuronopathy (53). In patients with isolated paraneoplastic sensory neuronopathy, no Hu antibody synthesis takes place in the CSF. In its pure form, subacute sensory neuronopathy starts with lower-limb paraesthesia, which may be very distressing. Clinical examination shows that all sensory modalities are disturbed, predominantly in the lower limbs. Symptoms and signs, which are bilateral but often asymmetrical, progress over weeks to few months, causing severe sensory ataxia, gait disorders, and, less commonly, pseudo-athetosic involuntary movements of fingers. Pathological examination shows neuronal loss and inflammatory changes in spinal ganglia extending to posterior spinal tracts.

2. Peripheral neuropathies associated with monoclonal paraproteinemia

In a general population with peripheral neuropathy of unknown origin, about 10% of patients have an abnormal monoclonal serum protein (54,55). In some patients, the M-protein may act as an antibody directed towards a myelin protein (P0 or myelin-associated glycoprotein) or a glycolipid (GM_1 or GD_{1b} ganglioside). In most patients, the monoclonal gammopathy is of undetermined significance (MGUS).

In some patients, M-protein and peripheral neuropathy may be associated with malignant diseases such as myeloma or Waldenström disease.

Osteosclerotic solitary myeloma represents less than 3% of myelomas. In osteosclerotic myeloma the relationship between M-protein and peripheral neuropathy is made compelling by the fact that 50–80% of patients develop a slowly progressive, usually demyelinating, polyneuropathy which may regress after tumour treatment (56). The M-protein is usually an IgG or IgA. Its serum and urine concentration is low, and its presence may be difficult to demonstrate. Rare patients with osteosclerotic myeloma and polyneuropathy also present gynaecomastia, hirsutism, hepatosplenomegaly, lymphadenopathy, and endocrinopathy, a condition named **POEMS** or **Crow–Fukase syndrome** (57).

In the most common **osteolytic multiple myeloma** the incidence of clinically symptomatic, usually mild sensory or sensory-motor neuropathy ranges from 3 to 10% (58). Electrophysiological studies indicate a predominantly axonal neuropathy. In about one-third of these patients, amyloid deposit is found in the peripheral nerves.

In **Waldenström's disease** a sensory-motor neuropathy resembling chronic inflammatory demyelinating polyneuropathy (CIDP) is the most common form of peripheral neuropathy, occurring in about 5% of patients. Single cases of Guillain–Barré-like syndrome have been observed in patients with Waldenström disease (59).

3. Neuropathies in carcinomas or lymphomas

Different forms of peripheral neuropathy have been described in patients with various malignancies. Their incidence has seldom been assessed systematically. Croft and Wilkinson examined prospectively 1465 patients with various carcinomas and 200 controls without cancer (60). The incidence of 'carcinomatous neuromyopathy' varied with tumour type: 2% for uterus, 4.4% for breast, 6.4% for prostate, 9.0% for stomach, and 14.2% for lung carcinoma. In lung cancer patients with so-called carcinomatous neuromyopathy, Croft and Wilkinson found that 19% had sensory-motor neuropathy. However, potential causes of peripheral neuropathy are numerous. In the absence of biological markers such as specific antibodies, it is difficult to decide whether a polyneuritis found in a cancer patient results from a specific remote effect of the tumour or from a non-specific toxic, metabolic, or nutritional disorder. In a prospective study where neuromuscular biopsy and electromyography were performed in 50 consecutive cancer patients, it was found that in the absence of clinical evidence of nutritional deficiency, there was no indication of clinical or even subclinical neuromuscular disorder (61). However, a high proportion of histological neuromuscular abnormalities were found in association with malnutrition. The possibility that polyneuropathies seen in patients with cancer are not related to malignancy by a specific mechanism is further supported by the study of Wilner and Brody (62). These authors found that the incidence of unexplained signs of a PNS lesion was at least as high among patients with chronic non-neoplastic pulmonary diseases as in patients with lung cancer.

In our opinion, the observations that most strongly suggest a relationship between PNS lesions and cancer were made in patients with lymphoma:

1. There seems to be a disproportionate incidence of lower motor neuron disease (with or without corticospinal tract lesion) in patients with various types of lymphoproliferative disorders (63), with or without monoclonal paraproteinaemia.

2. Guillain–Barré-like syndrome has been reported both in Hodgkin's disease and non-Hodgkin's lymphoma. Although the estimated incidence of 1–2% is based on very small series or single case reports (64,65), it seems nevertheless superior to the rate of 1 per million per month reported in the general population.

4. Neuropathies caused by paraneoplastic vasculitis

Oh (66) has collected from the literature 13 patients with paraneoplastic vasculitis involving the muscles and the peripheral nerves. Three patients had mononeuritis multiplex, five a symmetric, and five an asymmetric sensory-motor polyneuropathy. Four had small-cell lung cancer and three had lymphoma. The interest in recognizing these complications is due to their response to anticancer drugs, given either with or without glucocorticosteroids.

Investigations

The diagnostic algorithm shown in Fig. 8.4 is based on the distinction between patients who develop peripheral neuropathy after the diagnosis of the malignant disease has been made, and patients in whom the peripheral neuropathy is a presenting symptom.

Chemotherapy is the most common cause of peripheral neuropathy developing in cancer patients. Although the diagnosis is often obvious, several points need to be considered before it is accepted:

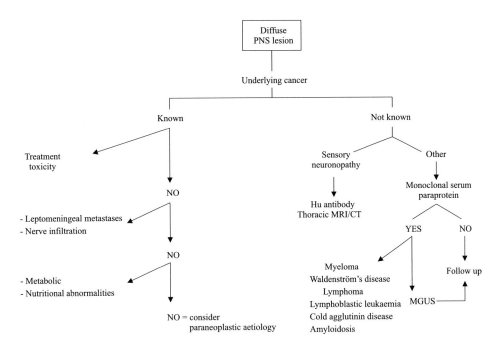

Fig. 8.4 Diagnostic algorithm in diffuse PNS lesions (MGUS, monoclonal gammopathy of undetermined significance).

1. The dose used must be sufficient unless factors enhancing nerve sensitivity are present. These factors include co-administration of other neurotoxic drugs, pre-existing neuromuscular diseases, and associated metabolic or toxic disorders such as diabetes or alcoholism.

2. The clinical features of the peripheral neuropathy should be evocative of neurotoxicity expected from the drug involved (see Table 8.3). For instance, weakness cannot be ascribed to cisplatin alone, and marked sensory changes are uncommon in vincristine neuropathy.

3. The neuropathy should develop during chemotherapy administration or shortly after its discontinuation.

When drug toxicity is ruled out, **neoplastic infiltration**, particularly leptomeningeal metastases involving spinal roots, becomes the most likely diagnosis. Its confirmation requires CSF examination and/or gadolinium-enhanced spinal MRI.

A paraneoplastic origin should be considered after ruling out not only chemotherapy toxicity and malignant infiltration, but also the common toxic and metabolic causes of peripheral neuropathy such as alcoholism, nutritional deficiency, or diabetes.

The diagnosis of paraneoplastic **subacute sensory neuronopathy** is made easy by its typical clinical presentation, and the possible finding of anti-Hu antibodies in the serum. In most patients the diagnosis of sensory neuronopathy precedes that of cancer and justifies the search for an underlying malignancy. The examinations should concentrate on the chest as 80% of associated cancers are small-cell lung carcinoma.

In the majority of patients presenting with peripheral neuropathy of unknown origin, the search for an underlying cancer will be fruitless since paraneoplastic diseases are rare and peripheral neuropathy is common, especially after the age of 50 years. Detection of a serum paraprotein is a simple and useful laboratory test. **M-protein** is found in several malignant illnesses, such as **myeloma, Waldenström's disease, lymphoma**, and **lymphoid leukaemia**, and in other conditions such as cold agglutinin disease or amyloidosis. In most patients, however, the monoclonal gammopathy will be of undetermined significance (MGUS). Patients with the diagnosis of MGUS must be followed up, as about 20% will develop a malignant plasma cell disorder. In **osteosclerotic myeloma** the levels of IgG or IgA in the serum and the urine may be low and sometimes difficult to detect. Considering the very high percentage of peripheral neuropathy seen in this disease, bone radiography is a worthy examination in patients with idiopathic polyneuritis.

Treatment

Neuropathies due to chemotherapy are managed by withdrawal of the neurotoxic drug, but drug discontinuation is justified only when the neuropathy becomes disabling. However, it is important to remember that symptoms and signs of peripheral neuropathy due to vincristine or cisplatin may progress for up to 2 months after drug discontinuation. The best prevention of chemotherapy-induced neuropathy is avoiding co-administration of even mildly neuro-toxic drugs. There is no efficacious protection against chemotherapy-induced peripheral neu-ropathy. One randomized and double-blind study has shown some efficacy of glutamic acid in patients treated with vincristine. However, the benefit was limited to Achilles reflex preser-vation and paraesthesia (67). The protective activity of cronassial (a ganglioside mixture) in vincristine-induced polyneuritis was observed in an experimental model but could not be confirmed in clinical trials (68). A modest protective activity of an ACTH analogue (ORG 2766) was demonstrated in patients treated with cisplatin (69–70). In experimental models nerve growth factor has been shown to decrease or to prevent the neurotoxicity of Taxol® (71) or suramine (72). However, none of these substances has gained routine clinical use.

The treatment of leptomeningeal carcinomatosis is considered in Chapter 12 (p. 261–268). Widespread infiltration of peripheral nerves by leukaemia or lymphoma cells is a sign of sys-temic spread of the disease and is treated accordingly. The reported cases are rare and do not allow evaluation of the specific response of malignant peripheral nerve infiltration to chemotherapy.

Paraneoplastic peripheral syndromes respond poorly to treatment of the primary tumour, to glucocorticosteroids, cytotoxic, or immunosuppressive drugs. The most striking response of peripheral neuropathy to anticancer treatment has been observed after resection or irradi-ation of osteosclerotic myeloma (73). POEMS syndrome may be controlled by long-term chemotherapy combining melphalan and prednisolone (74).

References

(1) Bouche P. (1992). In: Neuropathies périphériques. Bouche P, Vallat J-M (eds). Doin, Paris, pp. 42–72.

(2) Wasserstrom WR. (1995). Leptomeningeal metastases. In: Neurological complications of cancer. Wiley RG (ed). M. Dekker, New York, pp. 45–72.

(3) Ardichvili D, Henneaux J, Musin L. (1971). Carcinomatose méningée à localisation exclusivement spinale et à point de départ inconnu. *Arch Med Brux*, **27**, 655–663.

(4) Parsons M. (1972). The spinal form of carcinomatous meningitis. *Q J Med [New Series]*, **XLI**, 509–519.

(5) Lackowski D, Koberda JL, De Loughery TG, So Y. (1998). Natural killer cell leukemia as a cause of peripheral neuropathy and meningitis: Case report. *Neurology*, **51**, 640–641.

(6) McLeod JG. (1992). Peripheral neuropathy associated with lymphomas, leukemias, and polycythemia vera. In: Peripheral neuropathy, (3rd edn). Dyck PJ, Thomas PK (eds). W.B. Saunders, Philadelphia, pp. 1591–1596.

(7) Brunet P, Binet JL, De Saxce H. *et al.* (1981). Neuropathies au cours de la lymphadénopathie angio-immunoblastique. *Rev Neurol*, **137**, 503–515.

(8) Gherardi R. (1992). Neuropathies des maladies hématologiques (3). Lymphomes. In: Neuroapthies Périphériques. Bouche P, Vollat J-M. (eds). Doin, Paris, pp. 296–309.

(9) Desi M, Laroche L, Adams D *et al.* (1999). Neuromuscular involvement in patients with erythrodermic cutaneous T-cell lymphomas. *J Neurol*, **246**, 1/67 [abstract].

(10) Zuber M, Gherardi R, Imbert M *et al.* (1987). Peripheral neuropathy with distal nerve infiltration revealing a diffuse pleiomorphic malignant lymphoma. *J. Neurol*, **231**, 61–62.

(11) Olsson Y. (1984). Vascular permeability in the peripheral nervous system. In: Peripheral Neuropathy, Vol. 1, Dyck PJ, Thomas PK, Lambert EH, Bunge R (eds). Saunders Co, Philadelphia, pp. 579–597.

(12) Pace A, Bove L, Nistico C *et al.* (1996). Vinorelbine neurotoxicity: clinical and neurophysiological findings in 23 patients. *J Neurol Neurosurg Psychiatry*, **16**, 409–411.

(13) Hildebrand J, Coers C. (1965). Etude clinique, histologique et électrophysiologique des neuropathies associées au traitement par la vincristine. *Europ J Cancer*, **1**, 51–58.

(14) Sandler SG, Tobin W, Henderson ES. (1969). Vincristine-induced neuropathy. *Neurology*, **19**, 367–374.

(15) Nelimark RA, Peterson BA, Vosika GJ, Conroy JA. (1983). Vindesine for metastatic malignant melanoma. *Am J Med*, **6**, 561–564.

(16) Whitelaw DM, Cowan DH, Cassidy FR, Patterson TA. (1963). Clinical experience with vincristine. *Cancer Chemother Rep*, **30**, 13–20.

(17) Weiden PL, Wright SE. (1972). Vincristine neurotoxicity. *N Engl J Med*, **286**, 1369–1370.

(18) Michalak JC, Dibella NJ. (1976). Exacerbation of myotonia dystrophica by vincristine. *N Engl Med*, **295**, 283.

(19) Hildebrand J, Kenis Y. (1971). Additive toxicity of vincristine and other drugs for the peripheral nervous system. *Acta Neurol Belg*, **71**, 486–491.

(20) De Vita VT, Serpick AA, Carbone PP. (1970). Combined chemotherapy in treatment of advanced Hodgkin's disease. *Ann Intern Med*, **73**, 881–895.

(21) Stewart DJ, Maroun JA, Lefebvre B, Heringer R. (1986). Neurotoxicity and efficacy of combined vinca alkaloids in breast cancer. *Cancer Treat Rep*, **70**, 571–573.

(22) Watkins SM, Griffin JP. (1978). High incidence of vincristine-induced neuropathy in lymphomas. *Br Med J*, **1**, 610–612.

(23) Aisner J, Weiss HD, Chang P, Wiernik PH. (1974). Orthostatic hypotension during combination chemotherapy with vincristine (NSC-67574). *Cancer Chemother Rep*, **58**, 927–930.

(24) Robertson GL, Bhoopalam N, Zelkowitz LJ. (1973). Vincristine neurotoxicity and abnormal secretion of antidiuretic hormone. *Arch Intern Med*, **132**, 717–720.

(25) Lipton RB, Apfel SC, Dutcher JP *et al.* (1989). Taxol produces a predominantly sensory neuropathy. *Neurology*, **39**, 368–373.

(26) Iñiguez C, Larrodé P, Mayordomo JI *et al.* (1998). Reversible peripheral neuropathy induced by a single administration of high-dose paclitaxel. *Neurology*, **51**, 868–870.

(27) Hilkens PHE, Verweij J, Stoter G *et al.* (1996). Peripheral neurotoxicity induced by docetaxel. *Neurology*, **46**, 104–106.

(28) Filley CM, Graff-Radford NR, Lacy JR *et al.* (1982). Neurotoxic manifestation of podophyllin toxicity. *Neurology*, **32**, 308–311.

(29) Merwe AM, Van Den Bergh JA, Falkson HC. (1975). A clinical trial of the oral form of 4′-demethyl-epipodophyllotoxin-B-D ethylidene glucoside (NSC 141540). *Cancer*, **35**, 1141–1144.

(30) Leff RS, Thompson JM, Daly MB *et al.* (1988). Acute neurologic dysfunction after high-dose etoposide therapy for malignant glioma. *Cancer*, **62**, 32–35.

(31) Comis RL. (1986). Clinical trials of cyclophosphamide, etoposide and vincristine in the treatment of small-cell lung cancer. *Sem Oncol*, **13**, 40–44.

(32) EORTC Brain Tumor Group. (1981). Evaluation of CCNU, VM$_{26}$ and procarbazine in supratentorial brain gliomas. *J Neurosurg*, **55**, 27–31.

(33) Roelofs RI, Hrushesky W, Rogin J, Rosenberg L. (1984). Peripheral sensory neuropathy and cisplatin chemotherapy. *Neurology*, **34**, 934–938.

(34) Standefer JC. (1984). Cisplatin neuropathy, clinical, electrophysiologic, morphologic and toxicologic studies. *Cancer*, **54**, 1269–1275.

(35) Ecles R, Talt DM, Peckham MJ. (1986). Lhermitte's sign as a complication of cisplatin containing chemotherapy of testicular cancer. *Cancer Treat Rep*, **70**, 905–907.

(36) Rosenfeld CS, Broder LE. (1984). Cisplatin-induced autonomic neuropathy. *Cancer Treat Rep*, **68**, 659–660.

(37) Brunner KW, Young CW. (1965). A methylhydrazine derivative in Hodgkin's disease and other malignant neoplasms: Therapeutic and toxic effects studied in 51 patients. *Ann Intern Med*, **63**, 69–86.

(38) Samuels ML, Leary WB, Alexanian R *et al.* (1967). Clinical trials with *N*-isopropyl- (2methyl-hydrazino)-*p*-toluamide hydrochloride in malignant lymphoma and other disseminated neoplasms. *Cancer*, **20**, 1187–1194.

(39) Spivack SD. (1974). Procarbazine, drugs five years later. *Ann Inter Med*, **81**, 795–800.

(40) EORTC Brain Tumor Group. (1983). Misomidazole in radiotherapy of suprasensorial malignant brain gliomas in adult patients: a randomized double-blind study. *Europ J Cancer Clin Oncol*, **19**, 39–42.

(41) La Rocca RV, Meer J, Gilliatt RW *et al.* (1990). Suramin-induced polyneuropathy. *Neurology*, **40**, 954–960.

(42) Eisenberger MA, Reyno LM. (1994). Suramin. *Cancer Treat Rev*, **20**, 259–273.

(43) Borgeat A, De Muralt B, Stalder M. (1986). Peripheral neuropathy associated with high-dose Ara-C therapy. *Cancer*, **58**, 852–854.

(44) Legha SS, Slavik M, Carter SK. (1976). Hexamethylmelamine. An evaluation of its role in the therapy of cancer. *Cancer*, **38**, 27–35.

(45) Neijt JP, ten Bokkel Huinink WW, van der Burg ME *et al.* (1984). Randomized trial comparing two combination chemotherapy reginons in advanced ovarian carcinoma. *Lancet*, **2**, 594–600.

(46) Levin JA, Wiernik PH. (1976). A comparative clinical trial of 5-azacytidine and guanazole in previously treated adults with acute nonlymphocytic leukemia. *Cancer*, **38**, 36–41.

(47) Lubitz JA, Freeman L, Okun R. (1973). Mitotane used in inoperable adrenal cortical carcinoma. *JAMA*, **223**, 1109–1112.

(48) Lovelace RE, Horowitz SJ. (1993). Peripheral neuropathy in long-term diphenylhydantoin therapy. *Arch Neurol*, **18**, 69–77.

(49) Bono A, Beghi E, Bogliun G *et al.* (1993). Antiepileptic drugs and peripheral nerve function: a multicenter screening investigation of 141 patients with chronic treatment. *Epilepsia*, **34**, 323–331.

(50) Isaacs AD, Carlish S. (1963). Peripheral neuropathy after amitriptylin. *Br Med J*, **I**, 1739.

(51) Wijdicks EFM, Dahlke LJ, Wiesner RH. (1999). Oral cyclosporine decrease severity of neurotoxicity in liver transplant recipients. *Neurology*, **52**, 1708–1710.

(52) Posner JB. (1995). In: Neurologic complications of cancer. Davis, Philadelphia, pp. 353–385.

(53) Dalmau J, Graus F, Rosenblum MK *et al.* (1992). Anti-Hu-associated paraneoplastic encephalomyelitis/sensory neuropathy. A clinical study of 71 patients. *Medicine (Baltimore)*, **71**, 59–72.

(54) Kelly JJ Jr, Kyle RA, O'Brien PC, Dyck PJ. (1981). Prevalence of monoclonal protein in peripheral neuropathy. *Neurology*, **31**, 1480–1483.

(55) Ropper AH, Gorson KC. (1998). Neuropathies associated with paraproteinemia. *New Engl J Med*, **338**, 1601–1607.

(56) Kelly JJ Jr, Kyle RA, Miles JM *et al.* (1981). The spectrum of peripheral neuropathy in myeloma. *Neurology*, **31**, 24–31.

(57) Bardwick PA, Zwaifler NJ, Gill GN *et al.* (1980). Plasma cell dyserasia with polyneuropathy, organomegaly, endocrinopathy, M protein, and skin changes: the POEMS syndrome: report on two cases and a review of the literature. *Medicine (Baltimore)*, **59**, 311–322.

(58) Driedger H, Pruzanski W. (1980). Plasma cell neoplasia with peripheral polyneuropathy: A study of five cases and a review of the literature. *Medicine (Baltimore)*, **59**, 301–310.

(59) Taillan B, Pedinielli FJ, Blanc AP. (1985). Association maladie de Waldenström-syndrome de Guillain-Barré. *Press Méd*, **14**, 844.

(60) Croft PB, Wilkinson M. (1965). The incidence of carcinomatous neuromyopathy in patients with various types of carcinoma. *Brain*, **88**, 427–434.

(61) Hildebrand J, Coers C. (1967). The neuromuscular function in patients with malignant tumors. *Brain*, **90**, 67–82.

(62) Wilner EC, Brody JA. (1968). An evaluation of the remote effects of cancer on the nervous system. *Neurology*, **18**, 1120–1124

(63) Gordon PH, Rowland LP, Younger DS *et al.* (1997). Lymphoproliferative disorders and motor neuron disease: An update. *Neurology*, **48**, 1671–1678.

(64) Julien J. (1992). Neuropathies des maladies hématologiques: Maladie de Hodgkin. In: Neuropathies périphériques. Bouche P, Vallat JM (eds). Doin, Paris, pp. 310–315.

(65) Lisak RP, Mitchell M, Zweiman, B. *et al.* (1977). Guillain–Barré syndrome and Hodgkin's disease: three cases with immunological studies. *Ann Neurol*, **1**, 72–78.

(66) Oh SJ. (1997). Paraneoplastic vasculitis of the peripheral nervous system. *Neurologic Clinics*, **15**, 849–863.

(67) Jackson DV, Wels HB, Atkins JN *et al.* (1988). Amelioration of vincristine neurotoxicity by glutamic acid. *Am J Med*, **84**, 1016–1022.

(68) Favaro G, Di Gregorio F, Panozzo C, Fiori MG. (1988). Ganglioside treatment of vincristine-induced neuropathy. An electrophysiologic study. *Toxicology*, **49**, 325–329.

(69) Hovestadt A, van der Burg MEL, Verbiest HBC, *et al.* (1992). The course of neuropathy after cessation of cisplatin treatment, combined with Org 2766 or placebo. *J Neurol*, **239**, 143–146.

(70) Gerritsen van der Hoop R, Vecht CJ, Van der Burg MEL *et al.* (1990). Prevention of cisplatin neurotoxicity with an ACTH (4–9) analogue in patients with ovarian cancer. *N Engl J Med*, **322**, 89–94.

(71) Apfel SC, Lipton RB, Arezz JC, Kessler JA. (1991). Nerve growth factor prevents toxic neuropathy. *Ann Neurol*, **29**, 87–90.

(72) Russel JW, Windebank AJ, Podratz JL. (1994). Role of nerve growth factor in suramin neurotoxicity studied in vitro. *Ann Neurol*, **36**, 221–228.

(73) Davis LE, Drachman DB. (1972). Myeloma neuropathy. *Arch Neurol*, **37**, 507–511.

(74) Kuwabara S, Hattori T, Shimoe Y, Kamitsukasa I. (1997). Long-term melphalan-prednisolone chemotherapy for POEMS syndrome. *J Neurol Neurosurg Psychiatry*, **63**, 385–387.

9 Focal lesions of the peripheral nervous system

Introduction

The differential diagnosis of **focal** lesions involving the peripheral nervous system (PNS) have been separated from diffuse peripheral neuropathies because in cancer patients their causes are different. While diffuse neuropathies are mostly due to drug toxicity, focal PNS lesions are mainly caused by metastases, irradiation, or surgical trauma. Their early recognition is important as focal PNS may be the first manifestation of a hidden tumour. For instance, in 15% of patients reported by Jaeckle *et al.* (1) lumbosacral plexopathy was the presenting symptom of pelvic tumours. In patients known to have cancer, new PNS lesions usually indicate tumour recurrence or progression.

This chapter deals with focal lesions of spinal lower motor neurons, spinal roots, plexuses, and peripheral nerves. Injuries of cranial nerves are considered together with brainstem lesions in Chapter 6.

Clinical presentation

Thorough neurological examination of patients with focal lesions involving PNS is essential to localize the injury, and to make the distinction between lower motor neuron, radicular, plexus, or peripheral nerve damage. Clinical examination will guide complementary electrophysiological and radiological investigations. The main points of the neurological examination include:

1. Description and localization of **pain**. Neuropathic pain, which is often the presenting symptom in PNS injuries, is typically burning with shock-like paroxysms. It is usually of radicular or truncular distribution.

2. **Sensory** examination. This may show skin hyper- or hypoaesthesia indicative of the injured PNS structure. Neurophysiological examination may show decreased amplitude of sensory nerve action potential and slowing of sensory nerve conduction.

3. Evaluation of **muscle for atrophy** and **strength**. Muscle examination may be assisted by electromyographic (EMG) recording of muscles where the clinical deficit is uncertain. EMG may show a neurogenic pattern of motor unit potentials (Fig. 8.3) and fibrillations, and may also help to determine whether the lesion is radicular or more distally located. Other neurophysiological changes are decreased compound muscle action potential and slowing of motor nerve conduction.

4. **Fasciculations** and depression of **tendon reflexes** also favour the diagnosis of PNS lesion.

Main aetiologies

The main causes of focal PNS lesions in cancer patients are summarized in Table 9.1.

Neoplastic lesions

In cancer patients focal PNS lesions are most commonly caused by infiltration or compression of the nervous structures by primary or metastatic tumours, which more frequently involve spinal roots than peripheral nerves.

Primary tumours

Nerve-sheath tumours (**schwannoma** and **neurofibroma**) and **meningiomas** represent approximately 90% of all primary tumours involving **spinal** roots (2,3). Less common pathologies include ependymoma, dermoid and epidermoid tumours, lipoma, and sarcoma, and these tumours are mostly found in the lumbosacral region.

Schwannomas and neurofibromas are slowly growing, benign tumours. They generally present in the fourth decade and affect men and women equally. The diagnosis is usually made before the age of 20 years when they are found in association with neurofibromatosis (4,5). In patients with type 1 neurofibromatosis (NF1) neurofibromas tend to be multiple and present as two main subtypes. Dermal neurofibroma is a well-circumscribed, benign tumour. The plexiform variant produces diffuse enlargements of nerve trunks and it is almost pathog-

Table 9.1 Main causes of focal peripheral nerve lesions in cancer patients

Lesions	Causes
Neoplastic	Primary tumours
	Spinal root tumours
	Schwannoma, neurofibroma
	Meningioma
	Other
	Peripheral nerve tumours
	Metastases
	Leptomeningeal
	Epidural
	Brachial, lumbosacral plexopathy
	Peripheral nerve
Treatment related	Surgery
	Radiation therapy
	Chemotherapy (local)
Infectious	Herpes zoster
Vascular	Vasculitis
	Haematomas
Paraneoplastic	Entrapment neuropathy due to increased production of growth hormone
	Autoimmune (?) plexopathy

nomonic of NF1. Plexiform neurofibroma carries a 5% risk of malignant transformation. Multiple schwannomas are characteristic of type 2 neurofibromatosis (Fig. 7.8). Their propensity for malignant degeneration is lower than in plexiform neurofibroma. *De novo* malignant (grade 3) schwannomas of spinal roots and peripheral nerves have been observed, but are rare.

Intraspinal nerve-sheath tumours are distributed throughout the spinal axis, with a slight predominance in the thoracic segment. Radicular pain is a constant early presenting symptom, preceding signs of spinal cord compression by months to years. Pain may be exacerbated at night and in a recumbent position. When upper- or lower-limb roots are involved, neurological examination often demonstrates depressed tendon reflexes, hypoaesthesia, weakness, and muscle atrophy in the territory corresponding to the injured spinal roots. These features are less apparent when thoracic or abdominal roots are involved.

Spinal meningiomas are seen predominantly in the elderly and are more common in women than in men. The presence of radicular symptoms and signs depends on the tumour position, and radicular pain may not be a feature when posterior roots are spared.

Spinal schwannomas, meningiomas, and other intradural extramedullary tumours are best diagnosed by gadolinium-enhanced MRI (see Figs 7.8 and 7.9). If MRI is not accessible, CT myelography may be contributive and provides the opportunity to analyse CSF, which usually contains high protein levels, especially in schwannomas, which may produce very high protein concentrations even without CSF block.

Primary **peripheral nerve tumours** are rare. Most originate from nerve sheath. Peripheral schwannomas are most commonly located in head and neck nerves (6) or the anterior aspect of the upper limbs. Small peripheral nerve tumours are often asymptomatic. However, as they grow they tend to compress neural structures, causing paraesthesia, pain, hypoaesthesia, muscle atrophy, and weakness. In benign tumours, pain is often elicited by movements or percussion. In malignant tumours, pain tends to be spontaneous. MRI demonstrates tumour limits (Fig. 9.1), including the intraspinal extension (dumb-bell tumour, Fig. 7.7) which is frequent in proximally located nerve-sheath tumours. Ultrasound may be useful to delineate the tumour extent (Fig. 9.2).

Metastases

Focal metastatic PNS lesions mainly involve proximal structures such as cranial nerves (see Chapter 6, p. 112–113), spinal roots, and plexuses. Mononeuritis or mononeuritis multiplex caused by metastases to peripheral nerves are rare.

Spinal root lesions are very frequent in leptomeningeal and epidural metastases. In both conditions they are usually part of a more complex neurological disorder. In some patients with **leptomeningeal metastases** clinical deficit may be limited initially to a few spinal roots. However, meningeal metastases rapidly disseminate, causing widespread disease (see Chapter 1, p. 7–9). Unlike in leptomeningeal carcinomatosis, radicular symptoms and signs due to **epidural** metastases may remain circumscribed to one or a few spinal roots for weeks or months before causing manifestations of spinal cord compression (see Chapter 7, p. 134, 137–138). Radicular pain caused by epidural metastases is elicited or exacerbated by vertebral percussion, movement, straining, coughing, or sneezing. Rapid recognition of the 'radicular stage' is essential for successful therapy of epidural metastases (see Chapter 12, p. 268–272).

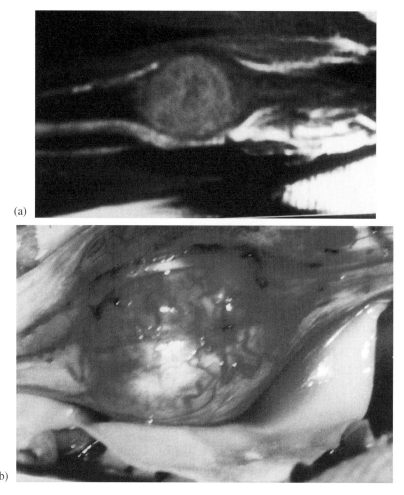

Fig. 9.1   (a) T_1WI MR scan of a schwannoma of tibialis posterior nerve; (b) same tumour viewed at operation (please see plate section). (Courtesy of Professor J. Noterman.)

Malignant brachial plexopathy occurs primarily in lung and breast carcinoma, and less commonly in lymphoma (7,8). The diagnosis of breast cancer usually precedes the development of the cancerous plexopathy, but in lung carcinoma **Pancoast's syndrome** may be the presenting manifestation of a tumour located in the superior pulmonary sulcus (9). The first manifestation of Pancoast's syndrome is reported pleural pain, often consisting of an aching sensation located at the anterior aspect of the chest and the shoulder (9,10). Pain is the initial manifestation of malignant plexopathies in over 90% of the patients. Ache may precede the development of neurological deficits by weeks or months, and is mostly located in the shoulder, axilla, and the inner aspect of the upper limb. Pain is initially moderate and dull but its intensity progressively increases and is often enhanced by the movements of the neck, shoulder, or arm. Both lung and breast cancers invade brachial plexus from below, injuring first T1

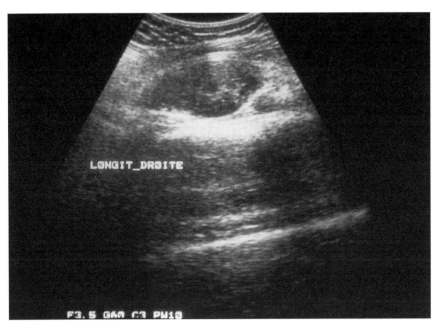

LONGIT_DROITE

F3.5 G6A C3 PW10

Fig. 9.2 Sciatic nerve fibrosarcoma demonstrated by ultrasound examination. (Courtesy of Professor J. Noterman.)

and C8 roots, causing weakness and atrophy of small muscles of the hand. Atrophy may be masked by oedema, especially in women with breast cancer. Motor deficit progressively extends to the wrist and elbow. Sensory signs are less frequent and less prominent. Clinical diagnosis of malignant brachial plexopathy is based on the presence of axillary, supra- or infraclavicular adenopathy or malignant infiltration of subcutaneous tissue at these sites. In patients without known malignancy, presenting with Pancoast's syndrome, a chest X-ray or CT scan needs to be performed to examine the lung apex and superior sulcus. In patients known to have cancer, malignant infiltration of plexus structures is best demonstrated by MRI or CT scan. They may show not only neoplastic tissue in contact with the brachial plexus (Fig. 9.3), but also adenopathy, and local malignant involvement of soft tissues or bone destruction. In about one patient out of three MRI and CT will demonstrate epidural extension of the tumour tissue. In doubtful cases a diagnostic biopsy may be performed (11).

Malignant **lumbosacral plexopathy** is most frequently associated with colorectal carcinoma, lymphoma, sarcoma, bladder, or prostate carcinoma. As in brachial plexopathy, unilateral pain is the usual initial manifestation (1,12). When the upper part of the plexus is involved, the pain is in the groin and anterior aspect of the thigh. In lower plexus lesions pain radiates to the posterior aspect of the thigh, leg, and ankle. Pain may be increased by sudden movement and may be worse in a recumbent position. Weakness, muscle atrophy, loss of tendon reflexes, and sensory changes occur later. Their distribution depends on the location of the plexus injury. MRI and CT scan features are similar to those of brachial plexopathy (Fig. 9.4).

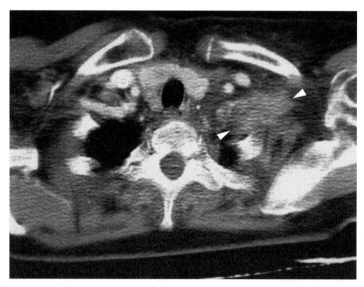

Fig. 9.3 Axial post-contrast CT scan in a patient with breast carcinoma and malignant brachial plexopathy. The malignant mass (arrows) is in close contact with the brachial plexus. (Courtesy of Dr M. Lemort.)

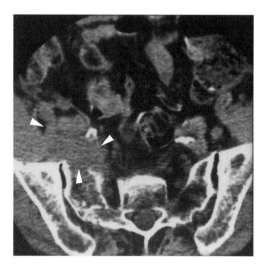

Fig. 9.4 Axial CT scan in a patient with non-Hodgkin's lymphoma and malignant lumbosacral plexopathy. The malignant mass (arrows) invades the presacral space, displaces forwards left iliac vessels, and causes cortical bone disruption. (Courtesy of Dr M. Lemort.)

Mononeuritis and **mononeuritis multiplex** due to single or multiple metastatic lesions of peripheral nerves are uncommon. Isolated cases, or small series of patients, have been reported in non-Hodgkin's lymphoma (13,14), leukaemia (15,16), osteosarcoma (17), or bone metastases (18). The most common example of metastatic mononeuritis in cancer patients is probably the entrapment of an intercostal nerve by rib metastasis, causing burning dysaesthesia and pain (19).

Treatment-related complications

Surgery and radiation therapy are the most common causes of focal PNS lesions caused by anticancer treatment. Focal neuropathies related to chemotherapy are unusual.

Surgery

Head and neck surgery mainly produce cranial nerve lesions (see Chapter 6, p. 118), but may also damage the cutaneous branches of the cervical plexus, causing dysaesthesia and pain in pre- and post-auricular areas and over the anterior shoulder and neck. Lesions of the sensory-motor supraclavicular nerves cause a predominantly sensory deficit extending from the jaw to the anterior and posterior aspects of the chest (20).

Radical mastectomy is followed by hypoaesthesia of the axilla and the upper median and posterior aspect of the arm, resulting from damage of cutaneous branch of second and third intercostal nerves. Pain may develop in these areas within weeks of surgery and is not associated with recurrent neoplastic disease. Serratus anterior nerve is injured in 5–10% of the patients, causing scapular winging (21).

Thoracotomy results in transsection of intercostal nerves, causing segmental thoracic sensory loss and painful dysaesthesia (19). Of 126 patients followed after thoracotomy by Kanner *et al.*, 63% presented immediate post-operative pain, which improved within 2 months. Persistent or recurrent pain around the thoracic scar is usually associated with tumour recurrence (22).

Surgery and **anaesthesia** may cause nerve compressions, mainly involving the upper limb and the brachial plexus. Most deficits are rapidly reversible. Haematomas are an additional cause of peripheral nerve lesion following surgery.

Radiation therapy

Radiation therapy may damage peripheral nerves and lower motor neurons. Peripheral nerve lesions are mostly due to an intense fibrosis of connective tissue surrounding the nerve and to vascular and axonal damage. In rare cases, nerve lesions are caused by radiation-induced tumours. Any peripheral nerve structure can be damaged, but brachial or lumbosacral plexuses are most commonly involved.

Post-radiation brachial plexopathy, occurs mainly in patients treated for lung or breast cancer, and occasionally after treatment of lymphoma. The incidence is correlated with total dose and dose per fraction, which reflects the duration of treatment, and field size (23). Post-radiation plexopathy was found in 73% of women irradiated with 6300 cGy, and in 15% irradiated with 5775 cGy (24). The doses of 5000 cGy given in 25 fractions or 4500 cGy in 20 fractions carry a 3% risk. The delay between irradiation and the onset of plexopathy ranges from a few months to over 10 years. Most cases have been observed between 2 and 6 years after irradiation (25,26).

First symptoms are dysaesthesia and paraesthesia. Pain is initially present in about 20% of patients and occurs in the course of the disease in 60%. Sensory changes and depression of tendon reflexes occur next, followed by weakness and atrophy. The upper trunk of the brachial plexus is more likely to be involved, as the amount of soft tissue surrounding it may be less and results in a higher radiation dose (27); however, this is not a constant finding. The disease usually progresses insidiously but is sometimes self-limiting. We have observed one patient with acute-onset brachial plexopathy attributed to post-radiation occlusion of subclavian artery (28). Radiological diagnosis of post-radiation plexopathy is based on the absence of neoplastic lesions surrounding the plexus and the loss of definition of muscle planes on MRI scan.

Post-radiation lumbosacral plexopathy is most frequently seen in patients with cervical, ovary, rectal, and prostate carcinoma (1,29). The incidence is also related to dose and dose per fraction, as most patients have been irradiated with more than 5400 cGy. The treatment of cervical carcinoma with intracavitary brachytherapy can considerably increase the local dose. The clinical features and the delay from irradiation are similar to those reported for brachial radiation plexopathy. However, because of the use of central irradiation fields, lumbosacral radiation plexopathies are bilateral in about 80% of cases.

Nerve-sheath tumours have been observed after irradiation with 2000–5400 cGy. Approximately half of the patients had type 1 neurofibromatosis. The majority of the tumours are malignant neurofibromas (30). The diagnosis of radiation-induced tumour is generally accepted if the tumour is histologically distinct from the primary malignancy and develops within the irradiation field after a delay of 10 years or more. However, shorter generation times have been reported.

Lower motor neuron lesions, causing weakness, atrophy, depression of tendon reflexes but preserving the sensory function, have been described after lumbosacral spine irradiation in patients with testicular cancer (31). The syndrome has been observed occasionally in patients with other malignancies (31,32). This rare syndrome may be either bilateral or unilateral (31) and occurs after a delay of a few months to over 20 years. With the current practice of small volume, low dose, para-aortic irradiation the risk is very small.

Chemotherapy

While chemotherapy is a frequent cause of peripheral polyneuropathy (see Chapter 8, p. 156–160), it seldom produces focal PNS lesions.

Castellanos *et al.* (33) observed nine cases of unilateral lumbosacral plexopathy, and two cases of mononeuritis, 48 hours after **cisplatin** infusion into the internal or external iliac artery. Only one patient made a partial recovery. The lesions were attributed to small-vessel injury. A case of painful and irreversible brachial plexopathy was also observed following intra-arterial injection of cisplatin (34).

Extravasation of **vincristine** causes a persistent, painful, predominantly sensory mononeuritis. Two cases of sensory-motor, predominantly proximal brachial plexopathy, clinically similar to neuralgic amyotrophy (Parsonage–Turner syndrome), have been observed in association with **interleukin-2** therapy (35).

Infections

Herpes zoster is the most frequent infection of peripheral nerves associated with cancer. The incidence rises from 0.5% in the general population to 9–25% in immunosuppressed patients with myeloma, chronic lymphocytic leukaemia, and lymphoma including Hodgkin's disease. Herpes zoster has a tendency to develop in previously irradiated dermatomes. It is characterized by pain distributed in one or several dermatomes and has generally three components:

a continuous burning pain, painful dysaesthesia, and electric-shock-like discharges. Papulovesicular skin lesions appear after 3–4 days in the corresponding dermatomes. Motor deficit may develop within a few weeks in the affected or neighbouring segments (36), and is generally reversible. Disseminated varicellas, which can be fatal (37), may follow localized disease, usually within a few days, and is more common in patients with immune suppression due to radiotherapy, chemotherapy, and glucocorticosteroids, or primary disease. **Postherpetic neuralgia** is a piercing, constant, burning pain. This is a troublesome complication that persists for 1 year after the cutaneous rash in about 5% of the patients, and is particularly common in the elderly.

Vascular lesions

Several previously considered causes of PNS lesions in cancer patients, including radiation therapy (28,38) and intra-arterial administration of cisplatin (33), may produce peripheral nerve lesions through vascular injury.

Haematomas may compress peripheral nervous structures such as the cauda equina, plexuses, or peripheral nerves. Haematomas are seen mainly in patients with coagulation disorders or after surgery. Subdural spinal haematoma damaging the cauda equina may follow traumatic lumbar puncture performed in thrombopenic patients.

Paraneoplastic lesions

Classic paraneoplastic neuropathies that posses specific antibody markers (see Table 4.2) do not cause focal PNS lesions. The best example of a remote effect of cancer causing focal PNS lesions is entrapment neuropathy associated with growth-hormone-secreting pituitary adenomas (see Chapter 11, p. 203). Reversible brachial plexopathy has been observed a few days to a few weeks after the initiation of radiation therapy in patients with Hodgkin's disease (39,40) and is considered to be a paraneoplastic (autoimmune) manifestation. Clinically the plexopathy resembles neuralgic amyotrophy.

Investigations

Accurate location of focal PNS injury is based on clinical and electrophysiological examination, which distinguishes four main lesion sites: lower motor neurons, spinal roots, the plexuses, and the peripheral nerves (Fig. 9.5).

1. Lower motor neuron lesion

Lower motor neuron lesions related to cancer are rare. Weakness, atrophy, and fasciculations without sensory changes, restricted to one leg or leg segment, have been reported occasionally after lumbosacral irradiation (31). In patients who did not have spinal irradiation, a degenerative versus paraneoplastic aetiology should be considered (see discussion, Chapter 7, p. 162).

2. Spinal root lesion

Spinal root lesions are either intradural or epidural. Vertebral compression and percussion is more painful in epidural than in intradural tumours, mainly because epidural neoplasms often

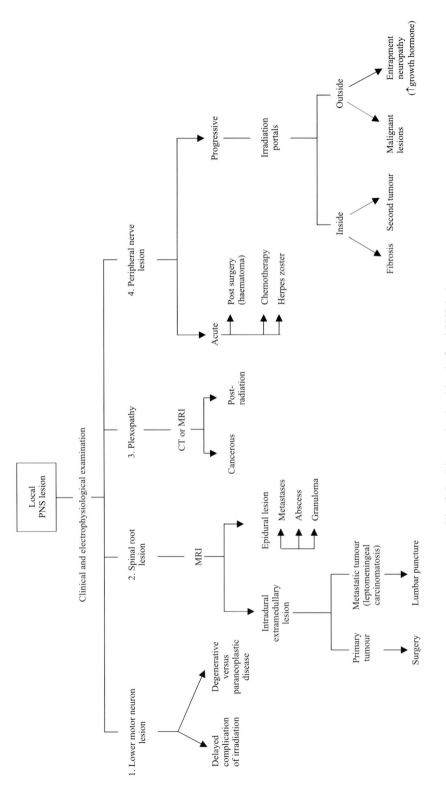

Fig. 9.5 Diagnostic algorithm in focal PNS lesions.

produce bone damage. The distinction between intra- and epidural mass lesion is best made by MRI. Patients with radiological evidence of a single **intradural extramedullary** mass usually undergo surgery, which either confirms tumour diagnosis or shows a less common infectious or granulomatous pathology. Leptomeningeal metastases rarely present as a single lesion clinically and radiologically limited to one or a few adjacent spinal roots; when this occurs, the diagnosis may be initially difficult, requiring repeated CSF examinations.

In patients with systemic cancer, the majority of **epidural** lesions are metastases with diagnostic radiological features (Figs 7.10 and 7.12). In patients not known to have an underlying malignant disease, it is appropriate to obtain tissue for histological diagnosis, particularly if there is no obvious, easily accessible primary site.

3. Plexopathy

Malignancy and radiation damage are the main causes of plexopathy in cancer patients. The distinction between the two aetiologies may be difficult. The principal characteristics of the two plexopathy types are summarized in Table 9.2 (brachial plexopathy) and Table 9.3 (lumbosacral plexopathy). The features favouring malignant plexopathy are neuropathic pain as the initial symptom, and clinical or radiological features of local tumour progression (Figs 9.3 and 9.4). In lumbosacral plexopathy bilateral lesions favour radiation injury. EMG recordings of myokymia (motor unit bursts) have been reported to be characteristic of post-radiation plexopathy (26,41), but these are not a constant feature. In case of doubt, biopsy

Table 9.2 Differential diagnosis between cancerous and post-radiation brachial plexopathy

Criteria	Cancerous	Post-radiation
Incidence	10 times more common	Related to irradiation dose
Delay from irradiation	Months to over 20 years, mean: several years	
Initial symptom	Pain in over 90%	Numbness, paraesthesia, pain in fewer than 20%
Progression rate	Slow	Insidious, may be self-limiting
MRI or CT	Local lesions in over 90%	Loss of planes, no focal lesions
EMG		Myokymia (motor unit bursts)

Table 9.3 Differential diagnosis between cancerous and post-radiation lumbosacral plexopathy

Criteria	Cancerous	Post-radiation
Primary tumour	Colorectal, sarcomas, lymphomas, bladder carcinoma	Cervical, ovarian carcinoma
Delay from irradiation	Variable	1–31 years; median 5 years
Initial symptom	Pain in over 80%	Weakness in about 50%
Signs	Bilateral in 10–25%	Bilateral in 80%
MRI or CT	Local lesions in over 90%	Loss of planes, no focal abnormalities
EMG		Myokymia (motor unit bursts)

should be performed as it is a safe procedure when carried out carefully (11). However, a negative exploration does not always exclude malignancy.

4. Peripheral nerve lesion

The cause of an acute focal peripheral nerve injury is usually obvious when it follows surgery, local chemotherapy, or herpes zoster. Demonstration of a deeply located post-surgical haematoma compressing a nervous structure may require CT or MRI.

   Progressive focal neuropathy within radiation portals suggests radiation fibrosis or radiation-induced second tumour. MRI (Fig. 9.1) and ultrasound (Fig. 9.2) may help in differential diagnosis. Most radiation-induced tumours occur after a delay of more than 10 years and often in patients with type 1 neurofibromatosis (NF1). Sarcomas can occur earlier and are not associated with NF1. Lesions occurring in non-irradiated areas may be caused by primary or metastatic tumours or non-neoplastic entrapment neuropathies, which are common in acromegalic patients (see Chapter 11, p. 203).

Therapy

The aim of management of PNS lesions associated with cancer is to relieve pain and to treat the underlying cause.

1. Treatment of pain

Pain is present in 30–60% of hospitalized cancer patients (42). It is predominantly, but not exclusively, neuropathic. For example, in patients with epidural metastases neuropathic pain caused by spinal root injury is often combined with somatic pain from vertebral metastases. Pain is frequently accompanied by anxiety, insomnia, fear, and depression. Treatment of pain cannot be dissociated from the management of these components, and often requires a multidisciplinary approach. Management of pain in cancer patients has been reviewed elsewhere (42,43). There are a few basic guidelines concerning the administration of analgesic drugs:

1. The choice of analgesic drug depends on pain intensity and, in general, should follow the analgesic ladder. **Non-opioid analgesics**, such as aspirin or paracetamol, are used to treat mild to moderate pain. Weak opioids, such as codeine (starting oral dose 60 mg) or topromaxol are used in patients with moderate pain or if non-opioids fail or cannot be tolerated (gastrointestinal bleeding or thrombopenia). **Morphine** remains the prototype of strong opioids and is the drug of choice for the treatment of severe pain in cancer patients. Morphine bioavailability leads to a wide inter-patient variation and, because of its short plasma half-life (3–4 hours), requires frequent regular administration. Long-acting opioids may be substituted once daily requirements have been established.

2. Analgesics should be administered regularly on an around-the-clock basis, to either suppress or keep the pain tolerable. To achieve this, one should be acquainted with the duration of the analgesic effect of each drug, which is usually considerably shorter than plasma half-life. Intravenous administration of an opioid has the fastest action (within 10–15 min), but also the shortest analgesic effect, and is rarely required.

3. The fear of **addiction** is not justified in cancer patients who are not drug abusers (44).

4. The limiting factors to prolonged use of opioids is **tolerance**. It results in dose escalation, necessary to maintain an adequate analgesia. Escalation may cause sedation, alteration of consciousness, and respiratory depression or constipation. **Physical dependence**, causing withdrawal syndrome at acute discontinuation, may develop after chronic administration of opioid antagonists.

5. Neuropathic pain may respond to tricyclic antidepressants rather than to opioids. The analgesic effect, which may be seen following relatively low daily doses, such as 25 mg amitriptyline, appears to be independent of the antidepressant effect. Amitriptyline is the drug of first choice in post-herpetic neuralgia.

6. **Non-steroidal anti-inflammatory** drugs are recommended as adjuvants to treat pain due to bone metastases. Their efficacy is attributed to the inhibitory effect on prostaglandins that are produced abundantly in these lesions.

7. Glucocorticosteroids may relieve pain in patients with epidural metastases (see Chapter 12, p. 269). However, chronic administration is limited by serious side-effects.

8. In patients with epidural, skull base, or plexus metastases, radiotherapy has a marked analgesic effect.

2. Specific anticancer treatments

The treatment of intradural and extradural **primary spinal tumours** is considered in Chapter 7 (p. 147–149), and the treatment of **leptomeningeal** and **epidural metastases** in Chapter 12 (pp. 261–268 and 268–272).

Malignant plexopathies and **metastases** involving **peripheral nerves** are first irradiated if sufficient dose is still appropriate. Radiation therapy may alleviate pain and its effect may be consolidated by chemotherapy and hormone therapy in patients with sensitive tumours.

There is little effective treatment available for **post-radiation plexopathy**. It has been suggested that decompressive surgery, consisting of liberation of nervous structures from the surrounding fibrosis, may be beneficial. However, it is not recommended as it may put at risk the already compromised blood supply of the nerve trunks. The use of hyperbaric oxygen is under investigation.

Both benign and malignant **nerve-sheath tumours** are notoriously radio- and chemoresistant. Resection is the main therapeutic option. Radiation therapy is used in incompletely resected malignant or recurrent tumours (45–47).

References

(1) Jaeckle KA, Young DF, Foley KM. (1985). The natural history of lumbosacral plexopathy in cancer. *Neurology*, **35**, 8–15.
(2) Levy W, Latchaw J, Hahn J *et al.* (1986). Spinal neurofibromas: a report of 66 cases and a comparison with meningiomas. *Neurosurgery*, **18**, 331–334.
(3) Namer IJ, Pamir MN, Benli K *et al.* (1987). Spinal meningiomas. *Neurochirurgia*, **30**, 11–15.
(4) Riccardi VM. (1981). Von Recklinghausen neurofibromatosis. *N Engl J Med*, **305**, 1617–1627.

(5) Hosoi K. (1931). Multiple neurofibromatosis (von Recklinghausen's disease) with special reference to malignant transformation. *Arch Surg*, **22**, 258–281.

(6) Bruner JM. (1987). Peripheral nerve sheath tumors of the head and neck. *Semin Diagn Pathol*, **4**, 136–149.

(7) Cascino TL, Kori S, Krol G, Foley KM. (1983). CT of the brachial plexus in patients with cancer. *Neurology*, **33**, 1553–1557.

(8) Thyagarajan D, Cascino T, Harms G. (1995). Magnetic resonance imaging in brachial plexopathy of cancer. *Neurology*, **45**, 421–427.

(9) Marangoni C, Lacerenza M, Formaglio F *et al.* (1993). Sensory disorder of the chest as presenting symptom of lung cancer. *J Neurol Neurosurg Psychiat*, **56**, 1033–1034.

(10) Attar S, Miller JE, Satterfield J *et al.* (1979). Pancoat's tumor: irradiation or surgery? *Ann Thorac Surg*, **28**, 578–586.

(11) Bagley FH, Walsh JW, Cady B *et al.* (1978). Carcinomatous versus radiation-induced brachial plexus neuropathy in breast cancer. *Cancer*, **41**, 2154–2157.

(12) Thomas JE, Cascino TL, Earle JD. (1985). Differential diagnosis between radiation and tumor plexopathy of the pelvis. *Neurology*, **35**, 1–7.

(13) Vital C, Vital A, Julien J *et al.* (1990). Peripheral neuropathies and lymphoma without monoclonal gammopathy: a new classification. *J Neurol*, **237**, 177–185.

(14) Reid AC, Bone I. (1981). Lymphoma presenting as mononeuritis multiplex. *Postgrad Med J*, **57**, 176–177.

(15) Stillman MJ, Christensen W, Payne R *et al.* (1988). Leukemic relapse presenting as sciatic nerve involvement by chloroma. *Cancer*, **62**, 2047–2050.

(16) Lekos A, Katirji BM, Cohen ML *et al.* (1994). Mononeuritis multiplex. A harbinger of acute leukemia in relapse. *Arch Neurol*, **51**, 618–622.

(17) Kramer ED, Lewis D, Raney B *et al.* (1989). Neurologic complications in children with soft tissue and osseous sarcoma. *Cancer*, **64**, 2600–2603.

(18) Roger LR, Borkowski GP, Albers JW *et al.* (1993). Obturator mononeuropathy caused by pelvic cancer. *Six cases. Neurology*, **43**, 1489–1492.

(19) Foley KM. (1984). Pain syndromes in patients with cancer. *Med Clin North Am*, **71**, 169–184.

(20) Swift TR. (1970). Involvement of peripheral nerve in radical neck dissection. *Am J Surg*, **199**, 694–698.

(21) Delmar AR, Minton JP. (1983). Complications associated with mastectomy. *Surg Clin North Am*, **63**, 1332–1352.

(22) Kanner RK, Martini N, Foley KM. (1982). Incidence of pain and other clinical manifestations of superior pulmonary sulcus (Pancoat's tumors). In: Advances of pain research and therapy. Bonica JJ, Ventafrida V (eds). Raven Press, New York, pp. 27–39.

(23) Westling P, Svensson H, Hele P. (1972). Cervical plexus lesions following postoperative radiation therapy of mammary carcinoma. *Acta Radiol Ther*, **11**, 209–216.

(24) Stoll BA, Andrews JT. (1966). Radiation-induced peripheral neuropathy. *Br Med J*, **1**, 834–837.

(25) Thomas JE, Colby MY. (1972). Radiation-induced or metastatic plexopathy. A diagnostic dilemma. *JAMA*, **222**, 1392–1395.

(26) Lederman RJ, Wilbourn AJ. (1984). Brachial plexopathy recurrent cancer or radiation? *Neurology*, **34**, 1331–1335.

(27) Kori SH, Foley KM, Posner JB. (1981). Brachial plexus lesions in patients with cancer: 100 cases. *Neurology*, **31**, 45–50.

(28) Gérard JM, Fanck N, Moussa Z, Hildebrand J. (1989). Acute ischemic brachial plexus neuropathy following radiation therapy. *Neurology*, **39**, 450–451.

(29) Thomas PK, Holdorff B. (1984). Neuropathy due to physical agents. In: Peripheral neuropathy. Dyck PJ, Thomas PK, Lambert EH, Bunge R (eds). WB Saunders, Philadelphia, pp. 1496–1504.

(30) Bernstein M, Laperrière N. (1991). Radiation-induced tumors of the nervous system. In: Radiation injury to the nervous system. Gutin PH, Leibel SA, Sheline GE (eds). Raven Press, New York, pp. 455–468.

(31) Lamy C, Mas JL, Varet B *et al.* (1991). Postradiation lower motor neuron syndrome presenting as monomelic amyotrophy. *J Neurol Neurosurg Psychiatry*, **64**, 648–649.

(32) Kristensen O, Melgard B, Schiodt AV. (1977). Radiation myelopathy of the lumbosacral spinal cord. *Acta Neurol Scand*, **56**, 217–222.

(33) Castellanos AM, Glass JP, Yung WKA. (1987). Regional nerve injury after intra-arterial chemotherapy. *Neurology*, **37**, 834–837.

(34) Samuels BL, Kahn CE, Messersmith RN *et al.* (1988). Brachial plexopathy after intraarterial cisplatin. *J Clin Oncol*, **6**, 1204.

(35) Loh FL, Herskovitz S, Berger AR, Swerdlow ML. (1992). Brachial plexopathy associated with interleukin-2 therapy. *Neurology*, **42**, 462–463.

(36) Thomas JE, Howard FM Jr. (1972). Segmental zoster paresis a disease profile. *Neurology*, **22**, 459–466.

(37) Merselis JG, Kaye D, Hook EW. (1964). Disseminated herpes zoster. A report of 17 cases. *Arch Intern Med*, **113**, 679–690.

(38) White DC. (1976). The histopathological basis for functional decrements in late radiation injury in diverse organs. *Cancer*, **37**, 1126–1143.

(39) Malow BA, Dawson DM. (1991). Neuralgic amyotrophy in association with radiotherapy for Hodgkin's disease. *Neurology*, **41**, 400–401.

(40) Lachance DH, O'Neill BP, Harper CM Jr *et al.* (1991). Paraneoplastic brachial plexopathy in a patient with Hodgkin's disease. *Mayo Clin Proc*, **66**, 97–101.

(41) Aho I, Sainio K. (1983). Late irradiation-induced lesions of the lumbosacral plexus. *Neurology*, **33**, 953–955.

(42) Foley KM. (1992). Management of cancer pain. In: Principles and practice of oncology, (4th edn). Devita VT, Hellman S, Rosenberg SA (eds). Lippincott, Philadelphia, p. 2417.

(43) Payne R, Foley KM. (1987). Cancer pain. *Med Clin North Am*, **71**, 153–352.

(44) Porter J, Jick H. (1980). Addiction is rare in patients treated with narcotics. *N Engl J Med*, **302**, 123.

(45) Ariel IM. (1988). Tumors of the peripheral nerves. *Semin Surg Oncol*, **4**, 7–12.

(46) Basso-Ricci S. (1989). Therapy of malignant schwannomas: usefulness of an integrated radio-logic surgical therapy. *J Neurosurg Sci*, **33**, 253–257.

(47) Campbell R. (1990). Tumors of peripheral and sympathetic nerves. In: Neurological surgery, (3rd edn). Youmans JR (ed). WB Saunders, Philadelphia, pp. 3667–3675.

10 Muscle disorders and fatigue

Introduction

With the exception of glucocorticosteroid myopathy, muscle and neuromuscular junction disorders are rare in neuro-oncological practice. In contrast, fatigue, which is a cardinal symptom in muscular diseases, is also one of the most frequent complaints in cancer patients. Specific muscle diseases, disorders of the neuromuscular junction, and feeling of fatigue are considered in this chapter.

Clinical presentation and electrodiagnostic investigations

Clinical features

Muscle **atrophy** and **weakness** are the most prominent features in primary muscle diseases. In most muscular diseases related to cancer, they predominate in the proximal segments of the lower limbs, and are bilateral. Patients may have difficulty in rising from a low chair or climbing stairs. In more severe cases the gait is impaired and shows a side-to-side waddle. **Muscle pain** and **tenderness** may be prominent features, but there are no sensory signs. Tendon reflexes are reduced in proportion to muscle atrophy.

Fatigue is one of the most prevalent symptoms in cancer, reported by as many as 3 out of 4 patients (1). Fatigue has been defined as 'a reduction in the force of contraction of muscle fibres as a result of repeated use or electrical stimulation' (2). This electrophysiological definition applies to the fatigue found in myasthenia gravis or Lambert–Eaton syndrome. In Lambert–Eaton syndrome the strength may improve after a short exercise, but fatigue will eventually appear if the effort is carried on.

However, the vast majority of cancer patients complaining of fatigue do not have a specific disorder involving muscles or neuromuscular junctions. More generally, fatigue is a state resulting from activity and requiring an increased recovery time (2). In a survey conducted by Vogelzang *et al.* (3) 63% of cancer patients felt that fatigue adversely affected their daily life more than pain, and only 19% reported the opposite. In the same survey, 61% of interviewed oncologists believed that pain adversely affected their patient's life more than fatigue, but most of them admitted that fatigue is overlooked and underestimated. Fatigue may be produced by a large number of physical and psychological disorders. In many patients several factors causing fatigue coexist and cannot be dissociated.

1. Fatigue is invariably reported during the administration of **chemotherapy** and **interferons**.

2. A feeling of fatigue is frequent during abdominal or thoracic **irradiation**, but is seldom reported by patients with limb irradiation. Fatigue due to anticancer treatments may be

long-lasting. For example it persists in one-third of lymphoma patients 1 year after completion of treatment.

3. Fatigue is a cardinal manifestation of anaemia, a multifactorial disorder, present in at least 50% of cancer patients. Correction of anaemia by erythropoietin improves both the fatigue score and appetite (4).

4. Other causes of fatigue are **infections** including viruses (Epstein–Barr virus (EBV), CMV, or hepatitis virus), **anorexia** and **nutritional disorders**, which contribute to diffuse muscle atrophy. **Insomnia, anxiety**, use of **sedative drugs** and **depression** often coexist in cancer patients and may participate to the feeling of fatigue. However, there is still some disagreement concerning the contribution of these factors to fatigue. For instance, Stone *et al.* (5) found that the prevalence of fatigue, which was very high, among palliative-care patients with cancer was significantly associated with pain, dyspnoea, anxiety, and depression but, rather surprisingly, not with anaemia and the administered doses of opioids or glucocorticosteroids.

Electrodiagnostic investigations

The main electrodiagnostic investigations used to explore the function of muscle and the neuromuscular junction are electromyography (EMG) and repetitive nerve stimulation (RNS).

In a resting state **EMG** may record **fibrillations**, which correspond to spontaneous single muscle-fibre potentials. Fibrillation potentials are short (less than 5 ms) and their amplitude is small (less than 200 µV). In muscle diseases considered in this chapter, fibrillations are most likely to be seen in patients with polymyositis or dermatomyositis. Fibrillations must be distinguished from **fasciculations**, which correspond to action potentials of the whole of (or possibly a part of) a motor unit. Spontaneous fasciculations do not occur in primary muscular lesions. Voluntary muscle contraction allows the recording of **motor unit potentials**. In primary muscular lesions the number of active muscle fibres per motor unit is decreased. Therefore the **myopathic** EMG pattern is characterized by a reduction in amplitude and duration of motor unit potentials, an early recruitment, and interference (Fig. 10.1). **Repetitive nerve stimulation** and recording of the corresponding compound muscle action potential (CMAP) explores the neuromuscular transmission. This test uses low (2–5 Hz) and high (20–50 Hz) stimulation rates. It is commonly employed to diagnose and to differentiate myasthenia gravis and Lambert–Eaton syndrome (Figs 10.2 and 10.3).

Motor and sensory nerve conduction velocities are unchanged in muscular diseases. Their determination helps to differentiate myogenic and neurogenic lesions (see Table 10.2).

Main aetiologies

The main diseases affecting muscles or neuromuscular junctions in cancer patients are summarized in Table 10.1.

Neoplastic lesions

Both primary and metastatic muscle tumours present as a more or less painful, circumscribed mass or a more diffuse muscle swelling. Weakness is rarely a prominent feature.

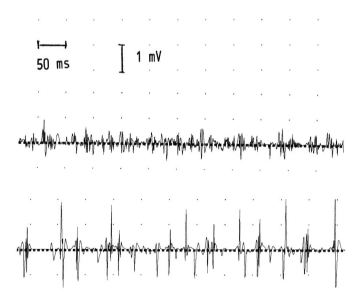

Fig. 10.1   Electromyographic recording in the deltoid muscle. The upper trace shows a myopathic pattern, charaterized by a reduction in amplitude and duration of motor unit potentials and early recruitment for a moderate effort. The lower trace shows the same recording in a matched control. (Courtesy of J.M. Caroyer.)

Rhabdomyosarcomas are the most common primary soft-tissue tumours, and occur mostly in children and young adults. In infants and children rhabdomyosarcomas are located primarily in the head and neck area. In young adults they tend to predominate in the muscles of the upper and lower limbs (6).

Several observations show that cancer cells originating from other organs may grow in muscle tissue. **Invasion of muscles by adjacent malignant tumours** occurs in the head and neck, lung and breast cancer, lymphoma, and sarcoma. Carcinoma originating from bladder mucosa tend to invade the detrusor muscle (7). Implantation of metastases in the abdominal wall may follow surgical or radiological percutaneous procedures (8), and it has been suggested that local production of growth factors stimulated by the wound favours the implantation. In all these situations, the diagnosis of muscle invasion is rarely clinically symptomatic and weakness is seldom a prominent feature.

Symptomatic **muscle metastases** are considered to be very rare, even in most aggressive malignancies. However, Herring *et al.* (9) identified skeletal muscle metastases in 15 patients, during a 10-year period, and 14 patients were referred with a diagnosis of soft-tissue sarcoma. The primary tumour was lung cancer in eight, melanoma or a non-identified tumour in two, gastrointestinal, bladder, or kidney carcinoma in one. Other primaries reported in the literature are lymphoma (10), breast, pancreas, or prostate cancer, and sarcoma. Muscle metastases may be the initial presentation of cancer. They affect any muscle, with a possible predilection for paraspinal and pelvic regions. Physical examination demonstrates a painless or tender mass or a more diffuse muscle swelling. Occasionally weakness may be present (10) and may mimic proximal myopathy clinically

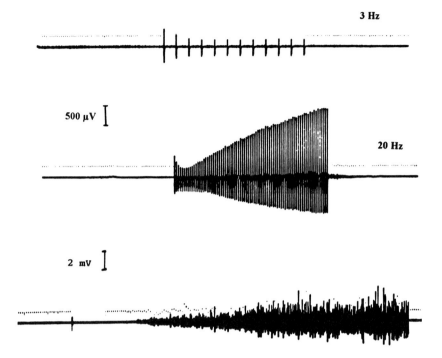

Fig. 10.2   Electromyographic abnormalities in a patient with small-cell lung carcinoma and Lambert–Eaton syndrome. Upper trace: low-rate repetitive stimulation at 3 Hz, showing a decrement of muscle compound action potentials (MCAP) in abductor digiti minimi. Middle trace: high-rate repetitive stimulation at 20 Hz, showing an increment of more than 200% in the same muscle. Lower trace: increment in MCAP following maximal sustained contraction of the muscle. (Courtesy of Dr N. Mavroudakis.)

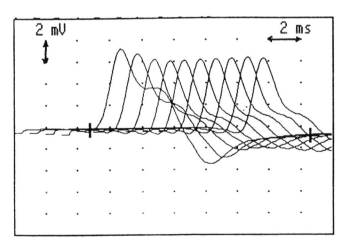

Fig. 10.3   Electrophysiological abnormality in myasthenia gravis. Decrement of muscle compound action potentials in adductor digiti minimi after low-rate stimulation (3 Hz) of the cubital nerve. (Courtesy of Dr N. Mavroudakis.)

Table 10.1   Main causes of muscle and neuromuscular junction lesions in cancer patients

Lesions	Causes
Neoplastic	Rhabdomyosarcoma
	Invasion from adjacent tumour
	Muscle metastases
Treatment related	Glucocorticosteroid myopathy
	Chemotherapy-related cramps
	Drug-related myasthenia gravis
Endocrine	Cushing's disease
	Cushing's syndrome
	TSH-secreting pituitary adenoma
Paraneoplastic	Lambert–Eaton syndrome
	Myasthenia gravis
	Polymyositis, dermatomyositis
	Carcinoid myopathy
	Acute necrotizing myopathy

TSH, thyroid-stimulating hormone.

and by EMG changes (11). Muscle metastases may be demonstrated by CT or MRI (Fig. 10.4) (12); however, their appearance is not specific. Based on both clinical and radiological criteria, the distinction between muscle metastases and soft-tissue sarcoma may be very difficult (9), requiring biopsy.

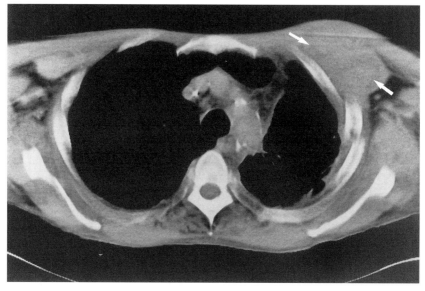

Fig. 10.4   Thoracic CT scan showing a carcinoma metastasis in the left pectoralis muscle (arrows). The primary site of the tumour was not identified. (Courtesy of Dr Th. Klopstock.)

Treatment-related myopathies

Glucocorticosteroid myopathy

As in Cushing's disease (see Chapter 11, p. 203) myopathy is a common and often disabling disorder in patients receiving glucocorticosteroids. This side-effect is particularly frequent in neuro-oncological practice, where prolonged administration of high-dose glucocortico-steroids may be required either to control vasogenic oedema surrounding a neoplastic brain lesion, or to treat epidural metastases (see Chapter 12, p. 224 and 269). Glucocorticosteroid myopathy was found in 19% of patients (11 out of 59) with intracranial malignancy or epidural metastatic compression reviewed retrospectively by Weissman *et al.* (13), and in 10.6% of adults (23 out of 216) with primary brain tumours reported by Dropcho and Soong (14). In a small series of prospectively followed brain tumour patients Batchelor *et al.* observed glucocorticos-teroid myopathy in as many as 60% of cases (15). These discrepancies in frequency of gluco-corticosteroid myopathy may be due to differences in treatment dose and duration, glucocorticosteroid structure (fluorinated glucocorticosteroids cause more severe muscle atrophy), and probably to inter-observer differences in diagnostic criteria. The onset delay also varies from one author to another. Eight of nine patients studied by Batchelor *et al.* (15) devel-oped weakness within 15 days, whereas in two-thirds of patients reviewed by Dropcho and Soong (14) the delay ranged from 9 to 12 weeks. Concomitant administration of phenytoin lowers the risk of myopathy, possibly by enhancing glucocorticosteroid catabolism in the liver; conversely, hypoalbuminaemia increases glucocorticosteroid toxicity (13).

The main feature of glucocorticosteroid myopathy is a symmetrical proximal weakness affecting the lower limbs more often and more markedly. Gait may be severely impaired and require assistance. Weakness of neck flexion is frequent. Less well-recognized symptoms are dyspnoea and reduction in ventilatory capacity. Many patients with glucocorticosteroid myopathy demonstrate other clinical features of Cushing's syndrome (see Chapter 11, p. 203). Glucocorticosteroid myopathy corresponds to an atrophy of type 2 (fast twitch) muscle fibres. EMG examination is usually normal even in symptomatic patients (14), but it may show a myopathic pattern of small and short motor unit potentials.

Chemotherapy-related cramps

Cramps are painful, usually involuntary muscle contractions. They have been observed in patients treated with cisplatin (16) or vincristine (17). Both drugs produce severe peripheral neuropathy, and the most likely mechanism of painful muscle contraction is peripheral nerve toxicity.

Drug-associated myasthenia

Many drugs may cause abnormalities of neuromuscular transmission similar to myasthenia gravis. The long list of these drugs includes antibiotics (18) such as neomycin and amino-glycosides, which are commonly used in cancer patients.

Endocrine disorders

Weakness and feeling of fatigue may complicate lesions of the hypothalamic–pituitary axis (see Chapter 11) or of endocrine glands. Proximal weakness, similar to that caused by

glucocorticosteroid administration, is seen in patients with Cushing's disease or ectopic production of ACTH. Proximal weakness also occurs in TSH-secreting pituitary adenoma.
Fatigability is a common complaint in patients with hypopituitarism, ACTH, glucocorticosteroid, TSH, and growth hormone deficiency. Excessive production of antidiuretic hormone
causes hyponatraemia and weakness.

Paraneoplastic diseases

Several paraneoplastic disorders may affect the neuromuscular junction or the muscle tissue.
Different pathogenic mechanisms have been identified. In Lambert–Eaton syndrome and in
patients with myasthenia gravis and thymoma or thymic carcinoma an autoimmune reaction
causes the neurological disorder. The pathogenic role of autoantibodies found in the stiff-person
syndrome is still somewhat unclear. Carcinoid syndrome is caused by tumour production of
serotonin. The relationship between polymyositis–dermatomyositis or necrotizing myopathy
and cancer is based on an allegedly increased frequency of association, and their pathogenesis
has not been elucidated.

Lambert–Eaton syndrome

Sixty to 70% of patients with Lambert–Eaton syndrome have an underlying cancer, mostly
small-cell lung carcinoma (SCLC). The prevalence of Lambert–Eaton syndrome in SCLC
patients is less than 2% (19). Other tumours occasionally associated with Lambert–Eaton syndrome include small-cell cancers located outside the lung, non-small-cell lung cancers (20),
lymphoma, and melanoma. Patients with non-neoplastic Lambert–Eaton syndrome are predominantly women presenting an increased incidence of other autoimmune disorders. In over
60% of patients neurological symptoms precede the diagnosis of cancer. The initial complaint
is weakness noted when rising from a low chair or climbing stairs. Muscle pain is present in
one-third of the patients (21). Weakness predominates in proximal segments of the lower limbs.
The upper limbs are involved in severe forms. Bulbar musculature is usually spared but respiratory muscles may be involved and may account for respiratory distress following anaesthesia (22). Typically, weakness is temporarily relieved by voluntary movements, but returns with
continued effort. Tendon reflexes may be decreased or abolished, mostly in the lower limbs.

   Cholinergic dysautonomia causing dry mouth and eyes, constipation, urinary retention,
and impotence occurs in half of the patients, mostly in severe cases (23,24). Some patients
with SCLC and Lambert–Eaton syndrome may present clinical and autoimmune features of
anti-Hu paraneoplastic syndrome (see Chapter 2, p. 38). The diagnosis of Lambert–Eaton
syndrome is confirmed by electrodiagnostic tests and the presence in the serum of antibodies
directed against voltage-gated calcium-channel protein.

   The classical triad of the repetitive nerve stimulation (RNS) test abnormalities involves:

(1) low CMAP amplitude at initial stimulation;

(2) decremental response at low-rate (2–5 Hz) stimulation; and

(3) incremental response (usually >200%) at high-rate (20–50 Hz) stimulation (HRS)
    (Fig. 10.2).

Although this pattern remains the most common, Oh has reported two others. All three
patterns are characterized by initially low CMAP, but vary in their response to HRS,

which may mimic myasthenia gravis in a small number of patients (25). HRS is often painful and may be replaced by maximal sustained voluntary contraction of the explored muscle (Fig. 10.2).

IgG directed against P/Q-type voltage-gated calcium channels are found in the serum of patients with paraneoplastic and non-paraneoplastic Lambert–Eaton syndrome. Although SCLC cells express calcium-channel protein in all patients, only 1–2% will develop Lambert–Eaton syndrome. The antibodies downregulate presynaptic calcium channels and decrease the liberation of acetylcholine 'packets'. The autoantibodies are considered to cause the disease because they are able to reproduce the electrophysiological abnormalities *in vitro* and in animals injected with IgG from Lambert–Eaton syndrome patients (26), and because Lambert–Eaton syndrome manifestations respond to immunosuppressive therapy (27,28) and to the treatment of the underlying tumour.

Myasthenia gravis

Myasthenia gravis may occur at any age, but is predominantly seen either in young women or during the fifth and sixth decade in males. The main manifestation is excessive fatigability; the weakness is increased by muscle activity. Clinical symptoms and signs may be either generalized or restricted to certain groups of muscles. Eye muscles are the first affected in about 60% of patients, causing an often asymmetrical ptosis and diplopia. Mastication and swallowing may become difficult, especially at the end of the meal. Speech fatigues, causing dysarthria. Impairment of respiratory muscles is a major life-threatening deficit. About 10% of patients with myasthenia gravis have thymoma or thymic carcinoma. Conversely about one-third of patients with thymoma develop myasthenia gravis. Myasthenia gravis is usually regarded as a paraneoplastic disorder when it occurs in patients with thymoma or thymic carcinoma but not thymic hyperplasia. Occasionally myasthenia gravis has been described in patients with Hodgkin's disease (29,30) or non-Hodgkin's lymphoma (31,32). Paraneoplastic myasthenia (due to a remote tumour effect) must be distinguished from ocular or bulbar 'myasthenic symptoms' caused by parasellar (33) or brainstem tumours (34), which occasionally mimic myasthenia gravis. Anti-acetylcholine receptor antibodies are found in up to 90% of patients with generalized, and in about 70% with ocular, myasthenia gravis. Their presence is highly specific of myasthenia gravis diagnosis (35). In addition to anti-acetylcholine receptor antibodies, 80–90% of patients with thymic tumours have anti-titin antibodies directed against striated muscles (36). Their presence allows differentiation of thymoma patients from those with thymic hyperplasia (37).

Electrodiagnostic tests are also helpful in the diagnosis of myasthenia gravis. Typical electrophysiological features include:

(1) normal or slightly reduced first-elicited CAMP;

(2) a decremental response to low-rate (2–5 Hz) RNS; and

(3) a lesser decrement to high-rate (>20 Hz) RNS (Fig. 10.3).

Such a pattern is expected to be found in over two-thirds of patients. The extreme figures of typical abnormalities vary from 41% (38) to 95% (39).

The **tensilon** (edrophonium) test is considered diagnostic if marked improvement of myasthenic symptoms and signs lasting up to 5 minutes is observed within 60 seconds following intravenous administration of 2–8 mg edrophonium.

Polymyositis, dermatomyositis

Polymyositis and dermatomyositis are acquired inflammatory muscle diseases. They affect all age groups but show peaks in late childhood and around the fifth decade. Dermatomyositis differs clinically from polymyositis by skin changes, typically consisting of heliotropic oedematous erythema of the upper eyelids, and a slightly raised red–purple rash involving the face (butterfly rash), the trunk, and the extensor surfaces overlying limb joints, mainly elbows and knees. Polymyositis–dermatomyositis occurring in cancer do not differ clinically from diseases seen in the general population. The diagnosis is usually based on criteria laid down by Bohan and Peter (40):

1. Progressive proximal, usually symmetrical, weakness of limb girdle and neck flexor muscles, with or without dysphagia.

2. Increased serum levels of muscle enzymes, particularly creatinine kinase (CK) and aldolase. However, approximately 10% of patients with a pathologically proven diagnosis show normal CK values, even during the acute stage (41).

3. A myopathic EMG pattern, with polyphasic short duration and low-amplitude motor unit potentials. Fibrillations are found in the majority of patients.

4. Evidence of inflammatory mononuclear infiltration, necrosis, degeneration, and regeneration of type 1 and 2 muscle fibres on muscle biopsy.

5. A more recent diagnostic criterion is the presence of myositis-specific autoantibodies, particularly Jo1 antibody directed against histadyl tRNA synthetase.

Patients who satisfy any four criteria have definite polymyositis. Patients may also complain of pain, either spontaneous or on grasping, but pain is rarely a presenting or a dominant symptom. About half of the patients present fever, anorexia and increased sedimentation rate.

At least 85% of patients with polymyositis or dermatomyositis do not develop cancer. Nevertheless, the classification of these diseases includes a category named 'associated with neoplasia'. In the absence of any paraneoplastic marker, the alleged association was based initially on anecdotal reports or small series of patients. Systematic studies yielded conflicting results and failed to confirm unequivocally the association between cancer and polymyositis or dermatomyositis (42–46). The excess of malignant diseases in patients with polymyositis–dermatomyositis could result from several biases, including more extensive evaluation for cancer of patients with polymyositis–dermatomyositis, referral to academic centres of patients having the association of muscle and neoplastic disease, and the possibility of cancer induction by immunosuppressive drugs used in the treatment of polymyositis–dermatomyositis. These biases were largely avoided in a nationwide study conducted in Sweden between 1963 and 1983 (47). The study, which includes 396 patients with polymyositis and 392 patients with dermatomyositis, demonstrated a moderately higher risk of cancer in both groups, as compared to the general population. The risk of ovary carcinoma was increased by nearly 17-fold in women with dermatomyositis. An increased mortality rate from cancer, considered to be a robust criterion of association, was found only in patients with dermatomyositis.

Carcinoid myopathy

Carcinoid tumours are located mainly in the digestive tract and the lung (48). They are thought to arise from neuroendocrine cells and to produce a variety of substances, including serotonin (metabolized to 5-hydroxyindole acetic acid, 5-HIAA), prostaglandins, kallikrein, and dopamine. When released into the systemic circulation these products cause **carcinoid syndrome**, which includes episodic flushing, wheezing, diarrhoea, valvular heart disease, and occasional myopathy. Muscle lesions produce a progressive, symmetrical, proximal weakness. The affected muscles are mildly wasted and tender to palpation. Cramps may occur at effort. Biopsy shows a predominantly type-2 fibre atrophy with little inflammatory change. Several observations indicate that serotonin, produced by carcinoid cells, causes the myopathic changes. In rats, muscle weakness may be induced by serotonin, and prevented by cyproheptadine, an antiserotonin drug (49). Carcinoid myopathy typically follows the diagnosis of the carcinoid tumour (50). Serum serotonin and urinary 5-HIAA, which are often markedly increased, contribute to the diagnosis.

Acute necrotizing myopathy

This is a very rare, clinically and pathologically distinct disease associated with a large variety of carcinomas, leukaemias, and lymphomas. The relationship between necrotizing myopathy and the underlying cancer has not been elucidated. Levin *et al.* (51) analysed the clinical and pathological features in four personal cases, and reviewed 26 additional patients from the literature. Patients usually present with an acute or subacute, symmetrical, predominantly proximal weakness. They may complain of myalgia. Serum creatinine kinase levels are usually very high. Pathological changes consist of widespread necrosis contrasting with very mild inflammation signs. Characteristically there is an intense alkaline phosphatase staining of muscle connective tissue.

Investigations

In cancer patients complaining of weakness, either central or peripheral nervous lesions are more common than muscular diseases. The main clinical and electrophysiological differences between central or peripheral nervous lesions, and muscular damage are summarized in Table 10.2. Once nervous lesions have been ruled out, a distinction must be made between **weakness** and **fatigue**. The diagnostic algorithm shown in Fig. 10.5 is based on this distinction. Many cancer patients complaining of weakness actually mean fatigability. In such patients the correct diagnosis may be missed or the degree of fatigue may be underestimated because the examination does not show weakness. In most cancer patients complaining of fatigability the neurological examination remains normal. Fatigue is extremely common in cancer patients (3–5), and its pathogenesis is often multifactorial. The feeling of fatigue may be related to anxiety, depression, pain, dyspnoea, anaemia, or diffuse muscle atrophy result-

Table 10.2 Differential diagnosis between muscular and neurogenic lesions causing weakness

Injured structure	Predominant weakness location	Sensory signs	Reflexes		Atrophy	EMG	Motor nerve conduction velocity
			Tendon	Plantar			
Muscles	Proximal (limb girdle)	Absent	Decreased in proportion to muscle atrophy	Flexor	Early, marked	Myogenic: Motor unit potential small, short Possibly fibrillations	Normal
Peripheral nerves or lower motor neurons	Distal	Frequent	Absent or decreased	Flexor	Early, marked	Neurogenic: Motor unit potential large and polyphasic Fibrillations Fasciculations	Decreased
Central motor pathway	Distal	Variable	Increased	Extensor	Late, slight	Normal	Normal

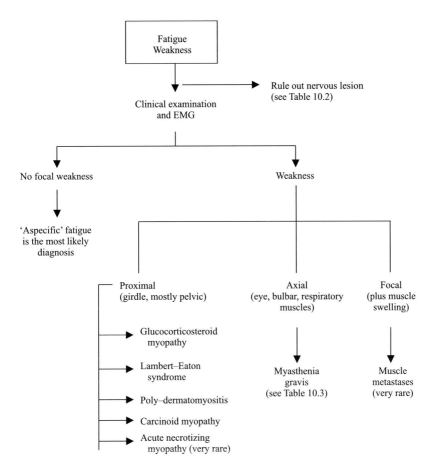

Fig. 10.5   Diagnostic algorithm of fatigue and muscle weakness in cancer patients.

ing from anorexia and malnutrition. Intensive chemotherapy, thoraco-abdominal irradiation, hypopituitarism, and excessive production of antidiuretic hormone may also contribute to increased fatigability.

In patients with demonstrable weakness, the differential diagnosis is based on weakness location, associated symptoms and signs, and laboratory investigations (Fig. 10.5).

The most common weakness location is pelvic girdle. **Glucocorticosteroid myopathy** is the most frequent cause of pelvic weakness in cancer patients. Its diagnosis is based on the patient's history and associated signs of hypercorticism. EMG is usually normal. Cushing's disease and Cushing's syndrome, which may cause clinically similar symptoms and signs, are comparatively rare.

The diagnosis of paraneoplastic **Lambert–Eaton syndrome** is based upon the association of pelvic weakness with signs of cholinergic dysautonomia. The diagnosis is confirmed by electrophysiological features, and the presence in the serum of IgG directed against voltage-gated calcium-channel protein. At least 50% of the cases of Lambert–Eaton syndrome are associated with SCLC. Therefore, in patients aged over 50 years, especially in smokers, with initially normal chest X-rays, CT or MRI, these examinations will have to be repeated during follow-up, as in most patients the diagnosis of Lambert–Eaton syndrome precedes that of the underlying cancer.

The combination of proximal weakness, cutaneous rash, and increased levels of serum creatinine kinase makes the recognition of **dermatomyositis** fairly easy. The diagnosis of **polymyositis**, which is less likely to occur as a paraneoplastic disease, may require muscle biopsy.

Other paraneoplastic manifestations causing predominantly proximal limb weakness are uncommon. Episodic flushing, wheezing, diarrhoea, and increased levels of serum serotonine and urine 5-HIAA are diagnostic of **carcinoid myopathy**. Scintigraphy with radiolabelled octreotide (a somatostatin analogue) may localize primary and metastatic carcinoid deposits (52). Biopsy is necessary to identify **acute necrotizing myopathy**, which remains a very rare disease.

Eye, bulbar, and respiratory muscles are predominantly affected in **myasthenia gravis**. In most patients the differential diagnosis between myasthenia gravis and Lambert–Eaton syndrome may be made on the basis of criteria summarized in Table 10.3. However, in males over 50 years of age, with atypical EMG, the distinction may be difficult.

Table 10.3   Differential diagnosis between Lambert–Eaton syndrome and myasthenia gravis

	Lambert–Eaton syndrome	Myasthenia gravis
Gender and peak age	Men in 5th or 6th decade	Young women
		Men in 5th or 6th decade
Associated tumours in paraneoplastic forms	SCLC ($\pm$60%)	Thymoma
		Thymic carcinoma ($\pm$10%)
Main location of fatigability/weakness	Eye, bulbar, respiratory muscles	Pelvic girdle
Autoantibodies	Anti-voltage-gated calcium-channel protein	Anti-acetylcholine receptors
		Anti-striated muscles in paraneoplastic forms
Electrodiagnostic (typical)	Low CMAP Decrement at LRS Increment at HRS	Decrement more marked at LRS than HRS
Main treatment	Specific antineoplastic therapy	Resection of thymoma
	3,4-Diaminopyridine (guanidine)	Glucocorticosteroids
	Plasmapheresis	Anti-acetylcholinesterase drugs
	Immunoglobulins	Plasmapheresis
	Immunosuppressive drugs	

Abbreviations: CMAP, compound muscle action potential; LRS, low-rate (2–5 Hz) repetitive stimulation; HRS, high-rate ($\geq$20 Hz) repetitive stimulation; SCLC, small-cell lung cancer.

Muscle metastases present most commonly as a more or less painful muscle mass or swelling with little or no weakness. Clinical presentation with weakness mimicking myopathy is exceptional (11). The diagnosis of muscle metastases is made by CT or MRI scan and may be confirmed by biopsy.

Therapy

Glucocorticosteroid myopathy improves after drug discontinuation or dose reduction, but it may take up to 1 year for the weakness to recover completely. Physical training may be useful, but the best prophylaxis is the use of the lowest possible dose for the shortest time. For instance, Weisman *et al.* have shown that in patients with brain metastases cerebral oedema was controlled during irradiation despite tapering dexamethasone, and that glucocorticosteroids could be discontinued at completion of radiation therapy (53).

Paraneoplastic **Lambert–Eaton syndrome** associated with SCLC may improve after successful treatment of the underlying tumour by chemotherapy and radiation therapy (54–56). However, this has been shown in a limited number of patients and the response of paraneoplastic Lambert–Eaton syndrome to the treatment of the underlying malignancy is not constant. Drugs that increase acetylcholine release are the first line of treatment of Lambert–Eaton syndrome in patients with cancer or with a high risk of lung cancer. 3,4-Diaminopyridine (10–20 mg four or five times daily) is as effective and is much better tolerated than guanidine (57). Paraneoplastic Lambert–Eaton syndrome responds to plasmapheresis and immunosuppressive drugs, including glucocorticosteroids (27) and immunoglobulins (58).

In **paraneoplastic myasthenia gravis** the removal of the thymic tumour is performed whenever the patient's condition permits surgical intervention. Plasma exchange or immunoglobulins improve myasthenic features for 2–4 weeks and may allow thymectomy in initially inoperable patients. The aim of surgical removal of thymoma is twofold: to prevent the risk of local neoplastic infiltration, which occurs in 10–20% of patients with thymoma, and to improve the clinical manifestations of myasthenia. A review by Hejna *et al.* (59) of articles published between 1965 and 1998 shows that there is no standard therapy of infiltrating (advanced) thymomas, apart from radical surgery. The issue of optimal adjuvant therapy is unsettled. The reviewed data (59) suggest that in invasive or subtotally resected tumours extended irradiation with 5000–6000 cGy lowers the rate of recurrence. However, it is uncertain whether radiation therapy is superior to chemotherapy. Malignant thymomas are chemosensitive and long-lasting remissions have been observed after administration of several drugs or drug combinations including glucocorticosteroids, cisplatin, anthracyclines, and cyclophosphamide (59). In patients with thymoma that respond poorly to surgery (60), the administration of glucocorticosteroids on alternate days, or of immunosuppressive drugs such as azathioprine at a dose of 2.5 mg/kg/day, should be considered for symptomatic relief of myasthenia gravis symptoms. The benefit of immunosuppressive therapy usually appears only after several months of treatment. In paraneoplastic myasthenia gravis the use of anti-acetylcholinesterase drugs is limited to symptomatic relief of mild generalized symptoms.

The response of **polymyositis–dermatomyositis** to treatment of the underlying tumour is inconstant. Patients with paraneoplastic polymyositis–dermatomyositis are treated like those without neoplasia. Glucocorticosteroids (prednisolone, 1 mg/kg/day) are the treatment of first choice. This dose is maintained until a significant clinical response is observed and serum creatinine kinase returns to normal values. Azathioprine (2.5 mg/kg/day) may be either combined with prednisolone or reserved for patients who do not respond to glucocorticosteroids. Intravenous immunoglobulin treatment has been recommended in polymyositis–dermatomyositis after failure of glucocorticosteroids and azathioprine (61).

A somatostatin analogue (octreotide, 150 µg three times daily), which binds to somatostatin receptors expressed by carcinoid tumours (62), is highly effective in relieving symptoms of the **carcinoid syndrome** and decreasing urinary 5-HIAA excretion, but radiological tumour regressions are rare (62).

The small number of reported cases does not allow evaluation of the effect of anticancer treatments on **muscle metastases**. Symptomatic muscle metastases will be treated like other systemic metastases, by radiation and chemotherapy. Certain resistant lesions may be removed surgically (9).

References

(1) Cella D. (1998). Factors influencing quality of life in cancer patients: anemia and fatigue. *Semin Oncol*, **25**, 43–46.
(2) Kimura J. (1987). Electrodiagnosis in diseases of nerve and muscle: principles and practice. Davis, Philadelphia, p. 628.
(3) Vogelzang NJ, Breitbart W, Cella D *et al.* (1997). Patient, caregiver and oncologist perception of cancer-related fatigue: results of a tripart assessment survey. *Semin Hematol*, **34**, 4–12.
(4) Leitgeb C, Pecherstofer M, Fritz E, Ludwig H. (1994). Quality of life in chronic anemia of cancer during treatment with recombinant human erythropoietin. *Cancer*, **73**, 2535–2542.
(5) Stone P, Hardy J, Broadley J *et al.* (1999). Fatigue in advanced cancer: a prospective controlled cross-sectional study. *Br J Cancer*, **79**, 1479–1486.
(6) Enzinger FM, Shiraki M. (1969). Alveolar rhabdomyosarcoma: An analysis of 110 cases. *Cancer*, **24**, 18–31.
(7) Moonen L, van der Voet H, de Nijs R *et al.* (1998). Muscle-invasive bladder cancer treated with external beam radiation: influence of total dose, overall time and treatment interruption on local control. *Int J Radiat Oncol Biol Phys*, **42**, 525–530.
(8) Soyer P, Pelage JP, Dufresne AC *et al.* (1998). CT of abdominal wall implantation metastases after abdominal percutaneous procedures. *J Computer Assist Tomogr*, **22**, 889–893.
(9) Herring CL Jr, Harrelson JM, Scully SP. (1998). Metastatic carcinoma to skeletal muscle. A report of 15 patients. *Clin Orthop*, **355**, 272–281.
(10) Grem JL, Neville AJ, Smith SC *et al.* (1985). Massive skeletal muscle invasion by lymphoma. *Arch Intern Med*, **145**, 1818–1820.
(11) Doshi R, Fowler T. (1983). Proximal myopathy due to discrete carcinomatous metastases in muscle. *J Neurol Neurosurg Psychiat*, **46**, 358–360.
(12) Williams JB, Youngberg RA, Bui-Mansfield LT, Pitcher JD. (1997). MR imaging of skeletal muscle metastases. *Am J Roentgenol*, **168**, 555–557.
(13) Weissman DE, Dufer D, Vogel V, Abeloff MD. (1987). Corticosteroid toxicity in neuro-oncology patients. *J Neurooncol*, **5**, 125–128.

(14) Dropcho EJ, Soong SJ. (1991). Steroid-induced weakness in patients with primary brain tumors. *Neurology*, **41**, 1235–1239.

(15) Batchelor TT, Taylor LP, Thaler HT *et al.* (1997). Steroid myopathy in cancer patients. *Neurology*, **48**, 1234–1238.

(16) Siegal T, Haim N. (1990). Cisplatin-induced peripheral neuropathy. Frequent off-therapy deterioration, demyelinating syndromes, and muscle cramps. *Cancer*, **66**, 1117–1123.

(17) Hildebrand J, Coers C. (1965). Etude clinique, histologique et électrophysiologique de neuropathies associées au traitement par la vincristine. *Europ J Cancer*, **1**, 51–58.

(18) Argov Z, Mastaglia FL. (1979). Disorders of neuromuscular transmission caused by drugs. *N Engl J Med*, **301**, 409–413.

(19) Erlington GM, Murray NMF, Spiro SG, Newsom-Davis J. (1991). Neurological paraneoplastic syndromes in patients with small cell lung cancer. A prospective survey of 150 patients. *J Neurol Neurosurg Psychiat*, **54**, 764–767.

(20) Ramos-Yeo YL, Reyes CV. (1987). Myasthenic syndrome (Eaton–Lambert syndrome) associated with pulmonary adenocarcinoma. *J Surg Oncol*, **34**, 239.

(21) Lambert EH, Rooke ED. (1965). Myasthenic state and lung cancer. In: The remote effects of cancer on the nervous system. Lord Brain, Norris FH (eds). Grune and Stratton, pp. 67–80.

(22) Laroche CM, Mier AK, Spiro SG *et al.* (1989). Respiratory muscle weakness in the Lambert–Eaton myasthenic syndrome. *Thorax*, **44**, 913–918.

(23) Heath JP, Ewing DJ, Cull RE. (1988). Abnormalities of autonomic function in the Lambert–Eaton myasthenic syndrome. *J Neurol Neurosurg Psychiatry*, **51**, 436–439.

(24) Khurana RK, Koski CL, Mayer RF. (1988). Autonomic dysfunction in Lambert–Eaton myasthenic syndrome. *J Neurol Sci*, **85**, 77–86.

(25) Oh SJ. (1989). Diverse electrophysiological spectrum of the Lambert–Eaton myasthenic syndrome. *Muscle and Nerve*, **12**, 464–469.

(26) Fukunaga H, Engel AG, Lang B *et al.* (1983). Passive transfer of Lambert–Eaton myasthenic syndrome with IgG from man to mouse depletes the presynaptic membrane active zones. *Proc Natl Acad Sci*, **80**, 7636–7640.

(27) Newsom-Davis J, Murray NMF. (1984). Plasma exchange and immunosuppressive drug treatment in the Lambert–Eaton myasthenic syndrome. *Neurology*, **34**, 480–485.

(28) Bain PG, Motomura M, Newsom-Davis J *et al.* (1996). Effects of intravenous immunoglobulin on muscle weakness and calcium-channel autoantibodies in the Lambert–Eaton myasthenic syndrome. *Neurology*, **47**, 678–683.

(29) Quilichini R, Fuentes P, Metge G *et al.* (1994). Syndrome myasthénique révélateur d'une maladie de Hodgkin. *Rev Neurol (Paris)*, **150**, 81–82.

(30) Abrey LE. (1995). Association of myasthenia gravis with extrathymic Hodgkin's lymphoma: complete resolution of myasthenic symptoms following antineoplastic therapy. *Neurology*, **45**, 1019.

(31) Bowen JD, Kidd P. (1987). Myasthenia gravis associated with T helper cell lymphoma. *Neurology*, **37**, 1405–1408.

(32) Campello Morer I, Marta Moreno E, Capablo Liesa JL *et al.* (1995). Miastenia grave y limfoma no hodgkiniano. *Neurologia*, **10**, 246–248.

(33) Moorthy G, Behrens MM, Drachman DB. (1989). Ocular pseudomyasthenia or ocular myasthenia 'plus': a warning to clinicians. *Neurology*, **39**, 1150–1154.

(34) Straube A, Witt TN. (1990). Oculo-bulbar myasthenic symptoms as the sole sign of tumour involving or compressing the brain stem. *J Neurol*, **237**, 369–371.

(35) Vincent A, Newson-Davis J. (1985). Acetylcholine receptor antibody as a diagnostic test for myasthenia gravis results in 153 validated cases and 2967 diagnostic assays. *J Neurol Neurosurg Psychiatry*, **48**, 1246–1252.

(36) Williams CL, Hay JE, Huiatt TW, Lennon VA. (1992). Paraneoplastic IgG striational autoanti-
     bodies produced by clonal thymic B cells and in serum of patients with myasthenia gravis and
     thymoma react with titin. *Lab Invest*, **66**, 331–336.

(37) Voltz RD, Albrich WC, Nägele A *et al.* (1997). Paraneoplastic myasthenia gravis: detection of
     anti-MGT 30 (titin) antibodies predicts thymic epithelial tumor. *Neurology*, **49**, 1454–1457.

(38) Sanders DB, Howard JF, Johns TR. (1979). Single-fiber electromyography in myasthenia
     gravis. *Neurology*, **29**, 68–76.

(39) Ozdemir C, Young RR. (1976). The results to be expected from electrical testing in the diagno-
     sis of myasthenia gravis. *Ann NY Acad Sci*, **274**, 203–222.

(40) Bohan A, Peter JB. (1975). Polymyositis and dermatomyositis. *N Engl J Med*, **292**, 344–347.

(41) Kimura J. (1987). Electrodiagnosis in diseases of nerve and muscle: principles and practice.
     Davis, Philadelphia, pp. 538–539.

(42) Arundell FD, Wilkinson RD, Haserick JR. (1960). Dermatomyositis and malignant neoplasms
     in adults: A survey of 20 years' experience. *Arch Dermatol*, **82**, 772–775.

(43) Barnes BE. (1976). Dermatomyositis and malignancy. A review of the literature. *Am Inter Med*,
     84, 68–76.

(44) Medsger TA Jr, Dawson WN Jr, Masi AT. (1970). The epidemiology of polymyositis. *Am J
     Med*, **48**, 715–723.

(45) Manchul LA, Jin A, Pritchard KI *et al.* (1985). The frequency of malignant neoplasm in patients
     with polymyositis–dermatomyositis: a controlled study. *Arch Intern Med*, **145**, 1835–1839.

(46) Lakhanpal S, Bunch TW, Ilstrup DM, Melton LJ. (1986). Polymyositis–dermatomyositis and
     malignant lesions: does an association exist? *Mayo Clin Proc*, **61**, 645–653.

(47) Sigurgeirsson B, Lindelöf B, Edhag O, Allander E. (1992). Risk of cancer in patients with der-
     matomyositis or polymyositis. A population-based study. *N Engl J Med*, **326**, 363–367.

(48) Kulke MH, Mayer RJ. (1999). Carcinoid tumors. *N Engl J Med*, **340**, 858–868.

(49) Patten B, Oliver KL, Engel WK. (1974). Serotonin induced muscle weakness. *Arch Neurol*, **31**,
     347–349.

(50) Lederman RJ, Bukowski RM, Nickerson P. (1987). Carcinoid myopathy. *Cleve Clin J Med*, **54**,
     299–303.

(51) Levin MI, Mozaffar T, Al-Lozi MT, Pestronk A. (1998). Paraneoplastic necrotizing myopathy.
     Clinical and pathological features. *Neurology*, **50**, 764–767.

(52) Lamberts SWJ, Bakker WH, Reubi JC, Krenning EP. (1990). Somatostatin receptor imaging in
     localization of endocrine tumors. *N Engl J Med*, **323**, 1246–1249.

(53) Weissman DE, Janjan NA, Erickson B *et al.* (1991). Twice daily tapering dexamethazone treat-
     ment during cranial radiation for newly diagnosed brain metastases. *J. Neurooncol*, **11**,
     235–239.

(54) Chalk CH, Murray NMF, Newsom-Davis J *et al.* (1990). Response to the Lambert–Eaton myas-
     thenic syndrome to treatment of associated small cell lung carcinoma. *Neurology*, **40**,
     1552–1556.

(55) Ongerboer de Visser BW, Boven E, Ten Bokkel Huinink WB. (1979). Eaton–Lambert syn-
     drome: electrophysiological normalization during chemotherapy. *Clin Neurol Neurosurg*, **81**,
     235–240.

(56) Jenkyn LR, Brooks PL, Forcier RJ *et al.* (1980). Remission of the Lambert–Eaton syndrome
     and small cell anaplastic carcinoma of the lung induced by chemotherapy and radiotherapy.
     Cancer, **46**, 1123–1127.

(57) McEvoy KM, Windebank AJ, Daube JR Low PA. (1989). 3,4 diaminopyridine in the treatment
     of Lambert–Eaton syndrome. *N Engl J Med*, **321**, 1567–1571.

(58) Bird SJ. (1992). Clinical and electrophysiologic improvement in Lambert–Eaton syndrome with
     intravenous immunoglobulin therapy. *Neurology*, **42**, 1422–1423.

(59) Hejna M, Haberl I, Raderer M. (1999). Non surgical management of malignant thymoma. *Cancer*, **85**, 1871–1884.

(60) Verma P, Oger J. (1992). Treatment of acquired autoimmune myasthenia gravis. A topic review. *Can J Neurol Sci*, **19**, 360–375.

(61) Dalakas MC. (1992). Clinical immunopathologic and therapeutic considerations of inflammatory myopathies. *Clin Neuropharmacol*, **15**, 327–351.

(62) Reubi JC, Kvols LK, Waser B *et al.* (1990). Detection of somatostatin receptors in surgical and percutaneous needle biopsy samples of carcinoid and islet cell carcinomas. *Cancer Res*, **50**, 5969–5977.

11 Endocrine disorders caused by lesions of the hypothalamic–pituitary axis

Introduction

Only endocrine disorders resulting from CNS lesions of the hypothalamic–pituitary axis, are considered in this chapter. Other mechanisms may cause endocrine disorders in cancer patients, and these diseases, which are beyond the scope of this chapter, include:

- hormone-producing tumours, such as insulinomas, adrenal carcinomas, or testicular choriocarcinomas;
- ectopic hormone secretion by tumours, particularly small-cell lung carcinoma (SCLC) (1,2) and carcinoid tumours;
- removal or irradiation of endocrine tissues such as thyroid, parathyroid, or adrenal glands;
- metastatic lesions involving endocrine glands, which may occasionally cause endocrine deficiencies.

Clinical manifestations

The activity of several hormones may be modified by cancer-related processes. Distinctive clinical features may indicate an excessive production or hormone deficiency.

Prolactin

Prolactin secretion is stimulated by prolactin-releasing factor (PRF) and inhibited by dopamine, both of which are produced by hypothalamic cells.

Excessive prolactinaemia produces the amenorrhoea–galactorrhoea syndrome in pre-menopausal women, with secondary or primary amenorrhoea or oligomenorrhoea. Galactorrhoea is frequent in women but occurs only rarely in men, in whom loss of libido and impotence are early features of excessive prolactinaemia. Prolactinaemia has been associated with increased incidence of depression and anxiety and with bone demineralization.

Prolactin deficiency is asymptomatic except during the post-partum period when it impairs lactation.

Growth hormone

Growth hormone (GH) production is stimulated by growth-hormone-releasing hormone (GHRH) and inhibited by somatostatin. Both are produced by parvocellular hypothalamic neurons.

GH excess produces gigantism before metaphyseal closure and acromegaly thereafter. The most conspicuous features of acromegaly are due to overgrowth of connective tissues and bones, causing progressive enlargement of hands, feet, and skull, and coarse facial features with thick lips, macroglossia, and prognathism. Arthropathies and arthralgia are common and may be disabling. Excessive sweating causing oily skin, and hypertrichosis are frequent. Cardiovascular complications present in about one-third of patients include hypertension, arrhythmia, and cardiomyopathy, and may be the cause of increased mortality. Carbohydrate intolerance is frequent, with overt diabetes in about 15% of the patients. Peripheral entrapment neuropathies, such as carpal tunnel syndrome, are due to hypertrophy of soft tissues and bones. **Gigantism** is considered in children whose height is three standard deviations above the age-specific mean height. Hypogonadism is a frequently associated sign.

GH deficiency causes growth retardation in children. In adults it is associated with loss of muscle mass and fatigability.

Corticotrophin (ACTH)

Pituitary secretion of ACTH is stimulated by corticotrophin-releasing factor (CRF) produced in the hypothalamus. ACTH stimulates the production of endogenous corticosteroids by the adrenocortical glands.

ACTH hypersecretion due to pituitary adenoma causes Cushing's disease, which should be differentiated from Cushing's syndrome where hypercorticism is either due to ectopic ACTH or to pharmacological doses of glucocorticosteroids. Cushing's disease affects women more frequently than men. The fully developed disease includes weight gain, mainly due to facial, nuchal, truncal, and intra-abdominal fat deposits. Other features are hypertrichosis, purple abdominal striae, predominantly proximal muscle wasting, hypertension and osteoporosis, and mental symptoms ranging from depression to psychosis. Hirsutism and menstrual abnormalities due to excessive adrenal androgen secretion are present in about 80% of women. Laboratory changes include hypokalaemia, polycythemia, and elevated blood sugar.

ACTH deficiency causes secondary adrenocortical insufficiency. The major clinical features of chronic insufficiency are fatigue, generalized weakness, anorexia, weight loss, and dehydration. Hyperkalaemia is not present in secondary adrenal insufficiency and hypoglycaemia is mild.

Thyroid-stimulating hormone

Production of thyroid-stimulating hormone (TSH) is stimulated by thyrotrophin-releasing hormone (TRH) produced by parvocellular neurons of the hypothalamus.

TSH excess, due to pituitary adenoma, is rare. Less than 1% of all pituitary adenomas produce TSH. The clinical signs of hyperthyroidism include emotional lability, nervousness, weight loss, heat intolerance, tachycardia, atrial fibrillation, tremor, and proximal weakness. The thyroid gland may be enlarged.

TSH deficiency causes fatigue, weakness, lethargy, cold intolerance, and constipation. On examination the skin may be dry and limb extremities may be swollen. Cognitive functions, particularly memory, may be altered.

Luteinizing hormone and follicle-stimulating hormone

The secretion of luteinizing hormone (LH) and follicle-stimulating hormone (FSH) is stimulated by gonadotrophin-releasing hormone (GnRH) produced in the hypothalamus

In children, episodic release of GnRH, LH, and FSH causes precocious puberty, which occurs in a variety of hypothalamic injuries, including tumours (especially suprasellar gliomas and hamartomas) and radiation therapy. Puberty is considered precocious when it starts before the age of 8 years in girls and before the age of 9 years in boys. In adults with FSH- and LH-producing adenomas, hypogonadism with or without hypopituitarism is the most common endocrine disorder, and may simply reflect the impairment of normal pituitary function.

Antidiuretic hormone

Antidiuretic hormone (ADH) is synthesized in clusters of hypothalamic cells, the axons of which end in the posterior lobe of the pituitary gland where ADH is liberated by an exocytotic (quantal) process.

ADH excess causes dilutional hyponatraemia, which generally becomes manifest by nausea, weakness, lethargy, somnolence, or seizures when serum sodium falls to 120 mEq/l or below.

ADH deficiency causes diabetes insipidus, a polyuric syndrome. Pituitary diabetes insipidus results from impairment of hypothalamic centres producing ADH. The predominant clinical features are polyuria (>3 litres/day), nocturia, almost permanent thirst, and hypernatraemia.

Endocrine laboratory investigations

Clinical suspicion of hormone hypersecretion or deficiency is confirmed by the determination of basal hormone levels and dynamic tests.

Prolactin

Prolactinoma diagnosis is based on serum prolactin level. However, elevated prolactin may occur during pregnancy, lactation, shortly after seizure or sexual intercourse. Hyperprolactinaemia may also be caused by drugs blocking dopamine receptors (phenothiazines, butyrophenones, metoclopramide, domperidone, sulpiride). Moderate hyperprolactinaemia may also be seen in patients with hypothyroidism, chronic renal failure, or cirrhosis. In the absence of other causes, prolactinaemia exceeding 200 ng/ml strongly suggests a hypothalamic or pituitary disorder. In macroprolactinomas, the prolactin level is usually well beyond 200 ng/ml. Moderate hyperprolactinaemia may be caused by pituitary microadenomas or other lesions.

Growth hormone

In normal individuals and in patients with GH-secreting adenoma, GH secretion is pulsatile. A single random GH determination may therefore not be diagnostic. Normal morning blood

GH concentration is less than 2 ng/ml. Basal morning GH levels of 10 ng/ml or more are highly suggestive of a GH-secreting adenoma. The diagnosis is usually confirmed by insulin growth factor 1 (IGF-1) levels and an oral glucose tolerance test.

IGF-1 has a longer half-life than GH and provides a better measure of the 24-hour GH production. IGF-1 may be increased during pregnancy or puberty. Failure to lower GH levels to less than 2 ng/ml by glucose ingestion also favours the diagnosis of GH-secreting adenoma.

Corticotrophin

The endocrine evaluation of ACTH-secreting tumours is important as 30% of ACTH-secreting pituitary adenomas cannot be visualized on MRI (3).

Excess cortisol is best assessed by 24-hour urine free cortisol and is confirmed by the lack of inhibition of corticosteroid production by low-dose (1 mg) dexamethasone. Once high cortisol is diagnosed, the site of hormone overproduction has to be established. Two tests help to differentiate between corticotrophic pituitary adenoma (Cushing's disease) and other causes of excess production (Cushing's syndrome). They are based on the assumption that pituitary adenomas retain a certain sensitivity to negative feedback, and remain sensitive to CRF. Thus, the diagnosis of Cushing's disease is suggested by more than 50% reduction in 24-hour urinary cortisol following high-dose dexamethasone (8 mg daily for 48 hours), or by a 50% increase in serum ACTH after an intravenous bolus of CRF (100 μg). However, there are exceptions to these criteria. If the tests are inconclusive, it may be useful to sample ACTH concentrations in inferior petrosal sinuses (IPSs). If pituitary adenoma is the source of ACTH, the concentration should be higher within the IPS than in peripheral blood. Bilateral sampling may also help to localize small, unilateral tumours. The sensitivity of IPS sampling may be increased by CRF administration.

Thyroid-stimulating hormone

TSH-secreting pituitary adenomas may be diagnosed by blood TSH and thyroid hormones (triiodothyronine (T_3) and thyroxine (T_4)). Hyperthyroidism in the presence of elevated or 'inappropriately normal' TSH is in favour of TSH-secreting pituitary adenoma.

Gonadotrophin

Endocrine identification of gonadotrophin (GnLH)-secreting adenoma is difficult. In men, high FSH and LH blood levels suggest gonadotrophic adenoma, but in women, particularly in post-menopausal individuals, the interpretation of FSH and LH blood levels is difficult.

Antidiuretic hormone

Pituitary diabetes insipidus results from an absence or reduction of ADH production. The so-called pituitary diabetes insipidus results from hypothalamic lesions and is very rare in pituitary tumours, except in metastases. Laboratory tests, aiming to demonstrate pituitary diabetes insipidus, are based on the inability to excrete hypertonic urine after osmotic challenge. The simplest way to produce hypertonicity is water deprivation, which should not raise plasma osmolarity above 290 mosmol/kg, and provides an adequate stimulus for ADH

Table 11.1   Main causes of endocrinopathies due to hypothalamic?pituitary axis lesions

Lesions	Causes
Neoplastic	1. Primary suprasellar tumours
	Suprasellar glioma
	Craniopharyngioma
	Hamartoma
	Meningioma
	Germ-cell tumours
	2. Pituitary adenomas
	3. Metastases
	Suprasellar
	Pituitary
Treatment related	Radiation therapy
	Surgery
	(Chemotherapy)
	Glucocorticosteroids
Vascular	Pituitary apoplexy
Paraneoplastic	Germ-cell tumours

release. The normal response is to produce urine of osmolarity greater than 800 mosmol/kg. The values are lower in patients with pituitary diabetes insipidus (4). Pituitary diabetes insipidus must be differentiated from renal diabetes insipidus and excessive liquid intake.

Main aetiologies

The most common causes of endocrine disorders in cancer patients are summarized in Table 11.1.

Neoplastic lesions

The hypothalamic–pituitary axis is the most common site of primary or metastatic tumours causing endocrine disorders. Tumours are either suprasellar or located in the pituitary sella. They may produce excess hormone secretion, hypopituitarism, or a combination of both.

1. Primary suprasellar tumours

The main primary suprasellar neoplasms are chiasma and hypothalamic gliomas, cranio-pharyngiomas, hamartomas, meningiomas, and germ-cell tumours. In addition to endocrine abnormalities, they may cause intracranial hypertension and a decline in consciousness (Chapter 1), cognitive changes (Chapter 2), and visual disorders (Chapter 5).

   Chiasma and hypothalamic gliomas (Fig. 5.4) are mostly tumours of young children or young adults (see Chapter 5, p. 82). Endocrine disorders were reported by Collet-Solberg *et al.*, in 68 children with hypothalamic–chiasma glioma followed for 3.6 years (5). Thirty-eight (56%) received cranial irradiation and 17 (25%) were operated on. Precocious puberty was found in 22% and was attributed to the effect of the tumour. Radiation therapy and surgery were considered to be the most likely causes of other endocrine disorders, such as GH deficiency and diabetes insipidus, observed in 38% and 16% of the patients, respectively (5). In the series of 124 patients with precocious puberty reported by Brauner *et al.* (6) chiasma glioma was the leading cause, found in 11 children. Endocrine disorders were also found in 56% of 33 patients with hypothalamic glioma reported by Rodriguez *et al.* (7).

In summary, whereas precocious puberty seems to be caused mainly by chiasma–hypothalamic glioma, other endocrine disorders and diabetes insipidus seen in patients with this tumour seem to be largely related to therapy.

Craniopharyngiomas (Chapter 5, p. 83, 84 and Fig. 5.5) usually arise in the suprasellar region, but some may be both supra- and intrasellar and few are purely intrasellar (8). The mechanism of endocrine disorders combines suprasellar and pituitary lesions. In children, the most common endocrine abnormalities are short stature (9) (mainly related to GH deficiency), hypothyroidism causing weight gain, fatigability, and poor intellectual performances, diabetes insipidus, and precocious or delayed puberty (10). The major cause of obesity in children with craniopharyngioma is direct hypothalamic damage. In adult women, the amenorrhoea–galactorrhoea syndrome is a common initial manifestation, and men may complain of impotence and develop hypopituitarism.

Hamartomas are formed by nodules of normally differentiated cells, found in an abnormal location. They may be regarded either as benign tumours or as malformations (11). Central nervous system hamartomas are most frequently found in the hypothalamus. Some neurons within hypothalamic hamartomas contain gonadotrophin granules (12), and may act as independent secretory units, causing precocious puberty (13). Hamartomas were the leading cause in 24 of 107 children with precocious puberty (14). Patients with hamartoma may exhibit gelastic epilepsy (bursts of laughing) (11). MRI is usually diagnostic (15,16), (Fig. 11.1).

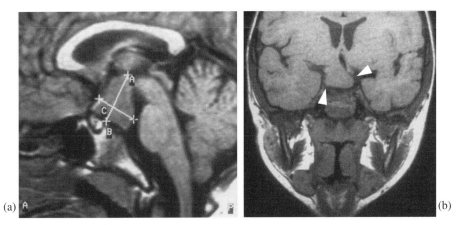

Fig. 11.1 Large hamartoma of the tuber cinereum. (a) Sagittal T_1WI MR scan (A × C). (b) Coronal T_1WI MR scan showing a mass isointense to grey matter (arrows) not enhanced by gadolinium. (Courtesy of Dr C. Christophe.)

Suprasellar meningiomas are primarily seen in women over 50 years of age, and they may arise from diaphragma sellae or extend to the suprasellar region from neighbouring structures such as the planum sphenoidale, tuberculum sellae, or the optic nerve sheath. They occasionally cause endocrine disorders by compressing the pituitary stalk.

The majority of intracranial **germ-cell tumours** are diagnosed during adolescence or early adulthood. Germinomas and mature or immature teratomas are the most common pathological types and arise in suprasellar or pineal (Chapter 6, p. 108) location. **Suprasellar germ-cell tumours** may present with endocrinopathies, which may precede visual symptoms and hydrocephalus. The most common endocrine manifestation is diabetes insipidus. Other hypothalamic–pituitary abnormalities include delayed or precocious puberty, usually subtle hypopituitarism, and growth failure. Fluctuations in blood pressure, heart rate, respiration, and temperature may also be seen (17).

2. Pituitary adenomas

Most pituitary adenomas arise in the anterior lobe. They account for 10–15% of intracranial tumours (18), and are mainly diagnosed in adults. Autopsy studies (19) have shown that the majority of pituitary adenomas remain undiagnosed during the patient's lifetime.

The classification of pituitary adenomas relates to the presence or absence of excess hormone secretion, and histologically relies on immunocytochemistry that allows identification of prolactin-, GH-, ACTH-, TSH-, LH-, and FSH-containing cells. About 70% of pituitary adenomas are endocrinologically active (20) and, in most patients, there is a good correlation between tumour immunocytochemistry, serum hormone levels, and clinical symptoms and signs. Prolactinomas are the most common type of secreting adenomas, accounting for 30–40% percent of all pituitary tumours. GH-secreting adenomas represent 15–20%, ACTH-secreting adenomas 10–15%, and TSH-secreting adenomas account for only 1% of pituitary adenomas. In most non-functional adenomas, electron microscopy does not demonstrate the granules seen in secretory tumours. Some, however, may secrete hormones that are either biologically inactive (α or β subunit) or of insufficient quantity to manifest endocrine syndromes. This group also includes most gonadotrophin adenomas because, unlike other functional adenomas, they are not characterized by a clinical endocrine phenotype.

Clinical features caused by pituitary adenomas include headaches, manifestations of excess or deficiency of hormone, and visual disturbances (Chapter 5, p. 86). **Headaches** are usually chronic and may lead to the diagnosis of tumour. They are attributed to stretching of the diaphragma sellae, but this mechanism does not explain headaches in patients with small tumours. Acute headache may indicate a sudden change in tumour size or intratumoural haemorrhage (pituitary apoplexy, see Fig. 1.3 and p. 212). The features of **endocrine syndromes** are considered above.

Microadenomas, defined as tumours of less than 10 mm in diameter, are usually detected by excessive hormone production. This is particularly the case in Cushing's disease and microprolactinomas. In **secreting macroadenomas**, the features of excess hormone may be combined with signs of hypopituitarism. **Non-secreting macroadenomas** manifest only hypopituitarism, which is assumed to result from direct damage to normal pituitary cells, the stalk, or the hypothalamus by tumour mass. With the exception of pituitary apoplexy, hypopituitarism caused by pituitary tumours tends to be progressive. However, pituitary cells show a remarkable functional resistance to chronic compression by tumour mass. GH secretion is the most fragile, followed by LH and FSH, which affect fertility and libido in both genders, and the menstrual cycle in women. TSH and ACTH function is impaired next. Diabetes insipidus due to insufficient production of ADH is very rare, even in large, primary pituitary tumours. In most patients, diabetes insipidus is due to a hypothalamic lesion impairing ADH production, and is usually the result of surgical damage.

Pituitary carcinomas   Despite their propensity to invade the floor of the sella (Fig. 11.2), the suprasellar cistern (Fig. 5.8), and the cavernous sinus, pituitary adenomas remain histologically benign. Few adenomas have been described as behaving in a malignant fashion. However, they can be invasive and disseminate along the cerebrospinal axis or outside the CNS to the liver, lung, bones, and lymph nodes (21). Pituitary carcinomas may be non-functional or produce ACTH (20%), GH (13%), or prolactin (11%). Their prognosis is poor, with a mean survival of 1.4 years (21).

3. Metastases

Suprasellar metastases may cause endocrine disorders which may be combined with visual or cranial nerve abnormalities. Endocrine disorders have been reported mainly in patients with acute leukaemia and in tumours spreading from the pineal region.

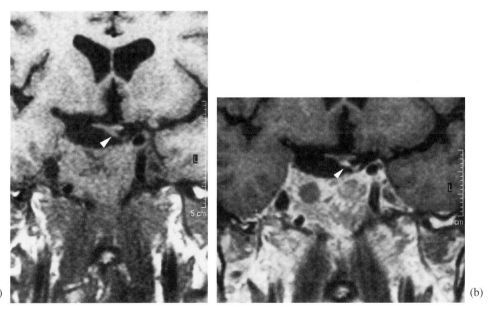

(a)   (b)

Fig. 11.2   Histologically benign macroprolactinoma invading the base of the skull and the cavernous sinus, mainly on the right side. (a) Precontrast coronal T_1W1 MR scan shows a heterogeneous mass without a sharp tumour–brain interface. (b) Intense, heterogeneous post-contrast enhancement. Note the shift of the pituitary stalk (arrow).

The **hypothalamic obesity syndrome** (22) combines hyperphagia, excessive weight gain, and frequent personality changes, such as irritability, and is attributed to an infiltration of the hypothalamic appetite centre by neoplastic cells. The syndrome may be the only sign of CNS recurrence of acute leukaemia, although it may be combined with other features of leptomeningeal disease and with diabetes insipidus resulting from leukaemic infiltration of the hypothalamic–pituitary axis (22).

Pineal tumours may metastasize to the suprasellar region. Diabetes insipidus was the most common sign in germinoma metastases, whereas visual symptoms predominated in teratoma seedings (23). Both germinomas and teratomas may cause signs of hypopituitarism (24).

Pituitary metastases were found at autopsy in 1.8% of cases in a series of 1000 cancer patients (25). Review of the literature up to 1979 reported 28 symptomatic for 150 asymptomatic patients, suggesting that a large proportion of pituitary metastases may remain undetectable and clinically asymptomatic (26). Breast carcinoma is the most common primary tumour, accounting for about 50% of pituitary metastases (27,28). They usually develop in patients with widespread dissemination, but they may be the first manifestation of malignancy (29). Lung carcinoma accounts for 20% of primary tumours (28), and other sites include gastrointestinal cancers, melanoma, germ-cell tumours, prostate carcinoma. The clinical presentation of pituitary metastases differs strikingly from that of pituitary adenomas (26). Diabetes insipidus, which is very rare in adenomas, was the initial symptom in 20 of 28 patients (71%) with pituitary metastases (26). Conversely, anterior pituitary insufficiency, which is common in adenomas, was initially observed in only two patients (7%) with metastatic lesions. The difference is attributed to the fact that metastases tend to develop first in the posterior lobe, usually preserving the anterior part of the gland.

Treatment-induced endocrinopathies

Radiation therapy of the hypothalamic–pituitary axis is a major cause of treatment-related endocrine disorders in cancer patients. Endocrine complications of surgery are less common and may be transient. The role of anticancer chemotherapy is not well established. The most common cause of Cushingoid features is the administration of glucocorticosteroids, which is particularly common in neuro-oncological practice.

Radiation therapy

Hypopituitarism may follow the irradiation of hypothalamic–pituitary axis (30). The incidence of the hormone deficiency is related to the total dose, dose per fraction, and irradiation volume (30). For a given total dose, larger fraction size and shorter treatment time increase the risk of hypopituitarism (31). Potentiation of radiation toxicity on hypothalamic–pituitary function by chemotherapy has not been demonstrated clearly, but remains possible.

The hypothalamus is considered to be more radiosensitive than the anterior pituitary (32,33). The relative radioresistance of the anterior pituitary has been postulated following the experience of pituitary implantation with yttrium-90, delivering high local doses, where 61% of treated patients had normal TSH and ACTH levels after 14 years (34). The delay in neuroendocrine dysfunction following irradiation has been observed in number of studies (30,35,36). However, endocrine changes may occur early (within a few months) and may reflect the degree of pre-existing damage and therefore functional reserve following irradiation. GH is usually the first anterior pituitary hormone affected by radiation, and is followed by deficiency of gonadotrophins and ACTH. TSH is the least likely and the last to be affected. Thyroid function may be affected by direct irradiation of the thyroid gland. Hyperprolactinaemia has been often observed after irradiation of the hypothalamus (32,36) and attributed to dopamine deficiency. The rise in prolactin peaks at 2 years following irradiation (30). Hypopituitarism following radiation therapy has been observed in patients treated for nasopharyngeal carcinoma, sellar and parasellar tumours, more distant primary brain tumours, and as prophylaxis in acute lymphoblastic leukaemia.

Radiation therapy is the primary therapy for **nasopharyngeal carcinoma** and the hypothalamic–pituitary axis may receive the full tumour dose of 6500–7000 cGy. Nasopharyngeal carcinomas may invade the pituitary region directly from below, and extensive neck node disease may require irradiation, which includes the thyroid. In patients irradiated for nasopharyngeal carcinoma, hypopituitarism and hyperprolactinaemia were found in both retrospective (37) and prospective studies (38). High-dose irradiation of inferomedial portions of the temporal lobes which lie within radiation ports may also cause prominent memory disturbance, personality changes, and complex partial seizures (39).

In **pituitary adenomas**, the issue of radiation-induced endocrine disorders is complicated by endocrine abnormalities related to the tumour, and surgery. In addition, the interpretation of gonadotrophin changes is difficult in patients with hyperprolactinaemia. Littley *et al.* reported abnormalities of hypothalamic–pituitary function in 165 adults treated for tumours of the pituitary region by external irradiation with 3750–4250 Gy, given in 15 or 16 fractions over 20–22 days (40); 140 had surgery before irradiation. Patients were followed prospectively for up to 10 years. Most deficiencies appeared within 3–4 years. After 10 years, approximately 50% of patients developed pituitary insufficiency, with GH production the most sensitive and TSH the most resistant.

In most **brain tumours**, the hypothalamic–pituitary axis is neither involved by the tumour nor is it injured during surgery. The hypothalamic–pituitary axis is damaged by wide-field irradiation; this is dose-dependent. After low-dose irradiation, endocrine disorders may be limited to GH deficiency; higher doses may produce additional abnormalities. The age of puberty is lower in children irradiated at younger age. In adults, the incidence of endocrine disorders has been underestimated (41). Recent studies (32,36) of brain tumour patients followed up to 11 (36) and 13 years (32) after brain irradiation have demonstrated an unexpectedly high frequency of hypothalamic–pituitary disorders, including hypothyroidism and gonadal dysfunction. Changes in adrenal function were either subtle or very rare. In one study (36) nine patients (29%) had hyperprolactinaemia.

Growth retardation has been documented in children receiving prophylactic cranial irradiation for **acute lymphoblastic leukaemia** (42,43), although most patients maintain normal growth after cranial irradiation with 1800–2400 cGy. The factors that contribute to growth deficit include GH deficiency due to cranial irradiation, precocious puberty due to irradiation of the hypothalamic–pituitary gonadal axis (44), and irradiation of the spine, causing fusion of epiphyses and lack of further spinal growth.

Surgery

Persistent endocrine disorders and diabetes insipidus requiring lifelong therapy may follow removal of suprasellar tumours. Endocrine disorders due to damage to the hypothalamus are particularly common after attempted radical resection of craniopharyngiomas, as these tumours tend to adhere to adjacent nervous structures (45). Transphenoidal resection of pituitary tumours may be complicated by transient diabetes insipidus.

Chemotherapy

Chemotherapy may enhance the neurotoxic effect of irradiation on the hypothalamic–pituitary axis, although such potentiation has not been documented adequately. Rare cases of syndrome of inappropriate secretion of antidiuretic hormone have been reported in patients treated with vincristine alone or in combination with cisplatin, but this may result from a toxic drug effect on peripheral receptors.

Glucocorticosteroids

Prolonged administration of glucocorticosteroids, aiming to reduce peritumoral vasogenic oedema, is probably the most frequent cause of Cushingoid features in neuro-oncology. The most common unwanted neurological side-effects include behavioural and psychiatric disorders (Chapter 2, p. 37), myopathy (Chapter 10, p. 197), or lipomatosis which may cause spinal compression (Chapter 7, p. 143). The most serious non-neurological side-effects include gastrointestinal bleeding, bowel perforation, avascular osteonecrosis (usually of the hip), increased incidence of opportunistic infections, and hyperglycaemia.

Vascular lesions

Pituitary apoplexy is an acute disorder due to haemorrhage into infarcted pituitary tumour, causing sudden clinical manifestations (Fig. 1.3). The expanding mass may compress the normal pituitary gland, the optic pathways, or the cavernous sinus, causing acute headache, panhypopituitarism, visual loss, and diplopia. In severe cases, bleeding may break into the subarachnoid space, producing vasospasm and altered consciousness.

Paraneoplastic diseases

Endocrine disorders caused by ectopic production of hormones, or hormone-like proteins, by systemic malignancies are beyond the scope of this chapter. Paraneoplastic endocrinopathies may cause metabolic encephalopathies, which are summarized in Table 1.5.

With the exception of pineal-region tumours, primary brain cancers do not secrete hormonally active proteins. Choriocarcinomas, and to a lesser extent germinomas, produce human chorionic gonadotrophins (hCGs), causing pseudo-precocious puberty in boys as hCG stimulates the testes to produce testosterone.

Investigations

The endocrine abnormalities considered in this chapter are limited to disorders due to dysfunction of the hypothalamic–pituitary axis. Their diagnosis is often delayed by months or years, probably due to the lack of specificity of symptoms such as loss of libido, depression, anxiety, fatigue, heat intolerance, and to the failure of the family circle to notice gradually evolving physical features such as an excessive weight gain or acromegalic changes. Visual field abnormalities may also remain unnoticed for a long time.

Endocrinopathies of hypothalamic–pituitary origin are caused by tumours, radiation therapy, or surgery. The main neoplastic lesions are compared in Table 11.2. MRI can identify and localize most tumours. However, even with high-resolution MRI, the distinction between optic chiasma and hypothalamic gliomas remains difficult, and microadenomas may be missed, particularly in Cushing's disease where MRI is normal in about 30% of patients. The nature of the tumoral lesion found in the hypothalamic–pituitary region tumours also depends on:

(1) patient's age and gender;

(2) endocrine disorders;

(3) presence of diabetes insipidus or precocious puberty;

(4) visual field abnormalities and the sequence of their development in relation to endocrine disorders; and

(5) accompanying clinical features (summarized in Table 11.2).

Although hormone determination plays a pivotal diagnostic role, several points should be stressed:

- hyperprolactinaemia may be induced by various drugs and metabolic disorders (see p. 204);

- single random GH determination is of poor value;

- the distinction between Cushing's disease and Cushing's syndrome may be difficult;

- serum TSH may be 'inappropriately normal' or even elevated with increased T_3 and T_4 levels in TSH-secreting adenomas;

- GnLH-secreting adenomas are often misdiagnosed as non-secreting tumours.

The diagnosis of treatment-related endocrinopathies is based on history. Most surgical complications appear shortly after operation and may be transient. Most radiation-induced endocrine disorders are delayed and progressive. The distinction between tumour- and treatment-induced endocrine disorders may occasionally be difficult, particularly in patients with suprasellar gliomas (5–7) or craniopharyngiomas (45).

Cancer patients with endocrine disorders not directly due to hypothalamic–pituitary axis dysfunction may have end-organ abnormality, such as surgical removal or irradiation of endocrine glands, or ectopic or paraneoplastic production of hormones or hormone-like proteins (1,2). Invasion of endocrine glands by malignancy is a rare cause of endocrine insufficiency. While adrenal gland metastases are very common in patients with disseminated breast cancer, they only exceptionally cause hypocorticism. These diseases are beyond the scope of this chapter.

Table 11.2 Differential diagnosis of hypothalamic–pituitary tumours

Tumours	Location	MRI/CT	Peak age/ gender	Endocrine abnormalities	Diabetes insipidus	Precocious puberty	Visual-field abnormalities	Other feature
Gliomas	Optic chiasma	Enlarged chiasma, may be exophytic	Children, Young adults	Also related to radiotherapy or surgery	Also related to radiotherapy or surgery	Mainly due to the tumour	Very frequent	± 30% associated neuro-fibromatosis
	Hypothalamus			Mostly in exophytic tumours				Diencephalic syndrome (≤ 2 years) Behavioural changes
Craniopharyn-giomas	Suprasellar (may be intrasellar)	Fairly typical MRI/CT	Children; Occur in adults	Frequent: ↓ GH (short stature) ↓ TSH (↑ weight)	Frequent	May occur	Frequent	Poor intellectual performance
Hamartomas	Tuber cinereum	Isointense on T_1 WI Hyperintense on T_2 WI	Children	–	–	Leading cause	–	Gelastic epilepsy
Germ-cell tumours	Suprasellar (and pineal region)	Suggestive	Adolescents; Young adults	↓ GH (short stature)	Frequent in germinomas	Ectopic hCG (in boys)	Usually follow endocrine abnormalities	Parinaud's syndrome Hydrocephalus
Meningiomas	Suprasellar (rarely intrasellar)	Extra-axial mass	40–60 years ♀:♂ ratio 2:4	Late, in ± 20% (hyperpro-lactineaemia)	Rare	–	Frequent optic atrophy	Frequent headache

Table 11.2 Differential diagnosis of hypothalamic–pituitary tumours *(continued)*

Tumours	Location	MRI/CT	Peak age/gender	Endocrine abnormalities	Diabetes insipidus	Precocious puberty	Visual-field abnormalities	Other feature
Pituitary microadenomas	Intrasellar	May be negative: 30% in Cushing's disease		Usually single hormone abnormality	Very rare even in larger tumours	–	–	–
Pituitary macroadenomas	Frequent extrasellar extension	Easily demonstrated	Adults	Single hormone abnormality + hypopituitarism Hypopituitarism only in non-functioning adenomas		–	Frequent	Headaches Cavernous sinus syndrome if lateral extension Hydrocephaly if major suprasellar extension
Metastases								
Acute leukaemia	Suprasellar infiltration	Gadolinium enhancement on MRI	Children	Obesity (hypothalamic syndrome)	Frequent	May be related to radiotherapy	In ± 10%	Other features of meningeal leukaemia
Carcinomas	Predominantly in posterior pituitary lobe	MRI often abnormal + bone destruction	Adults	Late, if present	Frequent	–	Late, if present	Systemic cancer (breast cancer in 50%)

Therapy

1. Pituitary adenomas

The main goal in the management of pituitary adenoma is restoration of endocrine status and correction of mass effect, particularly on the visual pathway. In many hormone-secreting adenomas, there is a correlation between tumour size, invasiveness, and hormone level. However, large tumours may also cause hypopituitarism. The aim of endocrine therapy is to lower hormone excess and, if necessary, to correct hormone deficit through hormone replacement therapy. Substantial progress has been made in microsurgery, medical treatment, and conformal radiation therapy of pituitary adenomas. Each technique has its own indications, merits, and drawbacks.

Microsurgery

Surgery offers rapid relief of mass effect and a reduction in hormone levels with the possibility of cure. Microsurgery is the primary treatment of choice in most patients with pituitary adenomas (20). The trans-sphenoidal approach, which is used in the majority of patients, avoids entering the intracranial compartment and allows resection away from critical structures surrounding the pituitary gland. This route is particularly suitable for smaller tumours confined to the sella. The transcranial approach is reserved for tumours with extrasellar extension, or for larger tumours that elevate the diaphragma sellae. Urgent surgery is necessary for pituitary apoplexy with haemorrhagic mass causing visual impairment, and in patients with adenomas that do not respond readily to medical treatment.

Medical treatment

Two types of agents, which may control excess hormone secretion, are currently available for the medical treatment of pituitary adenomas. Dopaminergic agonists, of which bromocriptine is the prototype, are very effective in the treatment of prolactinomas, producing a rapid drop in prolactin and reduction of adenoma size (46). Dopaminergic agonists may be useful in a small proportion of GH-secreting tumours, producing a modest and fluctuating reduction in growth hormone. Somatostatin analogues (octreotide) inhibit growth hormone and thyrotrophin release (47) and are used in the treatment of acromegaly.

Endocrine deficiencies, precocious puberty, or **pituitary diabetes insipidus** are treated by hormone replacement therapy.

Recombinant growth hormone is administrated at a daily dose of 0.006–0.03 u/kg of body weight and is used to allow the child to reach his or her height potential. However, GH administration is less effective in patients with radiation-induced GH deficiency than in idiopathic dwarfism. The role of GH administration in GH-deficient adults is debatable.

Thyroxine (50–100 μg/m^2) is administrated daily to patients with low T_3 and T_4 plasma levels, to correct hypothyroidism. Thyroxine may also be given to prevent overstimulation of the thyroid gland in patients where T_3 and T_4 are maintained within normal limits due to high TSH production.

The **hydrocortisone** requirement is about 30 mg/day in divided doses. In patients with ACTH deficiency, the supplemental doses of hydrocortisone are adjusted according to endogenous hormone production. They should be increased during intercurrent diseases, infections, or stress.

Gonadotrophin-releasing hormone analogues are used in precocious puberty to decrease the production of sex steroids and delay bone maturation and bone fusion. Delayed puberty is treated in girls by ethinylestradiol (2 μg/day p.o.) and in boys by testosterone (25–30 mg i.m. twice monthly).

Desmopressin, an analogue of antidiuretic hormone, is used in pituitary diabetes insipidus. It acts on V_2 receptors, and does not cause hypertension.

Radiation therapy

Fractionated external-beam radiation therapy to doses of 4500–5000 cGy in 160–180 cGy daily fractions is used in patients with unresectable residual or recurrent tumours. It produces excellent long-term tumour control and normalization of excess hormone levels, with acceptable long-term morbidity. In secretory tumours there is a considerable delay in the normalization of elevated hormone levels and the time to normalization is related to the starting value. Radiation therapy is very effective at arresting tumour growth in secretory and nonfunctional adenomas, but the minimal or no reduction in tumour size means that it is not effective in relieving the features due to a mass effect, such as visual field deficit. The side-effects of radiation therapy include delayed hypopituitarism, 1–2% risk of radiation optic neuropathy, and 1–2% risk of a second radiation-induced brain tumour at 10–20 years.

The sequence in which surgery, medical treatment, and radiation therapy are currently used in various pituitary adenoma types is summarized in Table 11.3.

In **prolactinomas** medical therapy with dopamine agonists is the treatment of first choice. It produces normalization of prolactin levels and of clinical abnormalities, and reduces tumour size in about 80% of adenomas. The use of dopamine agonists is limited by dose-dependent adverse effects, which include postural hypotension, nausea and vomiting, and confusional state with visual hallucinations. The second limitation is a lack of response, which occurs more often in large, haemorrhagic, or necrotic adenomas.

Surgery is indicated when medical treatment either fails or can not be tolerated. The timing of surgery depends on the rate of tumour progression and its mass effect and the delay should not exceed 1 year. Surgery is potentially curative. However, an international survey showed that normalization of serum prolactin after surgery was observed in 74% of 1518 patients with microprolactinomas and only 30% of 1022 patients with macroadenomas (48). The rate of recurrence after surgery is in the region of 20% (49,50).

The use of radiation therapy is offered to patients with recurrent or invasive tumours unresponsive to medical treatment, or to patients who can not or do not wish to undergo surgery.

GH-secreting adenomas are first treated by surgery, which achieves a lowering of GH below 5 ng/ml in 60–88% of patients (51,52). As in prolactinomas, the best surgical results are obtained in smaller tumours secreting lower GH levels. Although it is very rare, ectopic secretion of GHRH should be considered when MRI fails to demonstrate an adenoma and only shows pituitary hyperplasia.

Two different drugs currently used in medical treatment of GH-secreting adenomas are octreotide acetate and dopamine agonists. Octreotide is a potent somatostatin analogue

Table 11.3   Management of pituitary adenomas

Type of adenoma	First choice	Second choice	Third choice
Prolactinoma	Dopamine agonists (DAs)	Surgery if DAs fail, or not tolerated	Radiotherapy (invasive tumours)
	Surgery if mass effect or pituitary apoplexy (rare)		
Growth-hormone-secreting	Surgery (cures in ±70% microadenoma, ±40% macroadenoma)	Somatostatin analogues possibly combined to DAs	Radiotherapy (invasive tumours)
ACTH-secreting			
Cushing's disease	Surgery (±90% cures at 10 years)	Radiotherapy if incomplete resection or recurrence	Peripheral adrenal blockers
		Invasive tumours	(ketoconazole) or bilateral adrenalectomy (if all others fail)
Nelson's syndrome	Surgery (if macroadenoma)		
	Radiotherapy (prophylactic)		
TSH-secreting	Surgery	Radiotherapy	Somatostatin analogues
FSH- or LH-secreting	Surgery	Radiotherapy (if invasive tumours or if second surgery fails)	
Non-secreting	Surgery (aiming for mass reduction)	Radiotherapy in rapidly growing tumours	

Radiotherapy refers to conventional irradiation techniques.

capable of lowering GH levels to less than 10 ng/ml in one patient out of two, and to less than 5 ng/ml in one patient out of four (48), with reduction of tumour size in about 30% of patients. The administration of octreotide requires three daily subcutaneous injections, and is progressively replaced by long-acting formulations which may be administrated once every 2–4 weeks. Gallstones may develop in 10–20% of the patients. Bromocriptine (a dopamine agonist) reduces GH levels below 5 ng/ml in about 20% of the cases (53), and produces a limited reduction of tumour size in fewer than one-third of patients.

Radiation therapy is reserved for recurrent or incompletely removed tumours. Following radiation therapy the normalization of GH levels is delayed (54).

ACTH-secreting adenomas cause Cushing's disease. Most are microadenomas of less than a few millimetres in diameter. Finding the microadenoma is often difficult as approximately 30% can not be visualized by MRI. Transphenoidal surgery achieves cure in approximately 90% of ACTH-producing microadenomas (20,55). External radiation therapy is used to treat invasive or partially resected tumours. The most effective medical agents are peripherally acting adrenal blockers such as mitotane (ketoconazole), although they may cause adrenal insufficiency. Bilateral adrenal ablation is reserved for patients where all other therapeutic options have failed. Ten to 15% of patients undergoing bilateral adrenalectomy develop **Nelson's syndrome**, with enlarging corticotrophic pituitary adenoma which may be more invasive and fast growing than primary adenomas. Prophylactic pituitary irradiation has been recommended after bilateral adrenalectomy to prevent Nelson's syndrome, and conventional radiation therapy is given to patients with established Nelson's syndrome.

TSH is secreted by only 1% of pituitary adenomas. Their rarity may explain the frequent delay in diagnosis and large tumour size at diagnosis. Tumour resection is the treatment of first choice and may be curative in small tumours. However, its efficacy is limited by tumour size and invasiveness (56). In large tumours, the resection is usually subtotal and is followed by radiation therapy (56). Administration of somatostatin analogues (octreotide) has been suggested (57).

Twenty-five to 30% of pituitary adenomas are **clinically or biochemically non-functional**. This group probably also includes most **gonadotrophin-producing adenomas**. Surgery is the mainstay of therapy and aims to reduce the tumour mass effect on the normal pituitary gland and the optic pathways. The role of post-operative radiation therapy is debated. It improves long-term disease control but its effect on survival is not clear. It may avoid the need for second surgery. Radiation therapy is generally recommended for progressive and recurrent adenomas.

2. Craniopharyngiomas

Only a minority of craniopharyngiomas can be safely totally resected and most tumours are approached transcranially. The trans-sphenoidal approach may be used in rare tumours located below the diaphragma sellae. Craniopharyngioma adhere to the adjacent nervous structures, particularly the hypothalamus, and total removal is difficult even with careful microsurgical technique (45). Attempts to achieve total resection are associated with a high incidence of visual deficits, hypopituitarism, diabetes insipidus, and hypothalamic damage leading to hyperphagia and obesity. Partial resection is followed by adjuvant radiation to 5000 cGy in 160–180 cGy daily fractions to inhibit further tumour growth (58). Conventional external irradiation may cause visual and endocrine late effects as produced by radiotherapy for pituitary adenoma. Radiation therapy is best delayed or not used in younger children, to avoid potential cognitive impairment. Stereotactic techniques of irradiation allow for higher precision of treatment delivery and, for small tumours, more localized and focused irradiation. Single-fraction radiosurgery is damaging to the normal neural structures, particularly the optic chiasm and nerves, and is not recommended for the treatment of craniopharyngiomas. Fractionated stereotactic conformal radiation therapy is likely to become the treatment of choice for the majority of craniopharyngiomas, particularly in children. A recurrent cystic component of craniopharyngioma not controlled with radiation therapy may be treated with intracystic colloidal brachytherapy using ^{32}P (59), or yttrium.

3. Hypothalamic hamartomas

Both surgical resection and gonadotrophin-releasing hormone (GnRH) are able to reverse precocious puberty, the main clinical manifestation of hypothalamic hamartomas. The comparison of the two methods is difficult as it is based on small number of patients. Peduncular hamartomas appear most suitable for microsurgery, which may achieve lasting cures (60). However, Stuart *et al.* (61) have observed the recurrence of precocious puberty even after what was thought to be complete tumour removal, and they advise the use of GnRH as first-line therapy (61). This opinion has also been expressed by Mahachoklerwattana *et al.* (11).

References

(1) Keffer JH. (1996). Endocrinopathy and ectopic hormones in malignancy. *Hematol Oncol Clin North Am*, **10**, 811–823.
(2) List AF, Hainsworth JD, Davis BW *et al.* (1986). The syndrome of inappropriate secretion of antidiuretic hormone (SIADH) in small-cell lung cancer. *J Clin Oncol*, **4**, 1191–1198.
(3) Klibanski A, Zervas NT. (1991). Diagnosis and management of hormone-secreting pituitary adenoma. *N Engl J Med*, **324**, 822–831.
(4) Miller M, Dalakos T, Moses AM *et al.* (1970). Recognition of partial defect in antidiuretic hormone secretion. *Ann Inter Med*, **73**, 721–729.
(5) Collet-Solberg PF, Sernyak H, Satin-Smith M *et al.* (1997). Endocrine outcome in long-term survivors of low-grade hypothalamic/chiasmatic glioma. *Clin Endocrinol*, **47**, 79–85.
(6) Brauner R, Thibaud E, Pomarede R *et al.* (1982). Precocious puberty. Comment on the diagnostic conditions and etiological as facts. *Ann Endocrinol (Paris)*, **43**, 497–508.
(7) Rodriguez LA, Edwards MS, Levin VA. (1990). Management of hypothalamic gliomas in children: an analysis of 33 cases. *Neurosurgery*, **26**, 242–247.
(8) Bertherat J, Carel JC, Adamsbaum C *et al.* (1994). Endocrine evaluation and evolution of intrasellar craniopharyngioma (CPIS): study of 8 cases. *Arch Pediatr*, **10**, 886–893.
(9) Sorva R. (1988). Children with craniopharyngioma: Early growth failure and rapid postoperative weight gain. *Acta Paediatr Scand*, **77**, 587–592.
(10) Perilongo G, Rigon F, Murgia A. (1989). Oncologic causes of precocious puberty. *Pediatr Haematol Oncol*, **6**, 331–340.
(11) Mahachoklertwattana P, Kaplan SL, Grumbach MM. (1993). The luteinizing hormone-releasing hormone-secreting hypothalamic hamartoma is a congenital malformation: natural history. *J Clin Endocrinol Metab*, **77**, 118–124.
(12) Culler FL, James HE, Simon ML, Jones KL. (1985). Identification of gonadotropin-releasing hormone in neurons of a hypothalamic hamartoma in a boy with precocious puberty. *Neurosurgery*, **17**, 408–412.
(13) Judge DM, Kulin HE, Page R *et al.* (1977). Hypothalamic hamartoma. A source of luteinizing-hormone-releasing factor in precocious puberty. *N Engl J Med*, **296**, 7–10.
(14) Pescovitz OH, Comite F, Hench K *et al.* (1986). The NIH experience with precocious puberty: diagnostic subgroup and response to short-term luteinizing hormone releasing hormone analogue therapy. *J Pediatr*, **108**, 47–54.
(15) Kornreich L, Horev G, Blaser S *et al.* (1995). Central precocious puberty: evaluation by neuroimaging. *Pediatr Radiol*, **25**, 7–11.
(16) Robben SG, Oostdijk W, Drop SL *et al.* (1995). Idiopathic isosexual central precocious puberty: magnetic resonance findings in 30 patients. *Br J Radiol*, **68**, 34–38.
(17) Jennings MT, Gelman R, Hochberg F. (1985). Intracranial germ-cell tumors: natural history and pathogenesis. *J Neurosurg*, **63**, 155–167.

(18) Annegers JF, Coulam CB, Abboud CF *et al.* (1978). Pituitary adenoma in Olmstead County, Minnesota, 1935–1977: a report of an increasing incidence of diagnosis in women of childbearing age. *Mayo Clin Proc*, **53**, 641–643.

(19) Burrow GN, Wortzman G, Rewcastle NB *et al.* (1981). Microadenomas of the pituitary and abnormal sellar tomograms in an unselected autopsy series. *N Engl J Med*, **304**, 156–158.

(20) Thapar K, Kovacs K, Laws ER. (1997). Pituitary tumors. In: Cancer of the nervous system. Black P Mcl, Loeffer JS (eds). Blackwell Science, Cambridge Mass, pp. 363–403.

(21) Kaiser FE, Orth DN, Mukai K *et al.* (1983). A pituitary parasellar tumor with extracranial metastases and high, partially suppressible levels of adrenocorticotropin and related peptides. *J Clin Endocrinol Metab*, **57**, 649–653.

(22) Pochedly C. (1975). Neurologic manifestations in acute leukemia. II Involvement of cranial nerves and hypothalamus. *New York State Journal of Medicine*, **75**, 715–721.

(23) Nishio S, Inamura T, Takeshitai I. *et al.* (1993). Germ cell tumor: in the hypothalamo-neurohypophysial region: clinical features and treatment. *Neurosurg Rev*, **16**, 221–227.

(24) Fetell MR, Stein BM. (1986). Neuroendocrine aspects of pineal tumors. *Neurol Clin*, **4**, 877–905.

(25) Abrams HL, Spiro R, Goldstein N. (1950). Metastases in carcinoma. Analysis of 1000 autopsied cases. *Cancer*, **3**, 74–85.

(26) Max MB, Deck MDF, Rottenberg DA. (1981). Pituitary metastasis: Incidence in cancer patients and clinical differentiation from adenoma. *Neurology*, **31**, 998–1002.

(27) McCormick PC, Post KD, Kandji AD, Hays AP. (1989). Metastatic carcinoma to the pituitary gland. *Br J Neurosurg*, **3**, 71–79.

(28) Juneau P, Schoene WC, Black P. (1992). Malignant tumors in the pituitary gland. *Arch Neurol*, **49**, 555–558.

(29) Kistler M, Pribram HW. (1975). Metastatic disease of the sella turcica. *Am J Roentgenol Radium Ther Nucl Med*, **123**, 13–21.

(30) Littley MD, Shalet SM, Berdwell CG. (1991). Radiation and hypothalamic–pituitary axis. In: Radiation injury to the nervous system. Gutin PH, Leibel SA, Sheline GE (eds). Raven Press, New York, pp. 303–324.

(31) Littley MD, Shalet SM, Berdwell CG *et al.* (1989). Radiation-induced hypopituitarism is dose-dependent. *Clin Endocrinol*, **31**, 363–373.

(32) Constine LS, Woolf PD, Cann D *et al.* (1993). Hypothalamic–pituitary dysfunction after radiation for brain tumors. *N Engl J Med*, **328**, 87–94.

(33) Richards GE, Wara WM, Grumbach MM *et al.* (1976). Delayed onset of hypopituitarism sequelae of therapeutic irradiation of central nervous system, eye and middle ear tumours. *J Pediatr*, **89**, 553–559.

(34) Jadresic A, Jimenez LE, Joplin GF. (1987). Long-term effect of 90Y pituitary implantation in acromegaly. *Acta Endocrinol*, **115**, 301–306.

(35) Fuks Z, Glatstein E, Marsa GW *et al.* (1976). Long term effects of external radiation on the pituitary and thyroid glands. *Cancer*, **37**, 1152–1161.

(36) Arlt W, Hove U, Müller B *et al.* (1997). Frequent and frequently overlooked: Treatment-induced endocrine dysfunction in adult long-term survivors of primary brain tumors. *Neurology*, **49**, 498–506.

(37) Samaan NA, Vieto R, Schultz PN *et al.* (1982). Hypothalamic, pituitary and thyroid dysfunction after radiotherapy to the head and neck. *Int J Radiat Oncol Biol Phys*, **8**, 1857–1867.

(38) Lam KSL, Tse VKC, Wang GCL *et al.* (1985). Endocrine function in patients with nasopharyngeal carcinoma after external irradiation to the head and neck region. *Proc Roy Coll Phys Edinb*, **15**, 185–186.

(39) Woo E, Lam K, Yu YL *et al.* (1988). Temporal lobe and hypothalamic–pituitary dysfunctions after radiotherapy for nasopharyngeal carcinoma: a distinct clinical syndrome. *J Neurol Neurosurg Psychiatry*, **51**, 1302–1307.

(40) Littley MD, Shalet SM, Beardwell CG, Sutton ML. (1988). Factors affecting the development of radiation-induced hypopituitarism. *J Endocrinol*, **117**, 94A.

(41) Bouchard J. (1966). Radiation therapy of intracranial tumours. Long term results. *Acta Radiol Ther Phys Biol*, **5**, 11–16.

(42) Robison LL, Nesbit ME, Sather HN *et al.* (1985). Height of children successfully treated for acute lymphoblastic leukemia: a report from the late effects study committee of the children's cancer study group. *Med Pediatr Oncol*, **13**, 14–21.

(43) Sklar CA. (1977). Growth and neuroendocrine dysfunction following therapy for childhood cancer. *Pediatr Clin North Am*, **44**, 489–503.

(44) Leiper AD, Stanhope R, Kitchine P, Chessells JM. (1987). Precocious and premature puberty associated with treatment of acute lymphoblastic leukemia. *Arch Dis Child*, **62**, 1107–1112.

(45) Brada M, Thomas DG. (1993). Craniopharyngioma revisited. *Int J Radiat Oncol Biol Phys*, **27**, 471–475.

(46) Chiodini P, Liuzzi A, Cozzi R *et al.* (1981). Size reduction of macroprolactinomas by bromocriptine or lisuride treatment. *J Clin Endocrinol Metabol*, **53**, 737–743.

(47) Ezzat S, Snyder PJ, Young WF *et al.* (1992). Octreotide treatment of acromegaly: a randomized multicenter study. *Ann Intern Med*, **117**, 711–718.

(48) Zervas NT. (1984). Surgical results for pituitary adenomas: results of an international survey. In: Secretory tumors of the pituitary gland. Black PM, Zervas NT, Ridgeway EC *et al.* (eds). Raven Press, New York, pp. 377–385.

(49) Molitch ME. (1992). Pathologic hyperprolactinemia. *Endocrinol Metab Clin North Am*, **21**, 877–901.

(50) Post KD, Habas JE. (1990). Comparison of long-term results between prolactin-secreting adenomas and ACTH-secreting adenomas. *Can J Neurol Sci*, **17**, 74–77.

(51) Ross DA, Wilson CB. (1988). Results of transsphenoidal microsurgery for growth hormone-secreting pituitary adenoma in a series of 214 patients. *J Neurosurg*, **68**, 854–867.

(52) Tindall GT, Oyesiku NM, Watts NB *et al.* (1993). Transsphenoidal adenomectomy for growth hormone-secreting adenomas in acromegaly: outcome analysis and determinants of failure. *J Neurosurg*, **78**, 205–215.

(53) Jaffe CA, Barkan AL. (1992). Treatment of acromegaly with dopamine agonists. *Endocrinol Metab Clin North Am*, **21**, 713–735.

(54) Eastman RC, Gorden P, Glatstein E, Roth J. (1992). Radiation therapy of acromegaly. *Endocrin Metab Clin North Am*, **21**, 693–712.

(55) Mampalam TJ, Tyrrel JB, Wilson CB. (1988). Transsphenoidal microsurgery for Cushing's disease. A report of 216 cases. *Ann Intern Med*, **109**, 487–493.

(56) Greenman Y, Melmed S. (1995). Thyrotropin-secreting pituitary tumors. In: The pituitary. Melmed S (ed.). Blackwell Scientific Publications, Cambridge, MA, pp. 546–558.

(57) Chanson P, Weintraub B, Harris A. (1993). Octreotide therapy for thyroid-stimulating hormone-secreting pituitary adenomas. A follow-up of 52 patients. *Ann Intern Med*, **119**, 236–240.

(58) Weiss M, Sutton L, Marcial V *et al.* (1989). The role of radiation therapy in management of childhood craniopharyngioma. *Int J Radiat Oncol Biol Phys*, **17**, 1313–1321.

(59) Pollack IF, Lunsford LD, Slamovits TL *et al.* (1988). Stereotaxic intracavity irradiation for cystic craniopharyngioma. *J Neurosurg*, **68**, 227–233.

(60) Albright AL, Lee PA. (1993). Neurosurgical treatment of hypothalamic hamartomas causing precocious puberty. *J Neurosurg*, **78**, 77–82.

(61) Stewart L, Steinbok P, Daaboul J. (1998). Role of surgical resection in the treatment of hypothalamic hamartomas causing precocious puberty. *J Neurosurg*, **88**, 340–345.

12 Therapy of the main neurological malignant diseases

Introduction

This chapter is devoted to the management of the most common primary or metastatic tumours involving the nervous system. The chapter will deal with:

1. Methodological bases of treatment evaluation.
2. Therapeutic techniques.
3. Current therapies:
   - (a) primary tumours
     - (i) glioblastomas and anaplastic astrocytomas
     - (ii) oligodendrogliomas
     - (iii) grade 2 astrocytomas
     - (iv) medulloblastomas
     - (v) primary non-Hodgkin's lymphomas of the CNS;
   - (b) metastatic tumours
     - (i) brain metastases
     - (ii) leptomeningeal metastases
     - (iii) spinal epidural metastases.

Methodological issues

The interpretation of therapeutic results obtained in brain tumour trials is full of pitfalls. The understanding of basic methodological issues may avoid incorrect conclusions, and may help to better understand the literature. Anticancer therapy may be tested in three types of clinical trials described as phase I, phase II, and phase III.

Phase I trials

These trials are single-arm, uncontrolled, prospective studies aiming to investigate drug **toxicity** and to establish the **maximum tolerated** (safe) dose for a new treatment.

Phase II trials

Phase II trials are single-arm, uncontrolled studies designed to assess the degree of antitumour effect. A distinction is sometimes made between early and late phase II studies. In early phase II studies the treatment tested is relatively new, and emphasis is put on the evaluation of toxicity. In late phase II studies the unwanted effects of the tested therapy are usually known, and the primary aim is to evaluate the **therapeutic activity**. Brain tumour patients usually enter phase II trials at the time of clinical and radiological progression and/or recurrence.

In general, histological confirmation is not required at the time of recurrence in patients with glioblastoma and anaplastic astrocytoma, when post-radiation necrosis is unlikely. In patients with low-grade tumours, reassessment of pathology may reveal malignant transformation. The appearance of contrast enhancement on CT or MRI or increased glucose metabolism on positron emission tomography (PET) in previously non-enhancing and hypometabolic tumours is suggestive of malignant transformation. However, in the context of phase II trials, the diagnosis of recurrent tumour should ideally be based on repeated histology.

The **evaluation criteria** proposed by MacDonald *et al.*, summarized in Table 12.1, have gained wide acceptance (1). The radiological assessment is based on the evaluation of contrast-enhanced tumour area obtained by multiplying the largest cross-sectioned diameter by the perpendicular diameter. MacDonalds's criteria also standardize the duration of radiological changes and the administration of glucocorticosteroids, which may affect both clinical and radiological evaluation. In 1994, Grant *et al.* (2) proposed the addition of standardized functional tests to allow for more objective assessment of clinical change. In most malignant brain tumours only a few patients have a complete or partial response. Many authors consider stabilization of a progressive tumour as indicating a therapeutic response, but the value of the endpoint of a stable disease is questionable. Assessment of tumour stabilization requires a progression-free time.

Radiological criteria are essential in studies including recently operated patients. Most of them have no signs of clinical progression, and neurological improvement may be related to post-operative recovery itself. In such patients, the baseline CT or MRI must be performed within 48–72 hours of surgery. Subsequently, post-operative contrast enhancement due to neovascularization cannot usually be distinguished from residual tumour (3). The gradual resolution of post-operative enhancement can therefore be mistaken for a tumour response when the baseline CT or MRI is performed late, making many phase II studies uninterpretable.

Table 12.1   Evaluation criteria for phase II trials (MacDonald *et al.* 1990, ref. 1)

Change of 'size' of contrast-enhanced area on CT or MRI scan	Duration of 'size' change on subsequent imaging	Clinical changes	Gluco-corticosteroids	Response
Reduction 100%	≥1 month	Improved or stable	Off steroids	Complete
Reduction 50–99%[a]	≥1 month	Improved or stable	Stable or reduced	Partial
Increase ≥25%	Compared to previous scan	Worsened	Stable or increased	Progressive disease
All other situations				Stable disease

[a]A 50% reduction of tumour bi-dimensional area corresponds to a 65% reduction in tumour volume.
(Paul Kleihues, adapted from table 1.28, *Pathology and Genetics*, Tumours of the nervous system).

Phase II trials are **non-comparative** by nature. However, the tendency is to compare the results with other published data. Such a comparison is difficult and subject to considerable bias. The general management and care strategies vary in different places and times. The selection criteria by prognostic factors, such as age, performance status, histology, and prior treatment, vary and affect outcome. One of the major problems of analysis is patient exclusion, which may seriously influence the results. Most trials should be analysed by treatment intent rather than treatment delivered. In addition, there is frequently a discrepancy between scheduled and actually given doses, although most trial results reflect treatment that is possible to deliver in practice.

Phase III trials

Phase III trials are comparative prospective studies evaluating a new therapy by comparing its efficacy, in randomly assigned groups, either to a placebo or to standard therapy. Patients with brain tumours usually enter phase III studies at two different stages of disease. Most studies are initiated after the first neurosurgical procedure, which may be a diagnostic biopsy. The treatment tested at this stage is in the form of **adjuvant therapy**. **Neoadjuvant** treatment refers to chemotherapy given either before surgery or irradiation. Randomized studies can also be performed at the time of recurrence and the methodology is similar to that of phase II trials. However, very few randomized studies have been performed at this stage.

Brain tumour phase III trials are often co-operative. In multicentre studies, the pathological diagnosis requires external central neuropathology review. The need for pathology review is greater when dealing with lower-grade tumours. In the experience of the EORTC-BTG (Brain Tumour Group), the agreement between the local pathologist and the reviewer was 95% for glioblastoma, but only 60% for anaplastic astrocytoma or low-grade glioma. The usual **primary endpoints** in phase III trials are survival and time to progression (or progression-free survival). Survival is expressed in actuarial terms and the easily understandable comparative measure is usually median survival. Progression is diagnosed at the time of clinical deterioration and requires radiological confirmation. In EORTC-BTG studies, the time to progression paralleled survival in patients with malignant glioma. The importance of progression as an endpoint is that the progression-free survival usually reflects a single treatment episode, not confounded by subsequent salvage treatment which affects survival endpoint. In addition, in patients with malignant glioma progression corresponds to worsening clinical condition and progression-free survival reflects quality of life.

Patients entered into phase III trials are heterogeneous, and differences in therapeutic effect may be smaller than differences due to **prognostic factors** alone. Randomization eliminates bias in the assignment of treatment, but does not guarantee an even distribution of prognostic factors. **Stratification** at randomization for factors that are most strongly correlated with prognosis, aims to achieve an even distribution of these factors over the treatment arms. The main prognostic factors for survival identified for various tumour types in multivariate analysis are summarized in Table 12.2. They differ according to tumour type. Several attempts have been made to correlate cell proliferation with survival. Incorporation of bromodeoxyuridine (which allows an estimate of the percentage of dividing cells) correlates with survival in patients with low-grade astrocytomas (5), but the method is less useful in high-grade gliomas. Ki-67 antibody measures the percentage of cycling cells. Its indices are considerably lower in grade 1 and 2 gliomas than in high-grade tumours. A Ki-67 (or MIB-1)

Table 12.2 Main prognostic factors for survival in primary brain tumours

Tumour type	Tumour-related factors	Patient-related factors	Tumour- and patient-related factors	Reference
High-grade glioma	Pathology (glioblastoma versus grade 3 tumours)	Age[a]	Performance status	4
	Extent of resection		Neurological status	
Low-grade glioma	Mitotic index (5), glucose metabolism (6)	Age[a]	Performance status	7
	Enhancement on CT/MRI		Neurological status	
			Epilepsy (favourable factor)	
Oligodendroglioma	Extent of resection	Age[a]	Major neurological deficits	8,9
Ependymoma	Extent of resection			10
Medulloblastoma	Extent of resection	Age (patients ≤ 3 years old have shorter survival)		11,12
	Metastases, tumour size			
Primary cerebral lymphoma	Pathology	Age[a]		13

[a]Younger age is correlated with longer survival.

labelling index below 5% is a favourable prognostic factor in low-grade gliomas. However, the wide range of intra- and intertumour variability of Ki-67 indices in grade 3 and 4 gliomas limits its use as a survival predictor in high-grade gliomas (14).

Therapeutic techniques

This section outlines the main characteristics of currently used techniques in brain tumour therapy.

Neurosurgery

Neurosurgery has a diagnostic and therapeutic role in the in the management of most brain tumours. Pathology-based diagnosis is mandatory in most patients with a radiological diagnosis of brain tumour. We recommend biopsy even in patients who are not candidates for operation, because it may reveal an unexpected, sometimes curable pathology. In tumours with characteristic radiological appearance, such as chiasmal gliomas or diffuse brainstem gliomas in children, histological confirmation is not considered necessary. The histological structure of malignant brain tumours, especially gliomas, is heterogeneous, and grading is based on the most malignant component. Because of limited sampling, stereotactic biopsy tends to underestimate the pathological grade. This bias may be minimized by multiple biopsies using more than one trajectory, and by sampling preferentially contrast-enhanced regions on CT or MRI. To enhance the accuracy of diagnosis and tumour grading further, Levivier *et al.* have described a PET-guided stereotactic brain biopsy (15). In contrast-enhanced tumours, all the trajectories guided by [^{18}F]fluorodeoxyglucose-PET (^{18}FDG-PET) were diagnostic.

Optimal resection should achieve tumour removal without morbidity and is appropriate for selected malignant and low-grade tumours, with the exception of primary brain lymphomas, where surgery is only for diagnostic purposes. The use of the operating microscope and image-guided three-dimensional reconstruction has made tumour resection easier and more complete. During surgery, the microscope view of the operation site is projected on the computed tumour image (Figs 12.1 and 12.2), providing the surgeon with information about the progress of tumour resection (16).

Radiation therapy

Radiation can be delivered to brain tumours either by external-beam radiation therapy or by implantation of sources directly into the tumour, described as interstitial irradiation or brachytherapy.

External irradiation

Conventional external-beam radiotherapy is delivered in the form of high-energy photons, usually by a linear accelerator. The aim of modern radiotherapy is to give the maximum dose to the tumour with lowest dose to the normal brain. This is achieved through localized techniques, where radiation is directed on to the tumour. The region treated to a high dose is described as the **planning target volume**. This includes the tumour visualized on imaging, the surrounding region presumed to contain microscopic disease, and a margin for the tech-

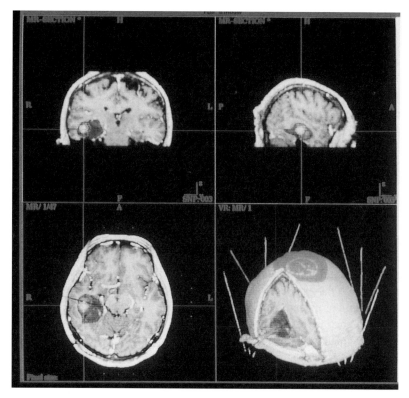

Fig. 12.1 Neurosurgical planning for resection of a right temporal anaplastic astrocytoma. The multiplanar view of T_1WI MR scan performed in stereotactic condition delineates the tumour (blue contour), the contrast-enhanced area (green contour), and the hypermetabolic area of ^{18}FDG-PET scan (red contour) (please see plate section). (Courtesy of Professor M. Levivier.)

nical inaccuracy of treatment delivery. Computer treatment planning provides a three-dimensional dose distribution, with the aim of achieving a homogeneous dose within the planning target volume (dose variation < 10%) and minimum dose to critical normal structures. Increasing the number of spatially distributed intersecting beams from two to three or four increases the dose differential between the target and normal brain. The usual arrangement for the treatment of average-sized benign as malignant tumours (4–8 cm) is to use three fixed fields. As the limitation to radiotherapy is the radiation tolerance of normal tissue, it is assumed that increasing the dose differential or dose gradient between the target and normal brain may allow for higher radiation doses with improved tumour control.

Radiation delivered through a high-precision localized technique of stereotactic radiotherapy, or stereotactic radiosurgery (when given in a single fraction), can increase the dose differential between the target and normal brain, but this is only the case for small target volumes of less than 4 cm diameter. Stereotactic irradiation requires a precise localization of the tumour, patient immobilization, and stereotactic treatment delivery, which can be achieved either with a multi-headed cobalt installation (gamma knife) or linear accelerator (Linac). Both deliver localized photon radiation with identical dose distribution. Localized irradiation can also be delivered with heavy particle beams, but this technique is restricted to a few centres.

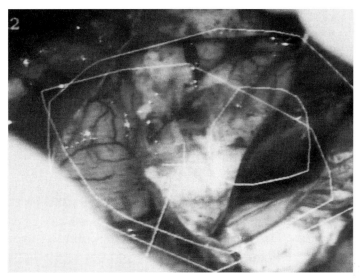

Fig. 12.2   The three contours defined in Fig. 12.1 are projected on the operation field during tumour removal (please see plate section). (Courtesy of Professor M. Levivier.)

Gamma knife is a cobalt unit consisting of 201 collimated cobalt-60 sources in a hemispherical arrangement. Secondary collimation allows spherical high-dose volumes ranging from 8 to 18 mm in diameter. For the treatment of a larger lesion, a number of small volumes need to be added and this is described as multiple isocentre treatment. The gamma knife is used for a single-dose treatment of small spherical and non-spherical lesions, generally not exceeding 3 cm in diameter.

Linac can deliver localized spherical irradiation by moving the radiation source in a number of arcs around the target. Non-spherical lesions can be treated by multiple non-coplanar fixed fields conforming to the shape of the lesion; this is described as stereotactic conformal radiotherapy. Linac allows the treatment of larger and non-spherical lesions, and the treatment can be given in multiple fractions.

For high-precision treatment delivery, the head needs to be immobilized in a fixation device. This can be either a fixed stereotactic frame, such as the Leksell frame or the Brown–Roberts–Wells frame, or relocatable device such as a relocatable stereotactic frame or a firmly fitting mask.

Interstitial irradiation or brachytherapy

Radioactive sources can be implanted directly into the tumour, delivering a high dose to small tumours with little irradiation to the adjacent brain. The most commonly used isotopes for interstitial radiation of brain tumours are iridium-192 (^{192}Ir) and iodine-125 (^{125}I). Low dose rate ^{125}I seeds can be used for permanent implantation, and high dose rate ^{192}Ir for a temporary implant. Sources are placed using stereotactically implanted catheters to achieve a uniform distribution throughout the tumour volume. High-dose interstitial brachytherapy is associated with a high risk of radiation-induced necrosis (17), particularly when used after previous external-beam radiotherapy. Necrosis may become clinically symptomatic and follow either a self-limiting or a progressive course. Clinically and radiologically necrotic lesions may be indistinguishable from recurrent tumours. They are surrounded by a vaso-genic oedema that responds to glucocorticosteroids. Persistent mass effect may require neu-rosurgical resection. Fluorodeoxyglucose-PET may help to differentiate tumour recurrence from radiation-induced necrosis. However, this distinction is not absolute (18).

Catheters placed for radioactive seeds have been used for inducing local hyperthermia in conjunction with brachytherapy. The rationale for combining hyperthermia with brachyther-apy is that heat inhibits the repair of radiation-induced DNA damage and may increase sen-sitivity to irradiation. Heat also causes cell death directly, depending upon time of exposure and temperature.

Boron neutron capture therapy and photodynamic therapy

Both methods are still experimental forms of local therapy. Boron neutron capture therapy (BNCT) is based on the local production of high LET (linear energy transfer radiation) charged particles which deposit energy very close to where they are generated. Bombarding non-radioactive ^{10}B (boron) with thermal neutrons generates α particles, which are highly ionizing. ^{10}B-compounds such as BSH ($Na_2B_{12}H_{11}SH$, mainly used in Japan and in a current EORTC trial) and BPA (*p*-boromophenylalanine, used in a trial in the US) selectively accu-mulate in brain tumours. The differential concentration determines that, following exposure to thermal neutrons, damage occurs in tumours with sparing of normal brain. (19).

Photodynamic therapy involves a selective tumour uptake of photosensitizers, which are haematoporphyrin derivatives that absorb light of an appropriate wavelength which is capable of penetrating tissues and activating photosensitizers. Differential damage due to light exposure is determined by the differential concentration of photosensitizers in tumour and normal tissue. This technique is detailed in Morstyn and Kaye (20).

Chemotherapy

Most chemotherapeutic drugs are administered systematically, either orally or intravenously. The effectiveness of brain tumour chemotherapy is limited by the intrinsic and acquired resist-ance, systemic toxicity of drugs, and also by the blood–brain barrier, which limits the penetra-tion of drugs to the CNS. Only small-sized lipophilic molecules readily cross the intact blood–brain barrier. To overcome or minimize the potential problem of drug penetration and of systemic toxicity, several alternative routes of drug administration have been developed.

Methods of bypassing the blood–brain barrier

Contrast enhancement of tumours on CT or MRI scans demonstrates that the blood–brain barrier (BBB) is damaged in large regions of malignant brain tumours. However, neoplas-tic cells commonly infiltrate normal brain beyond the area of contrast enhancement and such cells are protected by a largely intact BBB. The destruction of BBB in primary brain tumours is thus partial and the extent of damage varies in different parts of the tumour. The situation may be different in brain metastases, which have less tendency to infiltrate the brain parenchyma. Because the BBB restricts the entry of many drugs potentially active against malignant brain tumours, several methods are used to overcome or circumvent the BBB.

Opening of the blood–brain barrier

Intracarotid infusion of hypertonic solutions produces, in the perfused hemisphere, a reversible opening of the BBB. The duration of increased BBB permeability, first thought to last up to 2 hours, may in fact be only 5–10 minutes (21). Infusion of hypertonic solutions of either mannitol (20–25%) or glycerol (15%), causes shrinking of the endothelial cells and opening of the tight junctions of brain capillaries. Theoretically, according to Rapoport, the osmotic shock should produce a 50-fold increase in the uptake of hydrophilic drugs. In practice, the increase of BBB permeability is much greater in normal cortex than in the tumour. With the possible exception of primary CNS lymphoma (see p. 254), there is no indication that osmotic modification of the BBB is a useful adjunct to brain tumour chemotherapy. In addition, the procedure is not devoid of side-effects as it is associated with seizures and transient focal neurological deterioration.

Cereport (RMP-7, 1.5 µg/kg infused over 15 min), an analogue of bradykinin, has been shown to modify the permeability of the BBB through a receptor-mediated mechanism. It is likely that it selectively increases the permeability of apparently normal BBB in the peritumoral area infiltrated by neoplastic cells, due to differential receptor density (22). A phase II study testing RMP-7 and carboplatin in recurrent high-grade glioma has demonstrated a 61% rate of response or stabilization in chemotherapy naïve patients (23).

Local chemotherapy

Local chemotherapy that delivers agents directly into contact with brain-tumour cells, circumvents the BBB (24). The techniques include a drug injection into the tumour or tumour cavity, either during operation or via implanted catheters or pumps. However, direct injection has not been shown to be of clinical benefit. Drugs can be delivered locally by controlled-release drug-impregnated biodegradable polymers (25). Phase I–II studies of BCNU (carmustine)-impregnated polymers inserted following resection of recurrent disease demonstrated a modest efficacy in patients with malignant gliomas. Adjuvant phase III studies in patients with primary malignant gliomas are in progress.

Intraventricular or intrathecal administration

There is no barrier between CSF and brain parenchyma, and drugs exchange between the two compartments through diffusion along a concentration gradient. However, the use of the intrathecal route is limited to a few agents because of drug neurotoxicity, and the short distance of drug diffusion—limited to a few millimetres across normal nervous and tumoral tissue. Intraventricular or intrathecal administration is primarily used in the treatment of leptomeningeal metastases (p. 263–264).

Intra-arterial chemotherapy   The rationale for using the intra-arterial route is based on the assumption that, for a given drug dose, the concentration is higher in the tumour and lower in the systemic blood compartment when compared with systemic administration. This has been demonstrated for BCNU, cisplatin, and etoposide (VP16). However, intra-arterial administration is restricted to drugs that are extracted rapidly, have a high transcapillary permeability, and are rapidly metabolized or excreted, since the benefit is lost after the first blood passage. According to these criteria, nitrosoureas are theoretically more suitable for intra-arterial administration than platinum derivatives or VP16. While systemic toxicity of intracarotid chemotherapy is lower than that after systemic administration, local toxicity is higher (26). This is in the form of visual loss due to retinal damage when the tip of the catheter is placed below the origin of the oph-thalmic artery (Chapter 5, p. 91). The incidence of focal leucoencephalopathy is increased when the catheter is placed above the ophthalmic artery. The majority of focal leucoencephalopathies due to intra-arterial chemotherapy are subclinical and appear on CT or MRI as contrast-enhanced hypodense or hypointense white-matter lesions. The incidence of symptomatic leu-coencephalopathy is related to the type of the drug, drug dose, and the length of follow-up. In the phase III BTCG-study, severe leucoencephalopathy occurred in 10% of the patients (27). The occurrence of leucoencephalopathy is probably favoured by laminar streaming, which causes inhomogeneous drug delivery. Streaming is more important in patients receiving supra-ophthalmic or intracerebral selective infusion. Other neurological complications of intracarotid chemotherapy include seizures (Chapter 3, p. 51) and transient worsening of focal neurological deficits.

High-dose chemotherapy with brainstem cell rescue or bone-marrow transplantation   In patients with malignant brain tumours, bone marrow hardly ever contains neoplastic cells. Thus peripheral stem-cell or bone-marrow graft rescue with cells harvested before the administration of chemotherapy allows the administration of higher doses of anticancer drugs. Theoretically, higher doses increase CNS drug penetration and tumour cell kill. The procedure has been tested using several agents, including CCNU, BCNU, and VP16. Small phase II studies have demonstrated the feasibility of the procedure (28–32). But the benefit in terms of patient outcome is at best marginal. It remains uncertain whether larger doses, particularly of nitrosoureas, are more effective. High-dose chemotherapy may cause other end-organ toxicity not alleviated by stem-cell rescue, such as dose-related pulmonary fibrosis following nitrosoureas as well as renal or liver toxicity.

Immunotherapy and gene therapy   Biological treatment approaches may provide more selective cancer therapy. There are many preclinical studies based on increased understand-ing of tumour biology at the cellular and molecular level.

Immunotherapy has been tested. The reasons for the failure of previous immunotherapy protocols have largely been elucidated (33,34). Current strategies include vaccination, inhi-bition of local immunosuppressors, enhancement of the immune response, or use of tumour-specific monoclonal antibodies (35).

Gene therapy consists of a modification of the malignant cell genotype to impair tumour growth. Examples are reviewed by Chiocca and Breakefield (36) and by Ram and Oldfield (37).

At present, both immunotherapy and gene therapy remain experimental treatments, and are not considered further here.

Current therapy

Primary tumours

Supratentorial gliomas
The majority of glioma trials distinguish only between high-grade or malignant and low-grade gliomas. Malignant gliomas consist of glioblastomas (GBMs) and anaplastic astro-cytomas (AAs), which differ in prognosis and often in response to therapy. Anaplastic oligodendrogliomas have occasionally also been included but, due to their remarkable

chemosensitivity, they will be considered separately. Although there are clear differences between GBMs and AAs, they will be analysed together, as the majority of published trials have considered them as one entity.

Glioblastoma and anaplastic astrocytoma

Two-thirds of malignant gliomas are GBMs or grade 4 gliomas. While histologically GBMs are homogeneous, clinically they can be separated into two groups: primary or *de novo* GBMs, and secondary GBMs, which derive from a malignant transformation of low-grade glioma. The differences between the groups are listed in Table 12.3 and may also include different sensitivity to treatments. AAs, or grade 3 gliomas, account for 15–20% of all malignant gliomas. They occur in a younger age group and have a better prognosis than GBMs.

Surgery

Malignant gliomas extend beyond the contrast-enhancing area shown by CT or MRI scan (39,40), and cannot be excised in their entirety. However, extensive tumour removal is associated with prolonged survival in retrospective studies, and removal of tumour bulk mass improves the neurological deficit and quality of life. Although the benefit of resection extent has not been tested in prospective randomized trials, it is an important prognostic factor for survival in large prospective studies (41,42), and the amount of tumour removal is also a predictive factor for long-term survival (43,44). The extent of tumour resection is also of prognostic importance in children with AA or GBM (45,46). Although the benefit of tumour resection was found in patients with both GBM and AA, the impact is greater in the AA group (47).

Radiation therapy

Six-weeks of external irradiation with daily fractions of 180–200 cGy delivered 5 days a week prolongs the median survival of patients with malignant gliomas by 4–6 months (Table 12.4). The effect of radiation therapy is dose-dependent up to 6000 cGy (54), with no further improvement with higher doses to 7000 cGy (55). There is no information to suggest that radiation efficacy is different in GBM compared to AA. Current practice is to confine the planning target volume to the tumour as visualized by imaging plus a 2–3 cm margin, as the majority of malignant gliomas recur locally (56). Whole-brain radiotherapy is not generally practised, to minimize CNS toxicity. A radical 6-week course of radiotherapy may not be appropriate for elderly patients with a poor prognosis, severe disability, and low performance status, where

Table 12.3 Distinction between primary and secondary glioblastomas (from Kleihues *et al.* 1977, ref. 38)

	Primary GBM (*de novo*)	Secondary GBM (to low-grade glioma)
Clinical history	Few months	Several years
Mean age at diagnosis	55 years	40 years
Overexpression of epidermal growth factor receptors	58%	6%
p53 mutation	10%	71%

Table 12.4   Randomized trials testing radiation therapy in malignant gliomas

Scheduled treatment	Number of patients	Medial survival	Reference
Surgery alone	42	17 weeks	48
Surgery + 5000–6000 cGy	93	37.5 weeks*	
Surgery alone	17	5.4 months	49
Surgery + 5000 cGy	20	7.5 months*	
Surgery alone	38	6.1 months	50
Surgery + 4500 cGy	35	10.5 months*	
CCNU 130 mg/m^2/day every 8 weeks	22	6.6 months	51
CCNU + 5000 cGy	19	12.0 months*	
BCNU 80 mg/m^2 + vincristine 1.4 mg/m^2 on days 1 and 8 every 5–8 weeks	16	30 weeks	52
BCNU + 6000 cGy	17	44.5 weeks	
CCNU 100–130 mg/m^2/day every 6–8 weeks	27	8.4 months	53
CCNU + 5000 cGy	26	11.9 months	

Studies comparing surgery to surgery plus radiation therapy are summarized in the upper part of the table. Studies summarized in the lower part compare surgery plus adjuvant chemotherapy to surgery plus chemo- and radiation therapy.
*, statistically significant at $P \geq 0.05$.

prolonged treatment is unlikely to lead to useful functional improvement. In this setting it is reasonable to offer either a short palliative radiotherapy regimen, such as 3000 cGy in 6 or 10 fractions or supportive care alone.

Attempts have been made to increase the efficacy of radiation therapy through altered fractionation, use of radiosensitizers, and localized high-dose irradiation with interstitial or stereotactic radiotherapy.

Altered fractionation

Hyperfractionation refers to multiple, smaller than standard, daily doses which allow for an increased dose without exceeding the tolerance of the normal brain. Trials, testing increased radiation to 7200 cGy failed to show a survival benefit of hyperfractionation (57,58).

Accelerated fractionation aims to shorten the overall treatment time while delivering the same total dose. The superiority of this scheme over conventional radiation therapy has not been demonstrated in malignant gliomas (59).

Radiosensitizers

Radiosensitizers aim to increase damage to the tumour without increasing damage to normal tissue. Those tested in brain-tumour radiation therapy include electron affinic hypoxic sensitizers, nucleoside analogues, oxygen, ARCON, and radiosensitizing chemotherapy agents.

Sensitizers of **hypoxic cells**, such as nitromidazole derivatives (metronidazole, misonida-zole), failed to increase the efficacy of radiation therapy in randomized trials (60–62). Pyrimidine analogues such as 5-bromodeoxyuridine (BUdR) or 5-iododeoxyuridine (IUdR) which are **cell-cycle specific** sensitizers of dividing cells act independently of an oxygen effect. A suggested survival benefit of BUdR and IUdR in combination with 6000 cGy irra-diation observed in phase II studies (63,64) has not been confirmed in randomized trials. Platinum derivatives, which inhibit repair of sublethal radiation-induced DNA damage, did not potentiate radiation therapy of malignant gliomas in an EORTC trial (65). Other drugs, including Taxol® (paclitaxel), an inhibitor of microtubule depolymerization (66), and temo-zolamide remain untested in prospective randomized trials.

Interstitial radiotherapy or brachytherapy
An interstitial radiotherapy boost, adjuvant to external radiation therapy, was tested in several non-randomized phase II trials (67) with a median survival in patients with GBM ranging from 7 to 19 months (Table 4.1 in ref. 67). In the only fully published, prospective randomized study of brachytherapy boost in patients with newly diagnosed malignant gliomas, brachytherapy was not associated with a survival benefit (68). Following interstitial radiotherapy, a large proportion of patients require re-operation for focal radionecrosis. Currently there is no evidence that adjuvant brachytherapy improves survival in patients with GBM or AA. However, a role for brachytherapy in the treatment of selected patients with recurrent GBM or AA cannot be excluded (69).

Stereotactic radiotherapy
Stereotactic radiotherapy and radiosurgery are limited to patients with tumours not exceed-ing 3–4 cm in diameter. Patients with newly diagnosed and recurrent malignant gliomas have been treated with radiosurgery and stereotactic radiotherapy. Survival results are similar to those reported following brachytherapy (70), and it is not clear whether favourable results are related to treatment or to selection of patients with better prognostic factors. Fractionated stereotactic radiotherapy is associated with a lesser risk of radiation necrosis compared to brachytherapy or radiosurgery.

Summary
In summary, external-beam radiotherapy to 6000 cGy in 180–200 cGy daily fractions deliv-ered over 6 weeks to the tumour and a 2–3 cm margin remain the standard therapy for patients with malignant gliomas. So far, its efficacy has not been increased substantially by higher doses, altered fractionation, radiosensitizers, stereotactic radiotherapy, radiosurgery, or interstitial irradiation. Randomized studies of radiosurgery and fractionated stereotactic radiotherapy are currently under way.

Chemotherapy
In malignant gliomas chemotherapy has been tested either soon after the primary diag-nosis is made (as adjuvant or neoadjuvant chemotherapy) or at recurrence (salvage chemotherapy).

Adjuvant chemotherapy

Adjuvant chemotherapy is initiated in newly diagnosed tumours, usually during or shortly after the completion of radiation therapy. Two pivotal trials published in 1978 (48) and 1980 (71) have shown that in **adults** the administration of BCNU (80 mg/m^2 daily for 3 days every 6–8 weeks until recurrence), increased the number of survivors at 18 months by about 15% without prolongation of median survival. Based on these results, adjuvant BCNU became standard adjuvant therapy in the United States despite the overall negative results and the inability to select a group of potential responders who might benefit most. Despite many randomized phase III studies testing single agents and combination chemotherapy, the evidence for benefit is minimal and there has been little progress in developing new effective regimens. The suggestion for usefulness of chemotherapy comes from a meta-analysis of 16 published randomized trials involving more than 3000 patients (72). Patients treated with adjuvant chemotherapy following radiation had a modest 10% survival benefit at 1 year and 9% at 2 years. The analysis is flawed. It only includes published, not all performed, trials, and relies on the published results rather than using individual patient data. It is therefore not a true meta-analysis, is potentially biased, and the results are not conclusive. A recently completed randomized MRC trial of adjuvant chemotherapy, which included nearly 700 patients, failed to show a benefit for adjuvant PCV chemotherapy (procarbazine, CCNU, vincristine) in patients with malignant glioma (73). While it is suggested that patients with non-GBM malignant gliomas benefit from adjuvant PCV (74) or dibromodulcitol plus BCNU (75), the results so far are inconclusive and the analysis of the MRC study does not demonstrate a survival benefit for PCV chemotherapy in AA patients.

Only one study has tested the use of adjuvant **intra-arterial** chemotherapy with BCNU (27). The treatment was not superior to systemic administration in terms of survival but was more neurotoxic.

There is a suggestion that malignant gliomas are more chemosensitive in **children**. However the evidence that adjuvant chemotherapy is useful in children GBM is based on only one trial performed by the Children's Cancer Group (CCG), which demonstrated that adjuvant chemotherapy combining vincristine, CCNU, and prednisolone significantly prolongs the median survival. In addition, the 5-year event-free survival was 46% in children treated with adjuvant chemotherapy as compared with 18% in the controls (76). A further phase III trial failed to demonstrate the superiority of eight-drugs-in-one-day over CCNU, vincristine, and prednisolone in children with AA or GBL (46). However, chemotherapy alone appears to be surprisingly effective in infants aged less than 2 years with GBM.

Neoadjuvant chemotherapy

Neoadjuvant chemotherapy usually precedes irradiation and, in rare instances, gross surgical tumour removal. In **adults** several studies, including an EORTC-BTG trial, have demonstrated that radiation therapy can be delayed by 8–12 weeks by the administration of VM26 plus CCNU, although the benefit of neoadjuvant chemotherapy has not been demonstrated (77). National Cancer Institute (NCI) brain tumour consortia have initiated neoadjuvant studies of chemotherapy prior to irradiation, largely as a model to assess the efficacy of novel chemotherapeutic agents. In **children**, the main purpose of neoadjuvant chemotherapy is to delay irradiation. However, in malignant glioma its benefit remains unproven. Heideman *et al.* (78) have reported their 10-year experience with neoadjuvant chemotherapy, consisting of cisplatin and cyclophosphamide, in 41 patients with malignant glioma aged 0.2–20 years. No survival benefit was observed when compared to children who received post-irradiation adjuvant chemotherapy. The CCG treated 39 children under 2 years of age with an 'eight-in-one' chemotherapy. Only 24% of the children achieved a partial response and the survival, especially in children with GBM, was poor (79). In contrast, the Paediatric Oncology Group (POG) treated 10 children under 3 years with adjuvant cyclophosphamide and vincristine. The overall 5-year survival was 50%, and tumour reduction greater than 50% was observed in six patients after two chemotherapy cycles. Due to parental refusal, four children were not irradiated after 24 months of chemotherapy, and none developed recurrent disease at the time of publication (80).

Salvage chemotherapy

Several drugs have shown efficacy in recurrent malignant gliomas, leading to tumour regression or stabilization. Most information on salvage chemotherapy is based on phase II trials, with considerable variation in results due to varying criteria used for the assessment of the response and for patient selection.

Systemic administration is the most common means of drug delivery. Table 12.5 summarizes the results obtained with single-agent, first-line systemic chemotherapy in malignant gliomas. Nitrosourea derivatives remain for many neuro-oncologists the most active single agents, with 20–30% partial or complete response rate and 20–30% rate of stabilizations. However, the evaluation of the first, and still most commonly used, nitrosoureas such as BCNU and CCNU dates back to pre-CT scanning and the response data are therefore unreliable.

Three other drugs have been shown to be active in recurrent malignant glioma. Procarbazine has, for a long time, been considered as the most effective agent next to nitrosoureas (82). Its activity has been subsequently re-evaluated (88,89), showing a 20% partial response rate and 30% rate of stabilization. The response rate obtained with AZQ (diaziquone) varies widely between studies (90–94). Carboplatin has been evaluated as a single agent in several studies (95–97), with little objective response and some stabilization of disease for 4–6 months.

Temozolomide is an alkylating agent, which crosses the blood–brain barrier, currently administered orally at 150–200 mg/m^2/day $\times$ 5 every 4 weeks. It is well tolerated and the reported response rate is 5% for GBM and 35% for AA (98,99).

In **children**, particularly infants, malignant gliomas are considered to be more chemosensitive, although the data supporting this assumption are scarce. It is noteworthy that drugs such as vincristine and cyclophosphamide (100) or etoposide (VP-16) (101) that do not cross the intact blood–brain barrier readily have been used successfully in children with malignant gliomas.

Combination chemotherapy

Combination chemotherapy has been tested in the treatment of malignant gliomas in an attempt to improve efficacy. However, despite promising results from non-randomized phase II studies, the superiority of combination chemotherapy over single nitrosourea has not been established convincingly (102,103) in recurrent malignant gliomas.

Table 12.5 Systemic single-agent salvage chemotherapy in recurrent malignant gliomas in adults

Agent	Usual, scheduled doses (mg/m²)	Remissions		References
		%	Length (months)	
BCNU	80–130 × 3 or 2 every 6–8 weeks	47–60*	9	81,82
CCNU	120–130 every 6 weeks	19–44*	6–8	82,83
Methyl CCNU	130–170 every 6–8 weeks	50* (R = 18%, S = 32%)	8+	84
PCNU	90–100 every 6–8 weeks	69* (R = 27%, S = 42%)	6	85
HeCNU	130 every 5–6 weeks	55* (R = 20%, S = 32%)	9	86
Fotemustine	100 weekly × 3 then every 3 weeks	74* (R = 26%, S = 47%)	8	87
Procarbazine	150–200 daily for 3–4 weeks	50* (R = 20%, S = 30%)	6–8	88,89
AZQ (diaziquone)	10–40 weekly	6–52* (R = 24%, S = 28%)	5–9	90–94
Carboplatin	400–450 every 4 weeks	40–50* (most = S)	4–6	95–97
Temozolomide	150–200/day × 5 + every 4 weeks	60% (R = 35%, S = 25%)	5–6	98,99

*Tumour regression plus stabilizations.
R, regression rate; S, stabilization rate.

There are few studies separately reporting the rate of response of GBM and non-GBM, which suggest that non-GBM are more chemosensitive. However, the number of patients included in the phase II trials is usually small, and the level of statistical significance is seldom reached, with the exception of recently published temozolomide trials.

Intra-arterial chemotherapy

Intra-arterial chemotherapy has been evaluated in at least 1200 patients with malignant gliomas (104). Tested in a randomized study adjuvant setting, intra-arterial chemotherapy is not superior to systemic administration and is more toxic (27). On the basis of this evidence salvage intra-arterial chemotherapy with currently available drugs is not indicated because of the high incidence of eye and CNS toxicity without clearly superior outcome in terms of survival. The interest of intra-arterial **salvage chemotherapy** (Table 12.6) is the apparently higher rate of complete response compared to systemic administration, even in patients who failed on previous chemotherapy (108–111). Intra-arterial chemotherapy remains an investigational treatment and should be evaluated further with rigorous criteria using newer agents with mild neurotoxicity.

Treatment algorithm in glioblastomas and anaplastic astrocytomas

The main points of the algorithm (Fig. 12.3) are:

1. Optimal resection followed by external irradiation with 6000 cGy is the mainstay therapy in patients with GBM and AA and a reasonable life expectancy. Severely disabled and older patients should be offered limited intervention with palliative surgical and radiotherapy approaches.

2. Adjuvant brachytherapy has little proven benefit and a localized radiation boost with stereotactic irradiation is currently being evaluated in prospective randomized trials.

3. In AA the benefit of adjuvant chemotherapy of procarbazine–CCNU–vincristine or dibromodulcitol–nitrosourea combinations remains unproven.

4. In adults with GBL there is no proven benefit of adjuvant chemotherapy based on nitrosoureas. In the absence of criteria allowing the selection of potential responders, we do not use adjuvant chemotherapy in routine practice, but recommend the inclusion of patients in prospective trials testing new therapy.

5. In children there is a suggestion of benefit of adjuvant CCNU, vincristine, and prednisolone, based on one study (76).

6. Several drugs, including nitrosoureas and temozolomide, are active in recurrent GBM and AA.

Oligodendrogliomas

Oligodendrogliomas account for 5–10% of primary brain tumours in adults. From a pathological point of view, oligodendrogliomas raise several difficulties. The criteria distinguishing between well-differentiated (grade 2) and anaplastic (grade 3) oligodendro- gliomas are less clear than for other gliomas; aggressive forms may be pathologically well differentiated but clinically rapidly progressive, and mixed forms of oligoastrocytomas may be present. Mixed forms

Table 12.6 Intra-arterial chemotherapy in recurrent malignant gliomas in adults

Agent	Usual, scheduled doses (mg/m²)	ST	Number of responders/total		Response length (months)	References
			PR	CR		
BCNU	200–300 every 6–8 weeks	4/19	8/19	0/19	5	105
HeCNU	120 initial dose; every 6–8 weeks		9/53	17/53	8.5	106
Cisplatin	100, twice monthly		7/9			107
Cisplatin	60–120 every 4 weeks	6/20		6/20*	4 and 8	108
Cisplatin	58–100 every 4–6 weeks	0/12	1/12	0/12	6	109
Cisplatin	60 (one course)	14/35	12/35	0/35	4	110
AZQ (diaziquone)	10–20 every 4 weeks	4/20	2/20	0/20	3 and 8+	111
VP-16 (etoposide)	100–350 every 4 weeks	5/15	1/15	0/15	2–10	112
BCNU	≥100					
Cisplatin	60 } once + systemic	1/19		13/19*	4	113
VM-26 (teniposide)	175					
Cisplatin	150–200 } CCNU			10/12*	4–19+	114
BCNU	300					

*Partial plus complete responses.
ST, stable disease; PR, partial response; CR, complete response.

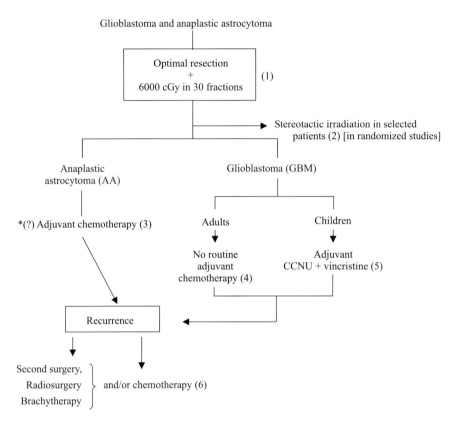

Fig. 12.3   Treatment algorithm in glioblastomas and anaplastic astrocytomas. *(?), unproven efficacy.

are more common than pure oligodendrogliomas and their classification varies between oligodendrogliomas in some centres, and mixed tumours or even astrocytomas in others. Over 50% oligodendroglial tumours are characterized by loss of one copy of 1p or 19q chromosome (115) and their chemosensitivity, which distinguishes these tumours from other gliomas.

Treatment of newly diagnosed oligodendrogliomas

Surgery
Surgery is considered appropriate treatment in resectable oligodendrogliomas. Although the role of surgery has not been tested prospectively, in retrospective analyses (116–119) optimal resection is the main prognostic factor for survival. Maximal resection may be of value in patients with low-grade and anaplastic oligodendrogliomas, provided they do not involve eloquent regions.

Adjuvant external irradiation
The use of adjuvant external irradiation with 4500–5400 cGy remains unproven (120–122), with some retrospective studies suggesting survival benefit (123–125). The groups most

likely to benefit from irradiation are patients with anaplastic, clinically aggressive, and/or partially removed tumours (119,123), and those with progressive unresectable tumours.

Neoadjuvant and adjuvant chemotherapy

Oligodendrogliomas are more chemosensitive than astrocytic tumours and chemosensitivity of anaplastic oligodendrogliomas is associated with the 1p chromosomal deletion. While treatment with procarbazine, CCNU, and vincristine (PCV) is increasingly given before irradiation, especially to patients with aggressive forms (126), a survival benefit of neoadjuvant chemotherapy has not been demonstrated. Two studies currently performed in North America and Europe are testing the use of adjuvant PCV in newly diagnosed, operated, and irradiated patients with anaplastic oligodendrogliomas.

Treatment at recurrence

Patients, especially with slowly progressive tumours located in surgically accessible areas, may benefit from second operation or radiotherapy if not previously given. Chemotherapy with PCV is a reasonable salvage option in previously untreated patients.

In 1988, Craincross and Macdonald reported eight patients with recurrent malignant oligodendrogliomas (127). Six received the PCV combination. One had a complete (CR) and five a partial response (PR) lasting 30+ to 78+ weeks. Several subsequent studies, summarized in Table 12.7, confirmed the efficacy of PCV in anaplastic oligodendrogliomas or oligoastrocytomas, as well as in low-grade oligodendrogliomas (133). In some studies the response was prompt, often observed after the first two courses of chemotherapy (128). Patients with CR had the longest duration of response (time to progression). Two different dosages of PCV—the standard or the intensive schedule (see the footnote of Table 12.7)—have been used. The intensive regimen is more toxic and is not clearly superior to the standard regimen. The chemosensitivity of oligodendrogliomas may not be limited to PCV, although other agents tested appear to be less active. Second-line chemotherapy with VP16 and cisplatin (135) or carboplatin (136), administered to patients with tumour progression following PCV therapy, show some activity.

Treatment algorithm in oligodendrogliomas

The main points of this algorithm (Fig. 12.4) are:

1. Clinically aggressive but pathologically low-grade tumours are treated along the lines of anaplastic oligodendrogliomas.

2. The benefit of neoadjuvant PCV in terms of survival length has not been demonstrated.

3. Adjuvant PCV is currently being tested in two prospective trials in patients with anaplastic oligodendrogliomas.

4. The nature of the best second-line chemotherapy is unknown.

5. A surveillance option may be offered to patients with quiescent tumours.

Low-grade or grade 2 astrocytomas

Grade 2 astrocytomas are well differentiated, poorly defined, infiltrating tumours characterized by increased cellularity and nuclear as well as cellular polymorphism. Vascular changes,

Table 12.7 Phase II trials testing PCV in oligodendrogliomas

Tumour characteristics	Patients: newly diagnosed (ND), recurrent (Rec)	Response				Duration	PCV schedule[b]: standard (S), intensive (I)	References
		CR	PR	SD	PD			
Aggressive[a]	8 Rec	2	6	0	0	15 months	S	128
	5 ND (evaluable)	3	1	0	1	18–48 months		
Anaplastic oligodendrogliomas	7 Rec	1	2	3	1	4–25+ months	S	129
Anaplastic oligoastrocytomas	7 ND	0	3	4	0	≤10 months		
	12 ND	2	3	7	0	>12 months	S	
Oligodendrogliomas or oligoastrocytomas	7 Rec	0	4	2	1	20–40 weeks	S	130
	14 ND	2	9	2	1	20–60+ weeks		
All types of oligodendrogliomas	17 Rec	2	8	6	1	6 months	S	131
Anaplastic oligodendrogliomas	24 (eligible)	9	9	4	2	CR = 25+ months PR = 14 months SD = 7 months	I	132
Low-grade oligodendrogliomas	1 Rec	1	7	0	0			133
	7 ND							
Oligodendrogliomas and oligoastrocytomas	52 Rec (retrospective study)	9	24	10	9	CR = 25 months PR = 12 months	S or I	134

Abbreviations: CR, complete response; PR, partial response; SD, stable disease; PD, progressive disease; Rec, recurrent; ND, newly diagnosed.
[a]Aggressive = enlarging, enhancing usually, but not always anaplastic.
[b]

PCV	Day	Standard intensity	Intensive
CCNU	1	110 mg/m^2 orally	130 mg/m^2 orally
Vincristine	8, 29	1.4 mg/m^2 iv	1.4 mg/m^2 iv
Procarbazine	8–21	60 mg/m^2 orally	75 mg/m^2 orally
Cycle repeated		Every 8 weeks	Every 6 weeks

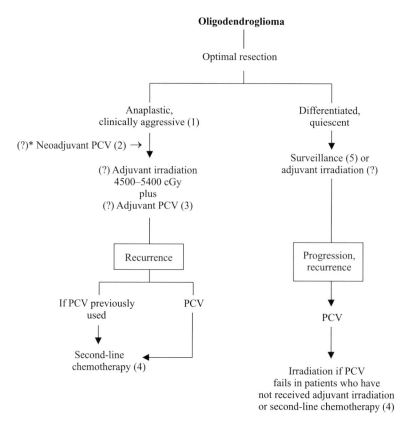

Fig. 12.4 Treatment algorithm in oligodendrogliomas. *(?), unproven efficacy; PCV, procarbazine, CCNU, vincristine.

mitoses, or necrosis are absent. The distinction between the fibrillary and astrocytic type is of no prognostic value. Patients with gemistocytic tumours have a worse prognosis (137). Pilocytic astrocytomas are grade 1 tumours with a 90% survival at 10 years. Because of their favourable prognosis, pilocytic astrocytomas should not be included in therapeutic trials together with grade 2 astrocytomas. The management of grade 2 astrocytomas is full of uncertainties and is one of the most controversial issues in neuro-oncology (138–140). Biopsy to establish the pathology is advisable, as in 25–50% of the cases the diagnosis based on clinical and radiological features may not be confirmed by the histological examination (141). However, repeated unenhancing MRI lesions in patients without progressive deficit, which remain unchanged on imaging 3 months apart, are strongly suggestive of low-grade glioma, although not indicative of precise histology.

Treatment of newly diagnosed grade 2 astrocytomas

Surgery

Surgery is not expected to be curative. Tumour resection is justified in patients with increased intracranial pressure, neurological deficits related to mass effect, and medically uncontrolled seizures. Age is the most powerful prognostic factor in grade 2 gliomas, suggesting that tumours occurring in older patients are more aggressive. From a retrospective review, Vecht (142) concluded that the treatment should be more aggressive in older patients, setting the limit for operation above the age of 35 years, although the benefit in this group has not been demonstrated in prospective studies. PET studies have shown that pathologically verified grade 2 gliomas containing areas of increased glucose metabolism (143) (Fig. 12.5) and contrast-enhanced tumours have a poorer outcome. Based on the assumption that surgery is of value in more aggressive tumours, we tend to advise surgical removal in these cases. In young asymptomatic patients with medically controlled seizures, the benefit of tumour resection in terms of survival or rate of malignant transformation has not been demonstrated, and has not been addressed prospectively. In the absence of such studies, the use of surgery has been assessed by comparing survival of patients who had total macroscopic removal with those who had partial tumour removal. The benefit was shown in some (144–147), but not all (148–150) analyses. The large number of prognostic factors in low-grade gliomas, and the change in life expectancy due to earlier diagnosis made possible by modern investigation techniques make such comparisons with historical controls highly unreliable and potentially misleading.

Adjuvant radiotherapy   The use of adjuvant radiotherapy is equally controversial. Its effectiveness is also based on retrospective studies with historical comparisons (151–152). Two prospective EORTC trials have addressed this issue. The first, comparing 4500 and 5400 cGy, showed no survival difference between the two treatments, with a 5-year survival rate of 58 and 59%, respectively (153). The second EORTC trial compared adjuvant 5400 cGy irradiation to irradiation at recurrence. The first analysis of this trial indicates that early irradiation does not prolong survival. The claim that radiation therapy can prevent or delay malignant transformation of low-grade into anaplastic astrocytoma is purely speculative.

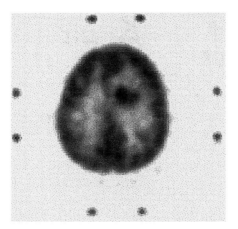

Fig. 12.5   Positron emission tomography after injection of [^{18}F]fluorodeoxyglucose in a woman with a predominantly hypometabolic low-grade astrocytoma infiltrating the left hemisphere. Stereotactic biopsy of the hypermetabolic nodule also revealed a low-grade tumour, but malignant transformation into a glioblastoma developed within 1 year. (Courtesy of Dr S. Goldman.)

Adjuvant and neoadjuvant chemotherapy   In **adults** adjuvant chemotherapy for grade 2 astrocytomas has received little attention, and its use remains unproven (154). A current Radiation Therapy Oncology Group (RTOG) study is testing the value of adjuvant PCV in incompletely resected low-grade gliomas.

In **children** neoadjuvant chemotherapy is increasingly used to control tumour growth and/or delay radiation therapy. This strategy has been used particularly in chiasmatic–hypothalamic gliomas, which are usually pilocytic astrocytomas (Chapter 5, p. 82). Its use has also been extended to brainstem gliomas (Chapter 6, p. 122) and hemispheric and diencephalic (155) grade 2 astrocytomas. The inclusion of pilocytic astrocytomas into some trials (156,157) makes it difficult to evaluate chemotherapy in truly grade 2 tumours. The observation that pilocytic astrocytomas are chemosensitive is noteworthy.

Treatment at recurrence

Almost all patients with grade 2 astrocytomas eventually show signs of tumour progression. When this occurs, all should have a second biopsy as about two-thirds of the tumours undergo malignant transformation. The management of secondary malignant gliomas does not differ from that of *de novo* malignant gliomas (see p. 233–239). The indications for surgery in patients with progressive but still grade 2 glioma are the same as for primary presentation. Radiation therapy is generally recommended, if it was not previously given to provide temporary growth arrest and, occasionally, reduction in tumour size. Chemotherapy may produce objective responses in grade 2 astrocytomas. From a literature review, Bloom (158) concluded that low-grade gliomas were more sensitive to nitrosourea-based chemotherapy than the more malignant forms. A 30% response rate to chemotherapy has been reported by Galanis *et al.* in low-grade gliomas recurring after radiation therapy (159).

Treatment algorithm in grade 2 astrocytomas

The main points of the algorithm (Fig. 12.6) are:

1. The cut-off for surgery at the age of 35 years is based on the review by Vecht (142).

2. The EORTC study evaluating early versus late irradiation showed no benefit in terms of overall survival.

Medulloblastomas

Medulloblastomas are the most common CNS tumours in childhood. They represent about 20% of brain neoplasms in children, but less than 5% in adults. Medulloblastomas are treated similarly in older children and in adults. In children under 2 years of age neoadjuvant chemotherapy is increasingly used to delay irradiation.

Treatment of newly diagnosed medulloblastomas

Surgery

Surgery has two main goals: tumour removal and restoration of normal CSF drainage, with normalization of the frequently present intracranial hypertension usually due to hydrocephalus. Medulloblastoma used to be staged according to Chang's criteria (160), separating patients with extensive tumours (T3 and T4) and metastases (M1–M4). Chang's staging is no

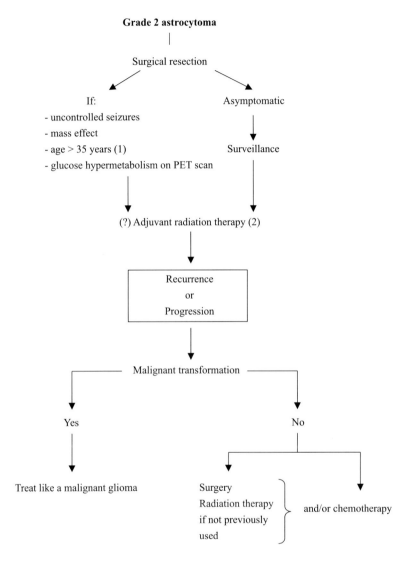

Fig. 12.6   Treatment algorithm in low-grade astrocytomas. (?), unproven efficacy.

longer employed as it is of no prognostic value other than the distinction between the presence or absence of disseminated disease (161). The T-stage system has been replaced by the
extent of surgical resection, primarily based on imaging.

The aim of surgery is radical resection. The presence of residual tumour is an adverse prognostic factor associated with a high rate of recurrence (162). While in the SIOP study (12)
the 5-year survival was similar in patients with subtotal or total resection (52.1% and 50.8%,
respectively), the extent of surgery was based on the surgeon's view without objective

imaging data. Using post-operative imaging, the extent of residual disease after surgery is a principal prognostic factor for disease control and survival, in addition to the presence of dis-seminated disease (161). The results indicate that as much tumour as possible should be removed, taking care not to damage critical areas, and the procedure should be carried out by experienced surgeons.

Adjuvant irradiation Adjuvant irradiation that encompasses the whole craniospinal axis remains the mainstay of medulloblastoma treatment, resulting in a 50–70% disease-free sur-vival at 5 years. Current recommended doses are 5600 cGy delivered in 160–180 cGy daily fractions (163–165) and 3500 cGy to the rest of the craniospinal axis. To decrease morbid-ity, several attempts have been made to reduce craniospinal irradiation to approximately 2400 cGy. A prospective randomized study in good-risk patients by the POG and CCSG showed a higher failure rate following 2300 cGy irradiation (166). A retrospective analysis of patients treated at the University of California SF, showed that craniospinal irradiation with less than 3000 cGy was associated with an increased risk of recurrence outside the posterior fossa (167). Single-arm studies suggest that in standard-risk patients reduced craniospinal dose com-bined with chemotherapy does not affect tumour control or survival, but the benefit in terms of decreased toxicity remains to be proven (168–170). Other studies aiming to reduce toxicity while maintaining efficacy are comparing 3600 cGy craniospinal irradiation with a combi-nation of 2300 cGy plus adjuvant chemotherapy in low-risk children. At present, it seems reasonable to maintain the dose of craniospinal irradiation at 3500 cGy in adults. In children 2400 cGy spinal irradiation is acceptable only if it is followed by chemotherapy.

Adjuvant chemotherapy Adjuvant chemotherapy has been tested in four prospective phase III trials (Table 12.8). None has shown benefit in unselected patients. The two major studies performed by SIOP (12) and CCSG (11) used similar treatment, and yielded similar results. There was no improvement in disease-free survival in patients who received adjuvant chemotherapy, but both trials identified similar high-risk subgroups who appeared to benefit from adjuvant treatment. An adjuvant therapy with vincristine–CCNU combination ± pred-nisolone may not be considered to be the most effective regimen, as the activity of nitrosoureas may be weak in medulloblastomas due to high levels of O^6-alkylguanine-DNA alkyltransferase (an enzyme that repairs DNA damage induced by alkylating agents) (171). Other regimens, including cisplatin or cyclophosphamide, have been tested and the favoured approach is a combination of CCNU, cisplatin, and vincristine given every 6 weeks in 8 cycles (172). In children with high-risk medulloblastomas, this adjuvant treatment yielded a 67% disease-free survival at 5 years in a selected group of patients from one institution (172) and multicentre studies suggest similar results. Thus the use of adjuvant chemotherapy may be revised in future years in view of the results obtained with more potent drug combinations.

Neoadjuvant chemotherapy Neoadjuvant chemotherapy is currently used in children before the age of 3 years. It aims to minimize the neuropsychological, endocrine and growth seque-lae of irradiation by delaying radiotherapy until the age of 3–4 years or until recurrence.

Neoadjuvant therapy was initiated by van Eys in 1976, using adjuvant MOPP combination. The results were updated by Ater *et al.* (175). Eight of the 12 children are still alive with no evidence of disease and six were never irradiated. In the Baby POG I protocol 62 children under 3 years of age were treated with two cycles of cyclophosphamide plus vincristine and cisplatin. Five-year survival was 60% in children with gross total resection and only 32% in children with subtotal tumour removal. The majority of children required radiotherapy, and progression-free survival after chemotherapy alone was poor (176). The CCG experience in 46 children under 18 months of age treated with an adjuvant 'eight-in-one' regimen was disappointing, with a 22% disease-free survival after 3 years. Better results were obtained in children with gross tumour resection and a few did not require irradiation (177). The German Paediatric Tumour Study Group (protocol HIT SKK 92) also attempted to avoid irradiation in children in complete remission after chemotherapy with cyclophosphamide, intravenous methotrexate, and intraventricular carboplatin and vincristine. Of 33 children included in the study, 12 were not irradiated (178). In several studies, failure of neoadjuvant chemotherapy occurred early, mostly within 6 months. In such patients, salvage radiation therapy is still appropriate (179).

Treatment at recurrence   A large number of phase II trials (Table 12.9) show that recurrent medulloblastomas respond to various drugs or drug combinations. These results suggest that carboplatin, cyclophosphamide and vincristine are among the most active agents, although none of the combinations offers curative treatment. Salvage therapy using high-dose chemotherapy in conjunction with autologous bone-marrow graft reported few long-term survivors but it is still experimental strategy, currently tested in prospective trials.

Treatment algorithm in medulloblastomas
The main points of this algorithm (Fig. 12.7) are:

1. Radical surgery and craniospinal radiotherapy with posterior fossa boost are the mainstay of curative therapy.

2. There is an increased tendency to delay craniospinal irradiation in children under 2–3 years of age.

3. The most active adjuvant and salvage chemotherapy regimens have not been established. CCNU–vincristine or CCNU, cisplatinum, and vincristine are frequently employed regimens.

4. The benefit of reducing spinal prophylaxis to about 2500 cGy by combining chemotherapy remains to be proven, and currently adults should receive 3600 cGy spinal irradiation.

Primary CNS lymphomas

Primary non-Hodgkin's lymphomas of the CNS (PCNSL) occur in the population of immunodepressed patients following organ transplantation and in AIDS. Sporadic PCNSL in immunocompetent individuals has also increased in incidence (189). Most cerebral PCNSLs are highly malignant and over 80% are B phenotype. The treatment of PCNSL in immunodepressed patients relates to the cause and the extent of immune deficiency and will not be considered here.

Assessment of tumour extension
About 50% of immunocompetent patients have multiple, usually periventricular, lesions (Fig. 2.2). The diagnosis of PCNSL is usually based on histological confirmation obtained by stereotaxic biopsy. The biopsy should be performed before the administration of gluco-

Table 12.8 Adjuvant chemotherapy in medulloblastoma

Study arm	Scheduled treatments (mg/m^2; unless specified otherwise)	Number of patients	Disease-free survival at 5 years (%)	Subgroups who benefit from chemotherapy	Reference
RT	50–55 Gy^a to posterior fossa in 7–8 weeks 35–45 Gy^a to rest of brain 30–35 Gy^a to spinal cord in 5–6 weeks	145	48	Partial (subtotal) surgery $P = 0.007$ Brainstem involvement $P = 0.001$	SIOP study (12)
RT + ChT	Same RT; ChT: VCR 1.5 weekly during radiation, plus CCNU 100 on day 1 + VCR 1.5 on days 1, 8, and 15 every 6 weeks; 8 courses	141	53	Advanced (T3 and T4) stages of disease $P = 0.001$	
RT	RT similar to the SIOP study	118	50	More extensive tumours (T3 and T4) $P = 0.006$	CCSG study (11)
RT + ChT	Same RT; ChT: VCR 1.5 weekly during radiation, plus CCNU 100 on day 1 + VCR 1.5 on days 1, 8, and 15 + prednisone 40/day for 14 days every 6 weeks	115	59		
RT	30–35 Gy to cerebrospinal axis plus 20 Gy to posterior fossa	43	59		GPO study (173)
RT + ChT	Same RT; ChT: PCZ 100 on days 1 and 2 + VCR 1.5 on days 2 and 8 + MTX 500 mg on days 2 and 8	51	59		
RT + ChT (maintenance)	Same RT, maintenance ChT: VCR 1.5+ CCNU 100 every 6 weeks for 7 months	15	59		

Table 12.8 Adjuvant chemotherapy in medulloblastoma *(continued)*

Study arm	Scheduled treatments (mg/m²; unless specified otherwise)	Number of patients	Disease-free survival at 5 years (%)	Subgroups who benefit from chemotherapy	Reference
RT	54-Gy (48 Gy if < 3 years) to posterior fossa	35	68	Children older than 5 years	POG study (174)
	35–40 Gy (25–35 Gy if < 3 years) to rest of brain				
	30 Gy (25 Gy if < 3 years) to spinal cord				
RT + ChT	Same RT, ChT:	36	57		
	Nit. Must. 3 on day 1, 8 every 4 weeks for maximum of 12 courses				
	VCR 1.4				
	Prednisone 40 on days 1–10				
	PCZ 50 mg on day 1				
	100 mg on day 2				
	100 mg on days 3–10				

ªDoses reduced by 5–10 Gy in children under 2 years.
RT, radiation therapy; ChT, chemotherapy; VCR, vincristine; PCZ, procarbazine; MTX, methotrexate; Nit. Must., nitrogen mustard

Table 12.9 Chemotherapy in recurrent medulloblastomas

Agent	Scheduled doses (mg/m^2) unless specified otherwise	Responders/Total			Length of remissions (months)	Reference
		ST	PR	CR		
Cisplatin	60 on days 1, 2 every 3–4 weeks	1/11	1/11	2/11		180
Cisplatin	60 on days 1, 2 every 3–4 weeks	1/10	2/10	2/10	4.5 and 7.5 for CR	181
Cisplatin	120 every 4 weeks	3/14	5/14	5/14	8+ (median)	182
Melphalan	8 × 5 every 4 weeks			1/5[a]	14+	183
Cyclophosphamide	50–80/kg on days 1, 2 every 4 weeks			7/7[a]	6+ (mean)	184
Vincristine	2-weekly × 5			5/5[a]	19–49	185
BCNU	100 (during maintenance)					
Methothrexate	500(iv), 12 (Ivt) weekly × 5					
Dexamethasone	8/day × 36					
Procarbazine	100 on days 1–14			10/16[a]	10+ (median)	186
CCNU	75 on day 1					
Vincristine	1.4 on days 1, 8					
CCNU	100 every 6 weeks		2/6	4/6	18.5 (mean)	187
Cisplatin	90 maximum					
Vincristine	1.5 8 courses					
Eight drugs in one day			5/9	1/9	2-year progression-free survival: 24%	188

[a]Partial plus complete responses.
ST, stable disease; PR, partial response; CR, complete response.

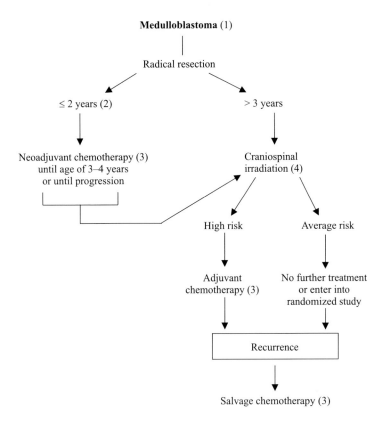

Fig. 12.7 Treatment algorithm in medulloblastomas.

corticosteroids, as 50% of patients with PCNSL respond to their administration, and occasionally the lymphomas disappear completely. In lymphomas, glucocorticosteroids have a cytolytic effect which may take place within 24 hours and compromise the pathological diagnosis. This cytolytic effect is usually transient, but it may persist for years, even after complete drug discontinuation (190). At diagnosis 10–30% of patients present CSF abnormalities characterized by moderately increased lymphocyte count, and high protein. Low glucose and oligoclonal fractionation of globulins occur in up to 20% of the cases. Approximately 10% of the patients have ocular (vitreous, retina, or choroid, Fig. 5.12) involvement. In patients with typical MRI or CT scan changes, and with retinal or vitreous lesions, biopsy is not mandatory, providing monoclonal lymphocytes are demonstrated in the CSF. In the absence of a history of systemic lymphoma and clinically detectable disease in lymph nodes, other staging investigations are not necessary.

Therapy

Surgery
Surgical resection adds little to survival compared to supportive care and should be discouraged (191,192).

Radiation therapy   Radiation therapy is less effective at controlling local disease in cerebral PCNSL than systemic lymphomas of similar pathology. While the response rate to irradiation is high, patients with primary brain lymphoma almost invariably relapse within or outside the high-dose volume, and a few (8%) outside the nervous system (193). Radiation therapy combined with glucocorticosteroids has increased the median survival from a few to 12–18 months (191,192,194). Retrospective studies suggest the lack of a dose–response relationship for doses above 4500 cGy, and intensification of irradiation does not improve survival (194). The current recommendation (195,196) is to treat the whole brain, including part of the orbit, with 4500 cGy in 180 cGy daily fractions, followed by a 1500 cGy boost to tumour volume. The whole orbit, including the eye, is irradiated with 2000–3000 cGy when ocular involvement is demonstrated. Spinal axis irradiation with 3000 cGy in 150 cGy fractions is recommended when spinal meninges are invaded macroscopically.

Chemotherapy

Single-arm studies of primary chemotherapy followed by radiation therapy suggest increased survival of PCNSL patients (197). Regimens achieving a median survival of about 40 months include high-dose methotrexate (MTX), and some contain drugs considered to cross the blood–brain barrier, such as hydroxyurea–procarbazine–CCNU–vincristine combination (198). De Angelis *et al.* (199) treated 31 patients with high-dose (1 g/m^2) systemic and intra-ventricular MTX, followed by irradiation and post-radiation cytosine arabinoside (3 g/m^2). The median survival was 42 months, with 55% of patients surviving at 3 years. Similar results were obtained by Glass *et al.* (200) with pre-irradiation high-dose (3.5 g/m^2) MTX. The CHOP combination (cyclophosphamide, Adriamycin®, vincristine, and prednisone), commonly used in systemic lymphomas given prior to irradiation, does not prolong survival (201).

In terms of CNS toxicity, the risk of combining high-dose chemotherapy with irradiation is serious, especially in older patients, where the incidence of leucoencephalopathy and severe dementia approaches 50% (202,203). The median survival after radiation therapy alone of patients over 60 years is only 7.6 months (194) and the alternative approach in older patients tested in prospective studies is primary chemotherapy alone. This approach is feasible, and high-dose methotrexate followed by maintenance chemotherapy may provide a high rate of complete responses without CNS toxicity (204–206), although currently without evidence of long-term survival benefit. These results are in agreement with the study of Neuwelt *et al.* (207) where intra-arterial MTX was used after disruption of the blood–brain barrier in conjunction with systemic cyclophosphamide and procarbazine. Patients did not receive radiation therapy and had a median survival of 44.5 months with little cognitive sequelae.

Treatment algorithm in PCNSL

The main points of the algorithm (Fig. 12.8) are:

1. Current optimum therapy in patients below 60 years of age is primary chemotherapy containing high-dose methotrexate followed by radiotherapy.
2. The optimum chemotherapy regimen has not been defined.
3. Newer approaches consider reduced doses of irradiation or avoiding radiotherapy, particularly in older patients.

Metastatic tumours

This section describes the management of metastases involving the brain, the leptomeninges, or the spinal epidural space. Not all metastases, however, are confined to a single site, as parenchymal brain metastases may disseminate via the CSF pathway into the leptomeninges. Leptomeningeal seedings may also extend into brain parenchyma following perivascular Virchow–Robin spaces.

CNS metastases cannot be considered in isolation. The survival of patients with CNS metastases depends largely on the extent and activity of primary tumour and systemic metastases, and the efficacy of therapy directed towards the control of CNS disease cannot be measured by survival alone. As the main aim of treatment of metastatic disease is palliation, effectiveness of treatment for CNS metastases should be assessed primarily in terms of symptom control, functional benefit (such as improvement in neurological deficit), and quality of life.

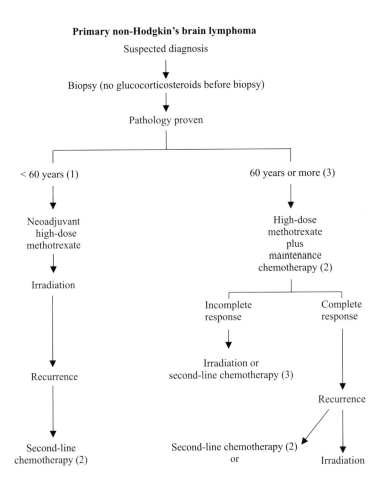

Fig. 12.8   Treatment algorithm in primary CNS lymphomas.

Brain metastases

Brain metastases are the most common malignant brain tumours in the adult, and the most frequent structural neurological complications seen in cancer patients (208). The distribution of primary cancers giving raise to brain metastases is given in Table 1.3. On MRI at least two-thirds of brain metastases are multiple at diagnosis (209). Lung cancer and melanoma metastases are more frequently multiple, while single metastases are more common in colorectal and renal carcinomas.

Supportive care

Brain metastases are often surrounded by a vasogenic **oedema** and this is largely responsible for neurological manifestations. Symptoms may be relieved within few days by gluco-corticosteroids. Glucocorticosteroid dosage has not been standardized and many clinicians initiate therapy with a daily dose of 16 mg dexamethasone or 80 mg methylprednisolone. However, a randomized study comparing 4, 8, and 16 mg dexamethasone daily, demonstrated equal outcome with less toxicity for the low dexamethasone dose (210). In the case of impending herniation, an initial loading with 100 mg dexamethasone has been recommended. In patients with signs of cerebral herniation, 20% intravenous mannitol solution may be used as an emergency treatment.

   Prolonged glucocorticosteroid use is associated with troublesome side-effects, that may be minimized by avoiding extended use of unnecessarily high doses. Even during radiation therapy, the daily dose of dexamethasone can be reduced from 8 to 2 mg and discontinued at completion of treatment. Weissman *et al.* reported that in 14 patients who completed radiation therapy, dexamethasone needed to be restarted within 30 days in only one (211).

   Epileptic seizures are the first manifestation of brain metastases in 15–25% of patients, and 15% more have seizures during the course of the disease. The treatment of symptomatic tumour-related seizures is considered in Chapter 3 (p. 57). We no longer use anti-epileptic prophylaxis in patients with brain metastases, although it has been recommended in patients with melanoma brain metastases (212).

Antineoplastic therapy

The choice of therapy for brain metastases is determined by several factors:

1. The extent and the control of the primary malignancy, which largely determine survival.
2. The pathology of the primary tumour.
3. The number and the location of cerebral lesions.

A meta-analysis of the RTOG studies defined four independent prognostic factors for survival in patients with brain metastases: (1) age, (2) extent of extracranial disease, (3) one versus several brain metastases, and (4) performance status. Patients with four favourable factors had a median survival of 7 months, and patients with only one favourable factor a median survival of 3 months (213).

   Patients with widespread, uncontrolled cancer and brain metastases therefore have a short life expectancy, and survival is unlikely to be significantly improved even by the most effective control of cerebral disease. The primary aim of treatment of brain metastases is to improve quality of life with minimal inconvenience and morbidity. A short course of palliative, whole-brain radiation therapy (WBRT) fulfils these requirements.

In patients whose primary tumour is either undiagnosed or controlled, the quality and the duration of survival are heavily related to the treatment of malignant brain lesions. There are a number of treatment options available for this group of patients.

Surgery

In patients with suspected brain metastases, surgery helps to confirm the histological diagnosis and may reveal an unexpected pathology (214). However, it is not appropriate in the context of known malignancy with a clear predisposition to CNS spread and within an expected time frame. The therapeutic benefit of surgery is based on two prospective and randomized studies (215,216) which have demonstrated that in selected patients with brain metastases surgical resection combined with post-operative WBRT is associated with better survival and CNS disease control than WBRT alone. However, one randomized trial did not confirm this observation (217). In the first randomized study of 48 patients comparing biopsy plus WBRT with complete resection followed by WBRT (12 daily fractions of 300 cGy), the patients who had resection had fewer local recurrences (20% versus 52%) and longer survival and functional independence (median 38 versus 8 weeks) (215). In the second study, 63 patients were randomized to resection plus WBRT or WBRT alone, consisting of 4000 cGy given in 10 days in two daily 200 cGy fractions. Patients in the surgical group had a prolonged median survival (10 versus 6 months), with a trend towards a longer functional independence. However, the benefit was only seen in patients with controlled systemic disease. In both studies the primary tumours were predominantly non-small-cell lung carcinomas, and all patients had single brain metastasis. In conclusion, while there is some uncertainty about the definite value of surgical resection in patients with accessible solitary metastases, the concensus view is that excision is the treatment of choice in patients who have controlled primary disease.

The value of surgery in patients with multiple brain metastases is debatable. Some studies suggest prolonged survival in patients where all lesions were surgically removed (218). However, the results could have been biased by selection of patients with favourable prognostic factors.

Radiation therapy

Less than one-third of brain metastases are single and at least half of them cannot be resected, due to the patient's general condition, progressive systemic disease, or tumour location. WBRT therefore remains the main treatment in the majority of patients with brain metastases. There is no survival or tumour control difference between regimens ranging from 2000 cGy in 5 fractions to 5000 cGy in 20 fractions, and short palliative fractionation is recommended. An RTOG study published in 1980 (219) showed no difference in survival, time to neurological progression, or rate of response between 2000 cGy in 5 fractions, 3000 cGy in 10 fractions, 3000 cGy in 15 fractions, 4000 cGy in 15 fractions, or 4000 cGy in 20 fractions. A second RTOG study (220), where only patients with minimal or controlled systemic cancer were randomized (a selection that makes survival evaluation a more meaningful criterion), found no difference between 3000 cGy in 10 fractions and 5000 cGy in 20 fractions. As a consequence, WBRT with 3000 cGy in 10 daily 300 cGy fractions became a standard therapy in many, but not in all, centres.

The use of hypoxic cell **radiosensitizers** (221) and **altered fractionation** has not demonstrated benefit in the treatment of brain metastases. **Re-irradiation** with 1500–2000 cGy is occasionally used for further brain recurrence, but there is no evidence that this is useful and the overall results are poor (222,223).

The survival benefit of **external** WBRT has not been demonstrated and, if present, is likely to be modest, with a prolongation in the region of 1–2 months. However, prolonged control of brain metastases with WBRT in patients with circumscribed or controlled systemic cancer is likely to prolong survival (224).

Post-operative WBRT often follows surgical resection of brain metastases. Its use, uncertain for a long time (see Table 1 in ref. 225), was assessed in a randomized multicentre trial that enrolled 95 patients with macroscopically totally resected single brain metastasis (225). Forty-nine patients received 5040 cGy WBRT over 5 1/2 weeks (140 cGy × 28 fractions). Recurrence of the tumour anywhere in the brain was found in 18% (9/49 patients) in the radiotherapy group, versus 70% (32/46 patients) in the control group (P < 0.001). Recurrences at the site of tumour removal or elsewhere in the brain were both statistically lower in the radiation therapy group. Irradiated patients were less likely to die of neurological causes, but the overall survival of 48 weeks in the radiation-therapy group and 43 weeks in the observation group were not statistically different. The authors interpreted the high rate of local recurrence in non-irradiated patients as an indication that surgery does not achieve microscopic tumour excision, and the recurrence in other parts of the brain in non-irradiated patients indicates an early and widespread dissemination of tumour emboli. They recommended post-operative WBRT to decrease neurological complications and neurological death. The failure to significantly prolong survival was attributed by Patchell et al. (225) to the progression of the systemic disease. A similar conclusion was reached by Smalley et al. in a non-randomized study comparing the outcome of 104 patients who received adjuvant WBRT with that of 118 patients treated only by resection of brain metastases. Only patients without active systemic cancer benefited from irradiation (226). However, it is permissible to arrive at an alternative conclusion. As additional WBRT does not prolong survival and is associated with morbidity, it could be reserved for patients with symptomatic progression of disease in the brain.

Prophylactic WBRT has been tested in several prospective and randomized trials that showed a significant reduction of brain metastases in patients with small-cell lung carcinoma, without effect on patients' survival (227–232). A recent meta-analysis including 987 patients with small-cell lung cancer in complete remission, who took part in seven trials comparing prophylactic cranial irradiation to no irradiation, showed a 5.4% increase in survival rate at 3 years in the treatment group (233). Unfortunately, the analysis does not report the rate of leucoencephalopathy and cognitive disorders. This worrying complication has been observed particularly in long-term survivors with brain metastases who have been treated by cranial irradiation and systemic chemotherapy (Chapter 2, p. 31, 33, 34). To minimize the risk of cognitive sequelae, prophylactic cranial irradiation should not be administered concurrently with chemotherapy, and probably not to elderly patients who are more prone to develop delayed post-radiation encephalopathy.

For non-small-cell lung cancer (NSCLC), a large co-operative study that included 1532 patients with complete surgical resection of the primary tumour led to the conclusion that 'prophylactic cranial irradiation would at best benefit a very small subset of patients' (234). The authors of this study do not believe that a randomized trial testing prophylactic WBRT in NSCLC is warranted. Currently there is no evidence that prophylactic cranial irradiation is of value in patients with NSCLC.

Stereotactic external radiation therapy

Linear accelerator or gamma knife radiosurgery is increasingly used to treat brain metastases. The use of stereotactic irradiation is limited to lesions less than 3–4 cm in diameter. In such lesions radiosurgery achieves immediate local tumour control in 80–90% of cases (235–240). The rate of local radionecrosis ranges from 0 to 7% and is related to lesion size and radiosurgery dose (241). Stereotactic irradiation can be used in patients with multiple brain metastases, although survival palliation benefit has not been demonstrated in comparison to WBRT, and is significantly shorter in patients with more than two metastases (242,243), with larger lesions, and infratentorial location (243). There has been no formal comparison between radiosurgery and surgery, and the choice of treatment depends on surgical accessibility and the availability of radiosurgical equipment (244,245). It seems unlikely that a prospective and randomized trial comparing surgery to radiosurgery will be performed in the foreseeable future.

Chemotherapy

Local treatment, such as surgery, stereotactic irradiation, or WBRT, is unlikely to prolong survival in many patients with brain metastases, as prognosis is frequently determined by the activity of systemic disease. The development of effective systemic therapy, including chemotherapy, is therefore essential for further progress. There are a number of limitations to the efficacy of chemotherapy. Many primary tumours are resistant to currently available drugs or develop resistance following exposure to chemotherapy. However, the potential limitation of poor drug penetration to the CNS due to the blood–brain barrier is largely theoretical, as most visible metastases enhance with contrast and therefore have a disrupted blood–tumour barrier. Clinical evidence summarized in Table 12.10 indicates that treatment efficacy is more likely to be related to tumour sensitivity rather than the drug's inability to cross the normal blood-brain barrier. In patients with chemosensitive tumours, brain metastases and extracranial metastatic disease respond equally to chemotherapy. The most chemosensitive brain metastases originate from germ-cell tumours (246,247) and choriocarcinoma (248), and chemotherapy, with the disappearance of brain as well as systemic disease, is the first-line treatment. The contribution of neurosurgery or radiosurgery in choriocarcinoma brain metastases is not clear, but is considered in patients with drug resistance and those with visible residual masses (248).

Breast carcinoma brain metastases respond to chemotherapy, as observed in a preliminary study (249) and confirmed in a series of 100 patients by Rosner et al. (250). The drug combinations and doses used (Table 12.10) were as those given in extracerebral disease despite

Table 12.10 Response of brain metastases to systemic chemotherapy

Primary tumour	Number of patients	Treatment	All responders (CR)	Median survival (months)	References
Germ-cell tumours	8	VCR, MTX (high dose), BLM + CDDP, VP-16, CP, ACM	7 (6)		246
Germ-cell tumours	12	Various drugs + irradiation	10 (8)	29.9 single metastasis / 13.7 multiple metastases	247
Choriocarcinoma	18	VP-16, MTX, ACM alternating with VCR, CP	13 (13)	All surviving median follow-up to 33 months	248
Breast carcinoma	11	CCNU, VCR, MTX	5	7	249
Breast carcinoma	52	CP, 5FU, P	27	CR: 39.5	250
Breast carcinoma	35	CP, 5FU, P, MTX, VCR	19 — Overall : 50 (10)	PR: 10.5	
Breast carcinoma	7	MTX, VCR, P	3	NR: 1.5	
Breast carcinoma	6	CP, ADM	1		
Breast carcinoma	22	CDDP, VP-16	12 (5)	14 + RT	251
Breast carcinoma	20	CP, MTX, 5FU	13 (2)	Overall: 5	252
Breast carcinoma	2	CP, ADM, 5FU	(>6 weeks)		
SCLC	9	VP-16 (high dose: 1.0–1.5 g every 4 weeks)	4 (1)	Few months	255
SCLC	26	VM-26 (150 mg/m² x 3 every 3 weeks)	11 (4)	R: 10, NR = 3	256
SCLC	8	VM-26 (120 mg/m² x 3 every 3 weeks)	3 (2)	R > 9	257
SCLC	19	CP, VCR, VP-16	10 (1)	7 + RT	258
SCLC (12 studies)	116	Various drugs including VP-16 or VM-26, CDDP or carboplatin	76% (43%) at diagnosis / 43% (18%) at relapse		259
SCLC	6	CDDP, 5FU	4 (2)	12+	261
Non-SCLC	10	CDDP, 5FU	4 (1)	9+	
Melanoma	39	Fotemustin (a nitrosourea)	10	6.5	262

Abbreviations: CR, complete response; PR, partial response; R, responders; NR, non-responders; ACM, actinomycin; ADM, Adriamycin®; BLM, bleomycin; CDDP, cisplatin; CP, cyclophosphamide; 5FU, 5-fluorouracil; MTX, methotrexate; VCR, vincristine; VM-26, teniposide; VP-16, etoposide; RT, radiation therapy; SCLC, small-cell lung cancer.

the fact that not all drugs used readily cross the normal blood–brain barrier. Half of the patients responded with 10% complete remission and 40% partial remission, which is equivalent to the systemic response rate, suggesting the similar effectiveness of chemotherapy on cerebral and systemic disease. Patients responding to chemotherapy had better survival than non-responders and this was also found in other studies (251,252). In addition, case reports have demonstrated clinical and radiological improvement of breast cancer brain metastases after administration of tamoxifen (253,254).

Several studies summarized by Kristensen *et al.* (259) have documented the sensitivity of small-cell lung cancer brain metastases to chemotherapy (255–259). The efficacy of chemotherapy was also demonstrated in a study of patients with predominantly non-small-cell lung carcinoma randomly allocated to WBRT given alone or in combination with two nitrosourea-based chemotherapy combinations (260). Responses have also been observed in phase II studies in patients with non-small-cell lung cancer (261) and melanoma brain metastases (262), although they reflected the limited chemosensitivity of these tumours.

Intra-arterial chemotherapy

Despite the evidence that intra-arterial infusion achieves higher tumour drug concentration than intravenous administration (263) this treatment modality is not recommend in patients with brain metastases. Microscopic metastases may be present in non-perfused territories, and intra-arterial chemotherapy is associated with a risk of CNS and eye toxicity, previously described for patients treated for primary tumours. In addition, the currently reported results are not clearly superior to those achieved with systemic chemotherapy.

Treatment algorithm in brain metastases

The main points of the algorithm (Fig. 12.9) are:

1. Performance status, age, and the extent and degree of control of the systemic malignant disease are the principal prognostic factors for survival, and largely determine therapeutic choice.

2. We favour radiosurgery in patients with small (one or two) brain metastases, in preference to surgery.

3. The choice of chemotherapy should be based on tumour pathology and presumed chemosensitivity in the context of acquired resistance due to previous chemotherapy exposure.

Leptomeningeal metastases

Leptomeningeal metastases occur in four main categories of malignant diseases:

(1) primary brain tumours, especially in childhood;

(2) acute leukaemias;

(3) non-Hodgkin's lymphomas; and

(4) solid tumours (see Table 1.4).

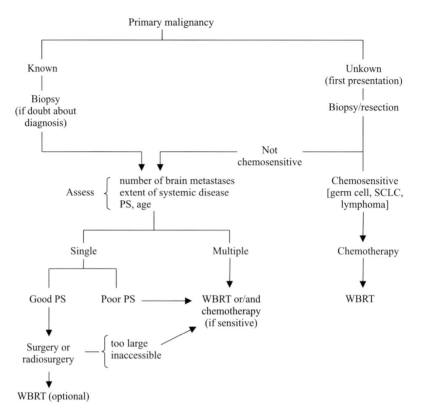

Fig. 12.9   Treatment algorithm in brain metastases. Abbreviations: PS, performance status; WBRT, whole-brain radiation therapy; SCLC, small-cell lung cancer.

These four groups differ considerably in their response to treatment. Three therapeutic modalities are used in the treatment of leptomeningeal metastases: radiotherapy, intra-CSF, and systemic chemotherapy.

Treatment modalities

Radiotherapy
Craniospinal irradiation to the whole CSF space is used as part of primary therapy in patients with a high risk of CSF seeding, such as medulloblastoma. In patients with established meningeal disease it is reserved as adjuvant treatment to consolidate complete microscopic remission following intrathecal chemotherapy in lymphoma and occasionally leukaemia. In this situation it is part of the curative treatment approach.

In the majority of patients with solid tumours external irradiation is limited to bulky radiological lesions or clinically symptomatic sites. The aim of external irradiation is to palliate symptoms, re-establish normal CSF flow in patients with CSF block, and relieve radicular pain.

Intrathecal irradiation has the theoretical advantage of limiting irradiation to the neuraxis, but it is seldom used in practice. The use of radioactive nuclides such as gold or yttrium is limited by toxicity. Radiolabelled monoclonal antibodies have been used experimentally and promising results were obtained in patients with medulloblastoma meningitis (264).

Chemotherapy

Systemic chemotherapy is able to act on neoplastic lesions located *in* and *outside* the leptomeninges. The considerations are similar to those for the use of systemic chemotherapy in patients with parenchymal brain metastases. Even hydrophilic drugs may achieve therapeutic concentrations in the CSF because the blood–brain barrier may either be altered by meningeal malignant infiltration or overwhelmed by high drug doses, such as 2–3 g/m^2 of cytosine arabinoside (Ara-C) and high-dose methotrexate (MTX) (265). Solid meningeal metastases are likely to behave as brain metastases.

Intra-CSF chemotherapy is used to circumvent the blood–brain barrier, and achieve therapeutic concentrations in the CSF. However, drugs such as MTX enter systemic circulation at a low, but persistent and potentially toxic concentration. Tumour penetration of intrathecally administered drugs is limited to a few millimetres and it is therefore unlikely to be a useful treatment for solid masses.

Intra-CSF chemotherapy is largely restricted to MTX, Ara-C, and thiotepa. The latter has a very short CSF half-life. They have a limited activity against most leptomeningeal metastases originating from solid tumours as they are not particularly effective in the systemic setting. Other drugs have been tested for intra-CSF use. Diaziquone (AZQ), an alkylating agent, was administered intraventricularly twice a week at a dose of 1 or 2 mg, or as a concentration × time ($C \times t$) schedule of 0.5 mg every 6 hours × 3 weekly (266). The dose-limiting factor was dose-related headache. ACNU, a nitrosourea, was shown to be safe up to 10 mg weekly when dissolved in 95 ml of artificial CSF and infused over 45 minutes (267). The use of mafosfamide, that breaks down in the CSF spontaneously to an active metabolite of cyclophosphamide, is limited to a total dose of 5 mg by severe headaches (268). Topotecan, an inhibitor of topoisomerase I, is currently under investigation.

Intraventricular administration through the Ommaya reservoir (or similar devices) is preferred to **intrathecal** injection, which requires repeated lumbar punctures. The intraventricular (Ivt) route offers several additional advantages:

(1) the drug distribution is more predictable (especially in the ventricles) and is more uniform;

(2) it allows administration of multiple daily injections ($C \times t$ schedule);

(3) it avoids inadvertent drug injection outside subarachnoid space; and

(4) it avoids subdural or epidural spinal haematoma in thrombocytopenic patients.

However, the implantation of an intraventricular reservoir is an invasive procedure associated with surgical morbidity, carries the risk of CNS infection, and predisposes to seizures (269).

Regardless of the route of administration, CSF chemotherapy requires normal CSF flow. This can be examined by an [^{111}In]DTPA radionuclide scan (270). In the presence of CSF block, local irradiation should precede intraventricular chemotherapy.

Treatment results

Treatment (Table 12.11) in meningeal metastases is used either prophylactically or as therapy for established disease. Prophylactic treatment aims to eradicate microscopic clinically asymptomatic seeding not detected by imaging or CSF examination. Salvage therapy aims to provide symptom control in patients with symptomatic disease.

Prophylactic treatment

Meningeal prophylaxis is used in primary brain tumours, mostly in children, acute leukaemias, and, rarely, non-Hodgkin's lymphomas (Table 12.11). Its benefit has been best demonstrated in medulloblastoma and acute lymphoblastic leukaemia.

In **medulloblastoma** prophylactic irradiation of the entire craniospinal axis is essential in all patients treated with radical radiotherapy with curative intent (see Fig. 12.7). The recommended prophylactic dose is 3500 cGy. High-risk patients (grade M1–M4) may benefit from higher doses, and new hyperfractionated and accelerated regimens are being tested. Lowering the irradiation dose to 2400 cGy in low-risk patients, combined with chemotherapy, is under investigation.

In **ependymomas** in the absence of demonstrable seeding there is no use of prophylactic irradiation of the spinal axis. The overall risk of meningeal seeding is less than 10%, but isolated meningeal relapse is rare (271) with the majority of CSF relapses occurring in patients with uncontrolled primary disease.

In **pineal or suprasellar germinomas**, meningeal dissemination occurs in more than 10–20% of patients (272–273). Prophylactic craniospinal irradiation with 3000 cGy may reduce the incidence of leptomeningeal seedings from 13 to 5% in histologically proven germinomas (274). However, this treatment is avoided increasingly (273,275,276) as the risk of seeding is lower in patients with negative CSF cytology and normal spinal and brain MRI. In addition, patients with isolated relapse may be effectively salvaged with subsequent treatment.

In **childhood acute lymphoblastic leukaemia** (ALL) CNS prophylaxis has reduced meningeal relapse from about 70% to less than 10%, and was the major step allowing a long-term cure in over 50% of children. The treatment has evolved over the years by replacing CNS irradiation with systemic chemotherapy in patients with low risk of meningeal seeding (277,278). In low-risk patients, intrathecal MTX combined with high-dose systemic MTX provides a protection equivalent to that achieved with irradiation (279,280). In high-risk children characterized by a leucocyte count over 50 000/mm^3, cranial irradiation is still recommended by some authors and the appropriate dose is under test. In other studies, cranial irradiation has been avoided through the use of extended intraventricular chemotherapy combining MTX, Ara-C and glycocorticosteroids, and intensive systemic chemotherapy (280,281). In some current ALL protocols for children, even Ivt and cerebrospinal irradiation are deleted, but not intrathecal chemotherapy. However, intensive chemotherapy including intrathecal administration is not without CNS

Table 12.11 Treatment in leptomeningeal metastases

Primary tumours	Prophylactic treatment		Salvage treatment modalities
	Use	Modalities	
Medulloblastomas	Standard procedure	Craniospinal RT: 3500 cGy; (?) 2500 cGy + ChT in low-risk patients	Standard or high-dose systemic ChT RT, if not previously used (Ivt ChT less commonly used)
Germinomas	Debatable	Craniospinal RT: 2400–3000 cGy	
Acute lymphoblastic leukaemia			
in children	Standard procedure	Low risk: extended Ivt ChT; Average risk: extended + intensive systemic ChT; High risk: cranial RT, extended Ivt, and systemic ChT	High-dose systemic ChT
in adults	Standard procedure	Cranial RT (1800–2400 cGy), high-dose and Ivt ChT	Extended Ivt ChT
Acute myeloblastic leukaemia	Controversial	High-dose ± Ivt Ara-C	Radiation therapy
Non-Hodgkin's lymphomas	Controversial; BI: lymphoblastic or Burkitt's lymphoma	Ivt MTX (4–6 doses); or high-dose systemic MTX; or Ara-C	Ivt ChT; Craniospinal RT of symptomatic areas
Solid tumours	Not used	–	Systemic ChT, especially if progressive systemic disease

Abbreviations: BI, best indication; ChT, chemotherapy; RT, radiation therapy, Ivt, intraventricular; (?), still questionable.

toxicity, and a long-term advantage in cognitive function in older children has not been demonstrated in comparison those treated with low-dose cranial irradiation.

In **adults**, progress made in the treatment of ALL has led to an increased rate of CNS relapse to 30–50% (282,283). The benefit of CNS prophylaxis in adults with ALL has been shown in several studies summarized by Gökbuget and Hoelzer (284). Prophylaxis combines high-dose MTX (1.5–3 g/m^2) as part of systemic leukaemia treatment, Ivt MTX or Ara-C, and cranial irradiation. Intraventricular chemotherapy starts during induction and continues during maintenance chemotherapy. Cranial irradiation is given to doses of 1800–2400 cGy in daily fractions of 180–200 cGy.

In **acute myeloblastic leukaemia** (AML), where systemic treatment is less effective, meningeal recurrence is less frequent than in ALL, and the benefit of meningeal prevention remains uncertain.

Comparison of two consecutive POG studies failed to show the benefit of cranial irradiation on event-free survival (285,286). The general consensus is that the use of intermediate to high-dose Ara-C with Ivt Ara-C decreases the incidence of meningeal relapse without significantly prolonging survival.

In **non-Hodgkin's lymphomas**, leptomeningeal involvement occurs in up to 20% of the patients. The main risk factors are high histological grade and advanced clinical stage (287). The benefit of meningeal prophylaxis is unproven and the appropriate type of prophylaxis is not defined (287,288). Patients with lymphoblastic or Burkitt's lymphoma with bulky disease and bone-marrow involvement (289) and patients with testicular and Waldeyer's ring presentation of diffuse large-cell lymphoma are at particularly high risk of meningeal relapse. A retrospective analysis of 553 patients with systemic non-Hodgkin's lymphoma failed to show any benefit of CNS prophylaxis in intermediate or high-grade tumours (288) with three or more intrathecal administrations of MTX 10 mg/m^2 or systemic high-dose Ara-C with or without intrathecal MTX.

Treatment of established meningeal disease

The primary aim of salvage therapy is to improve or stabilize neurological condition, achieve symptom control, and possibly prolong survival. As in patients with brain parenchymal metastases, survival is largely related to the control of systemic malignancy. Therefore the efficacy of salvage therapy is assessed primarily by its palliative benefit, which tends to parallel CSF clearing of neoplastic cells. However, CSF cytology is not a satisfactory endpoint as up to 40% of patients with leptomeningeal carcinomatosis at autopsy have negative CSF cytology (290). Treatment efficacy therefore cannot rely solely on quantitative changes in neoplastic cell count in the CSF.

Overt meningeal metastases require intensive treatment administrated urgently, as untreated patients rapidly lose consciousness and die. Radiation therapy, intra-CSF and systemic chemotherapy are often used concomitantly, and their individual contribution is difficult to separate. Intra-CSF drug administration is often regarded as the mainstay of treatment of leptomeningeal seedings. However, this assumption has been questioned (291).

Treatment of leptomeningeal leukaemia

Clinically symptomatic or asymptomatic meningeal leukaemia (≥5 blasts per mm^3 of CSF) may either be present at diagnosis or occur during or after cessation of antileukaemic therapy.

Meningeal leukaemia discovered at diagnosis is usually chemosensitive prior to the development drug resistance. It is not a poor prognostic factor in children with ALL treated with intensive systemic and intrathecal chemotherapy, including irradiation (292). Even avoiding irradiation does not seem to increase the rate of meningeal relapse (293).

In adults, however, most authors use additional CNS-directed treatment, with 3–5 doses of Ivt MTX followed by cranial irradiation and monthly Ivt maintenance therapy. This treatment negates the additional adverse prognosis of meningeal involvement at diagnosis (284), although the prognosis remains that of stage IV disease.

Meningeal ALL occurring during or within 6 months following completion of therapy carries a poor prognosis. Patients are often treated with craniospinal irradiation, intensive chemotherapy, and bone-marrow transplantation. Meningeal relapse occurring later is associated with better prognosis, and long-term survival may be achieved without bone-marrow transplantation.

In patients with meningeal AML Ara-C tends to be preferred to MTX, although the superiority of Ara-C has not been demonstrated convincingly.

In patients with acute leukaemia irradiation of the whole craniospinal axis with 1800–2400 cGy may contribute to bone-marrow toxicity and jeopardize the use of intensive systemic chemotherapy necessary to treat the frequently associated bone-marrow relapse. Extended Ivt chemotherapy and intensive systemic chemotherapy are often used combined with cranial irradiation alone.

Treatment of lymphomatous meningitis

The responsiveness to treatment of lymphomatous meningitis falls between that of acute leukaemia and solid tumours. The combination of intra-CSF MTX or Ara-C with external irradiation clears the CSF in up to 80% of patients (287,294–296). However, most clinical and CSF responses tend to be short lasting, with a 1-year survival rate of 12–16%. The poor prognosis is largely related to the progression of systemic disease, and favours the use of systemic chemotherapy. Siegal *et al.* reported 13 patients with lymphomatous meningitis treated by systemic chemotherapy and radiation therapy omitting intrathecal chemotherapy (297). Chamberlain and Kormanik treated 22 patients with lymphomatous meningitis (298), of which 16 with active systemic disease also had systemic chemotherapy The median survival was 10 months, but six patients treated with intensive chemotherapy and bone-marrow transplant did not have a superior outcome when compared to standard chemotherapy. These studies (297,298) support the use of systemic chemotherapy, especially in patients with extraneural lesions. They also confirm the neurotoxicity of brain irradiation combined with intensive systemic chemotherapy, with leucoencephalopathy on MRI in long-term survivors (297).

Treatment of leptomeningeal metastases of solid tumours

The prognosis of patients with leptomeningeal metastases from solid tumours is poor, due to the difficulty of eradicating meningeal disease in the context of progressive systemic cancer. The therapy has been derived from the treatment used in meningeal leukaemia and has not improved substantially over the past decades. Treatment is based on Ivt administration of MTX or Ara-C, which are poorly active in most solid tumours causing meningeal carcinomatosis, and on irradiation of symptomatic areas of the brain and spine.

MTX remains the drug of choice for Ivt administration. Because meningeal infiltration interferes with drug clearance, MTX concentration in the CSF is unpredictable.

Maintenance of MTX concentration close to the therapeutic level of 10^{-6} M requires monitoring. After the disappearance of neoplastic cells from the CSF, weekly Ivt administration is usually maintained until the clinical condition improves or stabilizes, and this is followed by monthly injections. The maintenance of Ivt therapy is based on the assumption that rapid relapse will follow treatment discontinuation. However, Siegal *et al.* (297) reported patients with prolonged response after stopping treatment and stressed the role of systemic chemotherapy. Systemic chemotherapy has several advantages. It is potentially active on the systemic malignant disease, has the potential to treat bulky meningeal lesions and to diffuse in the entire subarachnoid space, even in patients with CSF block. Lipophilic and hydrophilic drugs used in high (or very high) dose may reach therapeutic concentration in the CSF. However, the efficacy of systemic chemotherapy is limited by the intrinsic and acquired chemoresistance of the primary tumours, and its administration may be precluded or delayed by Ivt chemotherapy and craniospinal irradiation. The evaluation of treatment in meningeal carcinomatosis is complicated by the lack of standardization of treatment and evaluation criteria, and reliance on single-arm retrospective studies, which include a limited number of patients. With these limitations in mind, the published analysis of the literature (299) concerning the efficacy of intra-CSF chemotherapy associated with irradiation of selected areas of the craniospinal axis provides the following information.

1. Improvement or stabilization of the neurological status was observed in one- to two-thirds of patients with breast cancer leptomeningeal carcinomatosis treated in 11 trials. Responders had a mean or median survival of 5–6 months. Most patients who failed to respond survived 2 months or less. Fifteen per cent of patients survived 1–2 years.

2. The rate of response or stabilization also ranged from one- to two-thirds in patients with leptomeningeal carcinomatosis from small-cell or non-small-cell lung cancer investigated in 6 trials. The overall survival tended to be shorter than in patients with breast cancer, and 1-year survivors were exceptional.

3. The prognosis of patients with primary melanoma was dismal.

4. In a third of patients with miscellaneous primaries death was attributed to the progression of the systemic cancer.

5. Although there are no clear predictors of response, it seems that patients with controlled systemic breast or small-cell lung cancer are most likely to benefit from Ivt chemotherapy combined with irradiation of selected areas of the cerebrospinal axis.

Epidural metastases

The primary aim of epidural metastasis management is to relieve pain, and to prevent or restore spinal cord dysfunction. The degree of functional impairment may correlate with survival. The chance of surviving 1 year was 73% for patients with preserved or restored ambulation but only 9% for the non-ambulant (300). Patients with primary non-Hodgkin's lymphoma (301) or solitary vertebral plasmacytoma (302) presenting with spinal epidural location have a favourable outcome which correlates with extent of disease and local therapy.

Four treatment modalities are available to treat epidural metastases: glucocorticosteroids, radiation therapy, hormone- and chemotherapy, and surgery.

Glucocorticosteroids

The administration of glucocorticosteroids provides effective pain relief in two patients out of three, often within 24 hours,. The analgesic effect and arrest in progression of neurological signs are the primary indications for their use. The therapeutic effect may be due to anti-oedema activity of glycocorticosteroids, which is not related to the pathology of the underlying tumour. Glucocorticosteroids also have an oncolytic activity in lymphoma and myeloma, and in lymphoma this effect may be rapid. Many clinicians start glucocorticosteroids with an intravenous bolus of 100 mg dexamethasone. However, a prospective randomized trial showed the high dose is not superior to an initial intravenous bolus of 10 mg dexamethasone followed by 4×4 mg daily (303), and we prefer the lower dose. In patients with impaired ambulation, the risk of developing a rapid and severe pelvic amyotrophy is high and it is important to use glucocorticosteroids at the lowest possible dose for the shortest time.

There are no data indicating that in epidural metastases radiation therapy causes spinal oedema and worsens clinical signs. Therefore the protective use of glucocorticosteroids during irradiation is debatable.

External radiation therapy

Irradiation with 3000 cGy given in 10 fractions to the area including the metastatic lesion plus one to two vertebral bodies above and below is the mainstay therapy in most patients with epidural metastases.

Irradiation improves or completely relieves pain in about three patients out of four (304–306). In most series patients who have only pain do not become paraplegic after radiation therapy, and most remain ambulatory for the rest of their life (306–310). The effect of radiation therapy on neurological impairment depends upon the degree of the clinical deficit. The overall rate of improvement is around 40% (see Table 4 in ref. 311), but recovery of ambulation is only 5–10% in paraplegic patients (306,307,309). Another prognostic factor for the clinical response is tumour radiosensitivity. In one study 71% of paraparetic patients become ambulatory after irradiation if they had radiosensitive tumours, but only 34% with less radiosensitive cancers regained ambulation (306). However, even in patients with radiosensitive tumours, functional improvement does not generally start before the end of the first week of irradiation.

Many clinicians are reluctant to advise **re-irradiation** in patients who relapse locally because of fear of delayed radiation myelopathy (Chapter 7, p. 143). This risk depends on the initial dose, time from first radiotherapy, and the estimate of life expectancy, as well as the likelihood of obtaining worthwhile benefit. Schiff *et al.* (312) irradiated 54 patients with a median dose of 2425 cGy who have previously received a median dose of 3000 cGy. The benefits of re-irradiation were similar to the results obtained in patients with first irradiation. Only 12% of patients who were ambulatory after re-irradiation deteriorated before death, which could be ascribed either to radiation myelopathy or failure of treatment. The median survival after re-irradiation was 4.7 months. Re-irradiation used judiciously may therefore preserve ambulation, often with a limited risk of radiation myelopathy.

Chemotherapy and hormone therapy

Epidural metastases are not protected by a blood–CNS barrier, and may be treated as effectively as other systemic tumour locations by anticancer agents, including hydrophilic drugs. Tamoxifen and androgen suppressors may play a role in the treatment of epidural metastases originating from breast or prostate carcinoma. Cytotoxic agents may be effective in patients with lymphoma, neuroblastoma, Ewing's sarcoma, myeloma, germ-cell tumours, breast carcinoma, and small-cell lung cancer. However, the speed of the effect of chemotherapy depends on the predicted efficacy of each specific tumour type. Therefore, in patients with epidural metastases from common solid tumours such as breast or prostate, chemo- and hormone therapy should be used in combination with more rapidly effective treatments, such as radiation therapy or surgery.

In patients with highly chemosensitive tumours, such as lymphoma or testicular teratoma, with no or very mild neurological deficit, chemotherapy may be the initial treatment (313). This strategy will eliminate or delay the need for surgical decompression. In stage I and II non-Hodgkin's lymphoma, subsequent local radiotherapy is associated with improved survival.

Surgery

Two main approaches are used in the surgical treatment of epidural metastases.

Posterior laminectomy allows spinal cord decompression and the removal of tumour tissue located posteriorly and laterally. A **posterolateral** approach, which is also based on laminectomy, permits a more circumferential decompression of the dural sac but does not allow anterior stabilization. Several retrospective studies (306–308) and one small prospective study (314) failed to demonstrate a difference in neurological outcome between patients treated by laminectomy plus radiation therapy or radiation therapy alone. In addition, laminectomy carries an increased morbidity, and is associated with an increased risk of spinal instability, especially when vertebral body and pedicles are destroyed by the tumour. Laminectomy may still be indicated in patients with posteriorly located radioresistant metastases, and in patients who continue to deteriorate during or after irradiation. Laminectomy is also a useful diagnostic procedure. The claim that CT-guided needle biopsy is an equally efficacious diagnostic technique (315) needs confirmation.

The **anterolateral** approach seems more rational than posterior laminectomy (316) since, in most patients, the neoplastic process is located anteriorly and invades the vertebral body. This procedure allows the resection of destroyed and often collapsed vertebral bodies, decompression of nerve root or roots on the side of the surgical approach, replacement of the resected vertebral bodies, and anterior stabilization. However, anterolateral approach is a difficult surgical technique that carries a risk of major complications (317). It must be carefully planned, requires experienced surgeons, and should be only considered for patients in good general condition and with a reasonable life expectancy.

Treatment algorithm in spinal epidural metastases

The most important predictor for the effectiveness of treatment is the level of neurological function at the start of therapy. The outcome therefore depends on early diagnosis and prompt therapy, whichever treatment modality is chosen. The main points of the algorithm (Fig 12.10) are:

1. In patients known to harbour a systemic cancer, the diagnosis of epidural metastasis may be based on imaging alone.

2. When epidural metastasis is the first manifestation of cancer, pathological confirmation is required. Posterior laminectomy is the most commonly used technique, although CT-guided biopsy may offer an equally effective and less-invasive diagnostic procedure.

3. In lymphomas or teratomas presenting with spinal cord compression, glucocorticosteroids and chemotherapy are the first-line therapy when the neurological deficit is either absent or minimal.

4. In most radiosensitive tumours, radiotherapy is the first-line therapy, and may be combined with chemotherapy, usually given after completion of radiotherapy.

5. Patients with radioresistant tumour, collapsed vertebral body, or spine instability are the best candidates for an anterolateral approach in the light of their general condition and life expectancy.

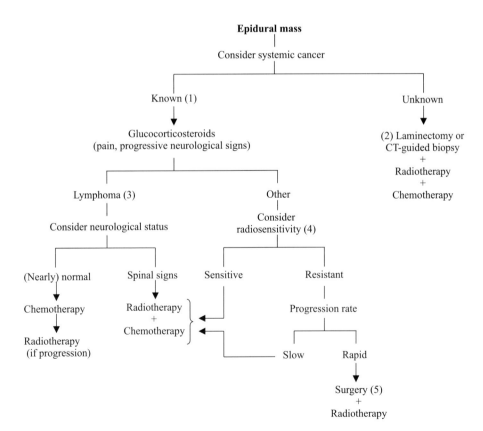

Fig. 12.10   Treatment algorithm in epidural metastases.

In patients with rapidly progressing paraparesis who have radioresistant tumour and can not undergo anterior surgery, there are two difficult decisions:

(1) Should laminectomy be performed before irradiation?

(2) When should laminectomy be performed in patients who continue to progress under irradiation?

These decisions rely largely on clinical judgement.

References

(1) MacDonald DR, Cascino TL, Schold SC, Cairncross JG. (1990). Response criteria for phase II studies of supratentorial malignant glioma. *J Clin Oncol*, **8**, 1277–1280.

(2) Grant R, Slattery J, Gregor A, Whittle IR. (1994). Recording neurological impairment in clinical trials of glioma. *J Neurooncol*, **19**, 37–49.

(3) Cairncross JG, Pexman JHW, Rathbone MP. (1985). Post-surgical contrast enhancement mimicking residual brain tumor. *Can J Neurol Sci*, **12**, 75.

(4) Byar DP, Green SB, Strike TA. (1983). Prognostic factors for malignant glioma. In: Oncology of the nervous system. Mahoney FI, Barthel DW (eds). Martinus Nijhoff, Boston, pp. 379–395.

(5) Hoshino T, Rodriquez LA, Cho KG *et al*. (1988). Prognostic implications of the proliferative potential of low-grade astrocytomas. *J Neurosurg*, **69**, 839–842.

(6) De Witte O, Levivier M, Violon PH *et al*. (1996). Prognostic value of positron emission tomography with [18F]fluorodeoxyglucose in low-grade gliomas. *Neurosurgery*, **39**, 470–477.

(7) Loiseau HP, Bousquet J, Rivel C *et al*. (1995). Astrocytomes de bas grade sus-tentoriels de l'adulte. *Neurochirurgie*, **41**, 38–50.

(8) Wilkinson IMS, Anderson JR, Holmes AE. (1987). Oligodendroglioma: An analysis of 42 cases. *J Neurol, Neurosurg Psychiatry*, **50**, 304–312.

(9) Shimizu KT, Tran LM, Mark RJ, Jelch MT. (1993). Management of oligodendrogliomas. *Radiology*, **186**, 569–572.

(10) Healey EA, Barnes PD, Kupsky WJ *et al*. (1991). The prognostic significance of postoperative residual tumour in ependymoma. *Neurosurgery*, **28**, 666–672.

(11) Evans AE, Jenkin RD, Sposto R *et al*. (1990). The treatment of medulloblastoma. Results of a prospective randomized trial of radiation therapy with or without CCNU, vincristine and prednisone. *J Neurosurg*, **72**, 572–582.

(12) Tait DM, Thonton-Jones H, Bloom HJG *et al*. (1990). Adjuvant chemotherapy for medulloblastoma: The first multicenter control trial of the International Society of Pediatric Oncology (SIOP I). *Europ J Cancer*, **26**, 464–469.

(13) Hochberg FH, Miller DC. (1988). Primary central nervous system lymphoma. *J Neurosurg*, **68**, 835–853.

(14) Deckert M, Reifenberger G, Wechsler W. (1989). Determination of the proliferative potential of human brain tumors using the monoclonal antibody Ki-67. *J Cancer Res Clin Oncol*, **115**, 179–188.

(15) Levivier M, Goldman S, Bidaut LM *et al*. (1992). Positron emission tomography-guided stereotactic brain biopsy. *Neurosurgery*, **31**, 792–797.

(16) Golfinos JG, Fitzpatrick BC, Smith LR, Spetzler RF. (1995). Clinical use of a frameless stereotactic arm: Results of 325 cases. *J Neurosurg*, **83**, 197–205.

(17) Leibel SA, Gutin PH, Davis RL. (1991). Factors affecting radiation therapy after interstitial brachytherapy of brain tumors. In: Radiation injury to the nervous system. Gutin PH, Leibel SA, Sheline GE (eds). Raven Press, New York, pp. 257–270.

(18) O'Neil A, Macapinlac H, De Angelis L. (1996 (abstract)). Positron emission tomography (PET) hypermetabolism with cerebral radionecrosis. *J Neurooncol*, **1**, 86.

(19) Soloway AH, Barth RF (eds). (1997). Boron neutron capture therapy of brain tumors. Current status and future prospects. *J Neurooncol*, **33**, 1–188.

(20) Morstyn G, Kaye AH (eds). (1990). Phototherapy of cancer. Harwood Academic, London.

(21) Zünkeler B, Carson RE, Olson J *et al.* (1996). Quantification and pharmacokinetics of blood–brain barrier disruption in humans. *J Neurosurg*, **85**, 1056–1065.

(22) Bartus RT. (1999). The blood–brain barrier as a target for pharmacological modulation. *Curr Opin Drug Discovery Develop*, **2**, 152–167.

(23) Gregor A, Lind M, Newman H *et al.* (1999). Phase II studies of RMP-7 and carboplatin in the treatment of recurrent high grade glioma. *J Neurooncology*, **44**, 137–145.

(24) Brem H (ed.) (1995). Local therapy of brain tumors. *J Neurooncology*, **26**, 89–158.

(25) Thompson RC, Brem H. (1999). Treatment of gliomas using polymer-drug delivery. In: The gliomas. Berger MS, Wilson CB (eds). Saunders Co, Philadelphia, pp. 555–563.

(26) Mahaley MS, Whaley RA, Blue M, Bertsch L. (1986). Central neurotoxicity following intracarotid BCNU chemotherapy for malignant gliomas. *J Neurooncol*, **3**, 297–314.

(27) Shapiro WR, Green SB, Burger PC *et al.* (1992). A randomized comparison of intra-arterial versus intravenous BCNU, with or without intravenous 5-fluorouracil, for newly diagnosed patients with malignant gliomas. *J Neurosurg*, **76**, 772–781.

(28) Hildebrand J, Badjou R, Collard-Ronge E *et al.* (1980). Treatment of brain gliomas with high doses of CCNU and autologous marrow transplantation. *Biomedicine*, **32**, 71–75.

(29) Hochberg FH, Parker LM, Takvorian T *et al.* (1981). High-dose BCNU with autologous bone marrow rescue for recurrent glioblastoma multiforme. *J Neurosurg*, **54**, 455–460.

(30) Phillips GL, Wolff SN, Fay JW *et al.* (1986). Intensive 1,3-bis (2-chloroethyl)-1-nitrosourea (BCNU) monochemotherapy and autologous marrow transplantation for malignant glioma. *J Clin Oncol*, **4**, 639–645.

(31) Giannone L, Wolff SN. (1987). Phase II treatment of central nervous system glioma with high-dose etoposide and autologous bone marrow transplantation. *Cancer Treat Rep*, **71**, 759–761.

(32) Fine HA, Antman KH. (1992). High dose chemotherapy with autologous bone marrow transplantation in the treatment of high grade astrocytoma in adults. Therapeutic rationale and clinical experience. *Bone Marow Transplant*, **10**, 315–321.

(33) Dubois CM, Ruscetti FW, Palaszynski EW *et al.* (1990). Transforming growth factor β is a potent inhibitor of interleukin 1 (IL-1) receptor expression: Proposed mechanism of inhibition of IL-1 action. *J Exp Med*, **172**, 737–744.

(34) Sawamura Y, Diserens A-C, de Tribolet N. (1990). *In vitro* prostaglandin E_2 production by glioblastoma cells and its effect on interleukin-2 activation of oncolytic lymphocytes. *J Neurooncol*, **9**, 125–130.

(35) Tada M, de Tribolet N. (1999). Tumor immunobiology. In: The gliomas. Berger MS, Wilson CB (eds). Saunders, Philadelphia, pp. 579–589.

(36) Chiocca EA, Breakefield XO. (1998). Gene therapy for neurological disorders and brain tumors. Humana Press, Totowa, New Jersey.

(37) Ram Z, Oldfield EH. (1999). Gene therapy for malignant brain tumors. In: The gliomas. Berger MS, Wilson CB (eds). Saunders, Philadelphia, pp. 157–163.

(38) Kleihues P, Burger PC, Plate KH *et al.* (1977). Glioblastoma. In: Pathology and genetics, tumours of the nervous system. Kleihues P, Cavenee WK (eds). IARC Library. Lyon, pp. 16–24.

(39) Burger PC. (1987). The anatomy of astrocytomas. *Mayo Clinic Proc*, **65**, 527–529.

(40) Halperin EC, Burger PC, Bullard DE. (1988). The fallacy of the localized supratentorial malignant glioma. *Int J Rad Oncol Biol Phys*, **15**, 505–509.

(41) Wood JR, Green SB, Shapiro WR. (1988). The prognostic importance of tumour size in malignant gliomas: A computed tomographic scan study by the Brain Tumor Cooperative Group. *J Clin Oncol*, **6**, 338–343.

(42) Simpson JR, Horton J, Scott C *et al.* (1993). Influence of location and extent on survival of patients with glioblastoma multiforme: results of three consecutive Radiation Therapy Oncology Group (RTOG) clinical trials. *Int J Radiol Oncol Biol Phys*, **26**, 239–244.

(43) Chandler KL, Prados MD, Malec M *et al.* (1993). Long-term survival in patients with glioblastoma multiforme. *Neurosurgery*, **32**, 716–720.

(44) Scott JN, Rewcastle NB, Brasher PMA *et al.* (1999). Which glioblastoma multiforme patient will become a long-term survivor. A population-based study. *Ann Neurol*, **46**, 183–188.

(45) Wisoff JH, Boyett JM, Berger MS *et al.* (1998). Current neurosurgical management and the impact of the extent of resection in the treatment of malignant gliomas of childhood: a report of the Children's Cancer Group Trial No. CCG-945. *J Neurosurg*, **89**, 52–59.

(46) Finlay JL, Boyett JM, Yates AJ *et al.* (1995). Randomized phase III trial in childhood high-grade astrocytoma comparing vincristine, lomustine and prednisone with eight-drugs-in-1-day regimen. *J Clin Oncol*, **13**, 112–123.

(47) Vecht ChJ, Avezaat CJJ, van Putten WLJ *et al.* (1990). The influence of the extent of surgery on the neurological function and survival in malignant glioma. A retrospective analysis of 243 patients. *J Neurol Neurosurg Psychiatry*, **53**, 466–471.

(48) Walker M, Alexander E Jr, Hunt W *et al.* (1978). Evaluation of BCNU and/or radiotherapy in the treatment of anaplastic gliomas. A cooperative clinical trial. *J Neurosurg*, **49**, 333–343.

(49) Trouillas P. (1973). Immunologie et immunothérapie des tumeurs cérébrales. *Etat Actuel Rev Neurol (Paris)*, **128**, 23–38.

(50) Kristiansen K, Hagen S, Kollevodt T *et al.* (1981). Combined modality therapy of operated astrocytomas grade III and IV. Confirmation of the value of postoperative irradiation and lack of potentiation of bleomycin on survival time: A prospective multicenter trial of the Scandinavian Glioblastoma Study Group. *Cancer*, **47**, 649–652.

(51) Reagan TJ, Bisel HF, Childs DS Jr *et al.* (1976). Controlled study of CCNU and radiation therapy in malignant astrocytoma. *J Neurosurg*, **44**, 186–190.

(52) Ciangfriglia F, Pompili A, Riccio A, Grassi A. (1980). CCNU-chemotherapy of supratentorial hemispheric glioblastoma multiforme. *Cancer*, **45**, 1289–1299.

(53) Shapiro WR, Young DF. (1976). Treatment of malignant glioma. *Arch Neurol*, **33**, 494–500.

(54) Walker MD, Strike TA, Sheline GE. (1979). An analysis of dose–effect relationship in the radiotherapy of malignant gliomas. *Int J Radiat Oncol Biol Phys*, **5**, 1725–1731.

(55) Chang CH, Horton J, Schoenfeld D *et al.* (1983). Comparison of postoperative radiotherapy and combined postoperative radiotherapy and chemotherapy in the multidisciplinary management of malignant gliomas. *Cancer*, **52**, 997–1007.

(56) Hochberg FH, Pruitt A. (1980). Assumptions in the radiotherapy of glioblastoma. *Neurology*, **30**, 907–911.

(57) Deutsch M, Green SB, Strike *et al.* (1989). Results of a randomized trial comparing BCNU plus radiotherapy, sterptozotocin plus radiotherapy, BCNU plus hyperfractionated radiotherapy, and BCNU following misonidazole plus radiotherapy in postoperative treatment of malignant glioma. *Int J Radiat Oncol Biol Phys*, **16**, 1389–1396.

(58) Horiot JC, van den Bogaert W, Ang KK *et al.* (1988). European Organization for Research on Treatment of Cancer trials using radiation therapy with multiple fractions per day. A 1978–1987 survey. *Front Radiat Ther Oncol*, **22**, 149–161.

(59) Brada M, Sharpe G, Rajan B *et al.* (1999). Modifying radical radiotherapy in high grade gliomas: shortening the treatment time through acceleration. *Int J Radiat Oncol Biol Phys*, **43**, 287–292.

(60) Wasserman TH, Stetz J, Phillips TL. (1981). Radiation Therapy Oncology Group clinical trials with misonidazole. *Cancer*, **47**, 2382–2390.

(61) Bleehen NM, Wiltshire CR, Plowman PN. (1981). A randomized study of misonidazole and radiotherapy for grade III and IV cerebral astrocytoma. *Br J Cancer*, **43**, 436–442.

(62) EORTC Brain Tumor Group. (1983). Misonidazole in radiotherapy of supratentorial malignant gliomas in adult patients: A randomized double-blind study. *Europ J Cancer Clin Oncol*, **19**, 39–42.

(63) Levin VA, Prados MD, Wara WM *et al.* (1995). Radiation therapy and bromodeoxyuridine chemotherapy followed by procarbazine, lomustine and vincristine for treatment of anaplastic gliomas. *Int J Radiat Oncol Biol Phys*, **32**, 75–83.

(64) Urtasun RC, Cosmatos D, Delrowe J *et al.* (1993). Iododeoxyuridine (IUdR) combined with radiation in the treatment of malignant glioma: A comparison of short vs long intravenous dose schedule (RTOG 86–12). *Int J Radiol Oncol Biol Phys*, **27**, 207–214.

(65) EORTC Brain Tumour Group. (1991). Cisplatin does not enhance the effect of radiation therapy in malignant gliomas. *Europ J Cancer*, **27**, 568–571.

(66) Wehbe T, Glantz M, Choy H *et al.* (1998). Histologic evidence of radiosensitizing effect of Taxol in patients with astrocytomas. *J Neurooncol*, **39**, 245–251.

(67) Sneed PK, Gutin PH. (1999). Interstitial radiation and hyperthermia. In: The gliomas. Berger MS, Wilson CB (eds). Saunders, Philadelphia, pp. 499–510.

(68) Laperriere NJ, Leung PM, Mc Kenzie S *et al.* (1998). Randomized study of brachytherapy in the initial management of patients with malignant astrocytoma. *Int J Radiat Oncol Biol Phys*, **41**, 1005–1011.

(69) Sneed PK, Larson DA, Gutin PH *et al.* (1994). Brachytherapy and hyperthermia for malignant astrocytomas. *Semin Oncol*, **21**, 186–197.

(70) Larson DA, Shrieve DC, Gutin PH. (1999). Radiosurgery. In: The gliomas. Berger MS, Wilson CB (eds). Saunders, Philadelphia, pp. 511–518.

(71) Walker MD, Green SB, Byar DP *et al.* (1980). Randomized comparisons of radiotherapy and nitrosoureas for the treatment of malignant glioma after surgery. *N Engl J Med*, **303**, 1323–1329.

(72) Fine HA, Dear KBG, Loeffler JS *et al.* (1993). Meta-analysis of radiation therapy with and without adjuvant chemotherapy for malignant gliomas in adults. *Cancer*, **71**, 2585–2597.

(73) Brada M, Thomas D, Bleehan N *et al.* (1998). Medical Research Council (MRC) randomised trial of adjuvant chemotherapy in high grade glioma (HGG) BR05. *J Clin Oncol (Proceedings of ASCO)*, **17**, 400a.

(74) Levin VA, Silver P, Hannigan J *et al.* (1990). Superiority of post-radiotherapy adjuvant chemotherapy with CCNU, procarbazine, and vincristine (PCV) over BCNU for anaplastic gliomas: NCOG 6G61 final report. *Int J Radiat Oncol Biol Phys*, **18**, 321–324.

(75) Hildebrand J, Shamoud T, Mignolet F and EORTC Brain Tumor Group. (1994). Adjuvant therapy with dibromodulcitol and BCNU increases survival of adults with malignant gliomas. *Neurology*, **44**, 1479–1483.

(76) Sposto R, Ertel IJ, Jenkin RDT *et al.* (1989). The effectiveness of chemotherapy for treatment of high grade astrocytoma in children: Results of a randomized trial. *J Neurooncol*, **7**, 165–177.

(77) EORTC Brain Tumour Group. (1987 (abstract)). Randomized comparison of radiotherapy versus VM-26 plus CCNU followed by radiotherapy in the treatment of supratentorial malignant brain gliomas in adult patients. Fifteenth International Congress of Chemotherapy, Istanbul.

(78) Heideman RL, Kuttesch JJ, Gajjar AJ, *et al.* (1997). Supratentorial malignant gliomas in childhood: A single institution perspective. *Cancer*, **80**, 497–504.

(79) Geyer JR, Finlay JL, Boyett JM *et al.* (1995). Survival of infants with malignant astrocytomas. A report of the Children's Cancer Group. *Cancer*, **75**, 1045–1050.

(80) Duffner PK, Krischer JP, Burger PC *et al.* (1996). Treatment of infants with malignant gliomas: the Pediatric Oncology Group Experience. *J Neurooncol*, **28**, 245–256.

(81) Walker M, Hurwitz B. (1970). BCNU (1,3-bis(2-chloroethyl)-1-nitrosourea (NSC-409962) in the treatment of malignant brain tumours. A preliminary report. *Cancer Chemother Rep*, **54**, 263–271.

(82) Wilson C, Gutin P, Boldrey E *et al.* (1976). Single agent chemotherapy of brain tumors. *Arch Neurol*, **33**, 739–744.

(83) EORTC Brain Tumour Group. (1981). Evaluation of CCNU, VM-26 plus CCNU and procarbazine in supratentorial brain gliomas. *J Neurosurg*, **55**, 27–31.

(84) Levine M, Walker M, Weiss H. (1974). Intravenous methyl-CCNU in the treatment of malignant gliomas (phase II). *ASCO Proc*, **15**, 167.

(85) Levin VA, Resser KJ, McGrath L *et al.* (1984). PCNU treatment for recurrent gliomas. *Cancer Treat Rep*, **68**, 969–973.

(86) Georges P, Przedborski S, Brotchi J *et al.* (1988). Effect of HeCNU in malignant supratentorial gliomas—a phase II study. *J Neurooncol*, **6**, 211–219.

(87) Frenay M, Giroux B, Khoury S *et al.* (1991). Phase II study of fotemustine in recurrent supratentorial malignant gliomas. *Europ J Cancer*, **27**, 852–856.

(88) Rodriguez LA, Prados M, Silver P, Levin VA. (1989). Reevaluation of procarbazine for treatment of recurrent malignant central nervous system tumors. *Cancer*, **64**, 2420–2423.

(89) Newton HB, Junck L, Bromberg J *et al.* (1990). Procarbazine chemotherapy in the treatment of recurrent malignant astrocytomas after radiation and nitrosourea failure. *Neurology*, **40**, 1743–1746.

(90) EORTC Brain Tumour Group. (1985). Effect of AZQ (1,4-cyclohexadiene-1,4-diacarbonic acid, 2,5-bis (1-aziridinyl-3,6-dioxo-diethylester) in recurring supratentorial malignant brain gliomas. A phase II study. *Europ J Cancer Clin Oncol*, **21**, 143–146.

(91) Taylor SA, McCracken JD, Eyre HJ *et al.* (1985). Phase II study of aziridinylbenzoquinone (AZQ) in patients with central nervous system malignancies: A Southwest Oncology Group study. *J Neurooncol*, **3**, 131–135.

(92) Decker DA, Al Sarraf M, Kresge C *et al.* (1985). Phase II study of aziridinylbenzoquinone (AZQ, NSC-182986) in the treatment of malignant gliomas recurrent after radiation. *J Neurooncol*, **3**, 19–21.

(93) Eagan RT, DiNapoli RP, Cascino TL *et al.* (1987). Comprehensive phase II evaluation of aziridinylbenzoquinone (AZQ, diaziquone) in recurrent human primary brain tumours. *J Neurooncol*, **5**, 309–314.

(94) Feun L, Yung W, Leavens M *et al.* (1984). A phase II trial of 2,5,diaziridyl 3,6-bis-(carboethoxy-amino) 1,4-benzoquinone (AZQ, NSC 182–986). *J Neurooncol*, **2**, 13–17.

(95) Poisson M, Pereon Y, Chiras J, Delattre JY. (1991). Treatment of recurrent malignant supratentorial gliomas with carboplatin (CBDCA). *J Neurooncol*, **10**, 139–144.

(96) Yung WK, Mechtler L, Gleason MJ. (1991). Intravenous carboplatin for recurrent malignant glioma: A phase II study. *J Clin Oncol*, **9**, 860–864.

(97) Warnick RE, Prados MD, Mack EE *et al.* (1994). A phase II study of intravenous carboplatin for the treatment of recurrent gliomas. *J Neurooncol*, **19**, 69–74.

(98) O'Reilly SM, Newlands ES, Glaser MG *et al.* (1993). Temozolomide: A new oral cytotoxic chemotherapeutic agent with promising activity against primary brain tumours. *Europ J Cancer*, **29A**, 940–942.

(99) Prados MD. (1999). Phase II and III trials with Temozolomide, including clinical trials in patients with brain tumors. Proc 90th Ann Mtg Am Assoc Cancer Res AACR, 40, p. 754, (abstract).

(100) Longee DC, Friedman HS, Albright RE *et al.* (1990). Treatment of patients with recurrent gliomas with cyclophosphamide and vincristine. *J Neurosurg*, **72**, 583–588.

(101) Chamberlain MC. (1997). Recurrent supratentorial malignant gliomas in children. Long-term salvage therapy with oral etoposide. *Arch Neurol*, **54**, 554–558.

(102) Levin VA, Wara WM, Davis RL *et al.* (1986). Northern California Oncology Group Protocol 6G91: Response to treatment with radiation therapy and seven-drug chemotherapy in patients with glioblastoma multiforme. *Cancer Treat Rep*, **70**, 739–743.

(103) Shapiro WR, Green SB, Burger PC *et al.* (1989). Randomized trial of three chemotherapy regimens and two radiotherapy regimens in postoperative treatment of malignant glioma. *J Neurosurg*, **71**, 1–9.

(104) Dropcho EJ. (1999). Intra-arterial chemotherapy for malignant gliomas. In: The gliomas. Berger MS, Wilson CB (eds). Saunders, Philadelphia, pp. 537–547.

(105) Greenberg HS, Ensminger WD, Chandler WF *et al.* (1984). Intra-arterial BCNU chemotherapy for treatment of malignant gliomas of the central nervous system. *J Neurosurg*, **61**, 423–429.

(106) Poisson M, Chiras J, Fauchon F *et al.* (1990). Treatment of malignant recurrent glioma by intra-arterial, infra-ophthalmic infusion of HECNU 1-(2-chloroethyl)-1-nitroso-3-(2-hydroxyl-ethyl) urea. A phase II study. *J Neurooncol*, **8**, 255–262.

(107) Lehane DE, Bryan RN, Horowitz B *et al.* (1983). Intra-arterial cis-platinum chemotherapy for patients with primary and metastatic brain tumours. *Cancer Drug Delivery*, **1**, 69–77.

(108) Feun LG, Wallace S, Stewart DJ, *et al.* (1984). Intracarotid infusion of cis-diamminedichloroplatinum in the treatment of recurrent malignant brain tumours. *Cancer*, **54**, 794–799.

(109) Newton HB, Page MA, Junck L, Greenberg HS. (1989). Intra-arterial cisplatin for treatment of malignant gliomas. *J Neurooncol*, **7**, 39–45.

(110) Mahaley MS Jr, Hipp SW, Dropcho EJ *et al.* (1989). Intracarotid cisplatin chemotherapy for recurrent gliomas. *J Neurosurgery*, **70**, 371–378.

(111) Greenberg SH, Ensminger WD, Layton PB *et al.* (1986). Phase I-II evaluation of intra-arterial diaziquone for recurrent malignant astrocytomas. *Cancer Treat Rep*, **70**, 353–357.

(112) Feun LG, Lee YY, Yung WK *et al.* (1987). Intracarotid VP-16 in malignant brain tumours. *J Neurooncol*, **4**, 397–401.

(113) Stewart DJ, Grahovac Z, Benoit B, *et al.* (1984). Intracarotid chemotherapy with combination of 1,3-bis (2-chloroethyl)-1-nitrosourea (BCNU), cis-diaminedichloroplatinum (cisplatin), and 4'-0-demethyl-1-0-(4,6-0-2-thenyliodeme-B-D-glucopyranosyl) epipodophyllotoxin (VM-26) in the treatment of primary and metastatic brain tumours. *Neurosurgery*, **15**, 828–833.

(114) Kapp JP, Vance RB. (1985). Supraophthalmic carotid infusion of recurrent glioma: rationale, technique and preliminary results for cisplatin and BCNU. *J Neurooncol*, **3**, 5–11.

(115) Bigner SH, Rasheed BKA, Wiltshire R *et al.* (1999). Morphologic and molecular genetic aspects of oligodendroglial neoplasms. *Neurooncology*, **1**, 52–60.

(116) Ludwig CL, Smith MT, Godfrey AD, Armbrustmacher VW. (1986). A clinicopathological study of 323 patients with oligodendrogliomas. *Ann Neurol*, **19**, 15–21.

(117) Celli P, Nofrone I, Palma L *et al.* (1994). Cerebral oligodendroglioma: Prognostic factors and life history. *Neurosurgery*, **35**, 1018–1035.

(118) Lindegaard KF, Mørk SJ, Eide GE *et al.* (1987). Statistical analysis of clinicopathological features, radiotherapy, and survival in 170 cases of oligodendroglioma. *J Neurosurg*, **67**, 224–230.

(119) Shaw EG, Scheithauer BW, O'Fallon JR, *et al.* (1992). Oligodendrogliomas: The Mayo Clinic experience. *J Neurosurg*, **76**, 428–434.

(120) Bullard DE, Rawlings CE III, Phillips B, *et al.* (1987). Oligodendroglioma: an analysis of the value of radiation therapy. *Cancer*, **60**, 2179–2188.

(121) Kros JM, Pieterman H, Van Eden CG, Avezaat CJ. (1994). Oligodendroglioma: The Rotterdam–Dijkzigt experience. *Neurosurgery*, **34**, 959–966.

(122) Nijjar TS, Simpson WJ, Gadalla T, MacCartney M. (1993). Oligodendroglioma: The Princess Margaret Hospital experience (1958–1984). *Cancer*, **71**, 4002–4006.

(123) Wallner KE, Gonzales M, Sheline GE. (1988). Treatment of oligodendrogliomas with or without postoperative irradiation. *J Neurosurg*, **68**, 684–688.

(124) Shimizu KT, Tran LM, Mark RJ, Selch MT. (1993). Management of oligodendrogliomas. *Radiology*, **186**, 569–572.

(125) Gannett DE, Wisbeck WM, Silbergeld DL, Berger MS. (1994). The role of postoperative irradiation in the treatment of oligodendroglioma. *Int J Radiat Oncol Biol Physics*, **30**, 567–573.

(126) Paleologos NA, MacDonald DR, Vick NA, Cairncross JG. (1999). Neoadjuvant procarbazine, CCNU, and vincristine for anaplastic and aggressive oligodendroglioma. *Neurology*, **53**, 1141–1143.

(127) Cairncross JG, MacDonald DR. (1988). Successful chemotherapy for recurrent malignant oligodendroglioma. *Ann Neurol*, **23**, 360–364.

(128) Cairncross JG, MacDonald DR, Ramsay DA. (1992). Aggressive oligodendroglioma: A chemosensitive tumor. *Neurosurgery*, **31**, 78–82.

(129) Kyritsis AP, Yung WKA, Bruner J *et al.* (1993). The treatment of anaplastic oligodendrolgiomas and mixed gliomas. *Neurosurgery*, **32**, 365–371.

(130) Glass J, Hochberg FH, Gruber ML *et al.* (1992). The treatment of oligodendrogliomas and mixed oligodendrogliomas-astrocytomas with PCV chemotherapy. *J Neurosurgery*, **76**, 741–745.

(131) Soffietti R, Chio A, Mocellini C *et al.* (1994 (abstract)). Response of oligodendroglial tumors to PCV chemotherapy. *Neurology*, **44** (suppl. 2):A309–A310.

(132) Cairncross JG, MacDonald D, Ludwin S *et al.* (1994). Chemotherapy for anaplastic oligodendrogliomas. National Cancer Institute of Canada Clinical Trials Group. *J Clin Oncol*, **12**, 2013–2021.

(133) Mason WP, Krol GS, De Angelis LM. (1996). Low-grade oligodendroglioma responds to chemotherapy. *Neurology*, **46**, 203–207.

(134) van den Bent MJ, Kros JM, Heimans JJ *et al.* (1998). Response rate and prognostic factors of recurrent oligodendroglioma treated with procarbazine, CCNU, and vincristine chemotherapy. *Neurology*, **51**, 1140–1145.

(135) Peterson K, Paleologos N, Forsyth P *et al.* (1996). Salvage chemotherapy for oligodendroglioma. *J Neurosurgery*, **85**, 597–601.

(136) Soffietti R, Chio A, Mocellini C *et al.* (1995 (abstract)). Treatment with carboplatinum of oligodendroglial tumors recurrent after PCV chemotherapy. *Neurology*, **45** (suppl. 4):A261.

(137) Scerrati M, Roselli R, Iacoangeli M *et al.* (1996). Prognostic factors in low grade (WHO grade II) gliomas of the cerebral hemispheres: role of surgery. *J Neurol Neurosurg Psychiatry*, **61**, 291–296.

(138) Cairncross JG, Laperriere NJ. (1989). Low-grade glioma: to treat or not to treat? *Arch Neurol*, **46**, 1238–1239.

(139) Shaw EG. (1990). Low-grade gliomas: to treat or not to treat? A radiation oncologist's viewpoint. *Arch Neurol*, **47**, 1138–1139.

(140) Shapiro WR. (1992). Low-grade gliomas: when to treat? *Ann Neurol*, **31**, 437–438.

(141) Kondziolka D, Lunsford LD, Martinez AJ. (1993). Unreliability of contemporary neurodiagnostic imaging in evaluating suspected adult supratentorial (low-grade) astrocytoma. *J Neurosurg*, **79**, 533–536.

(142) Vecht ChJ. (1993). Effect of age on treatment decision in low-grade glioma. *J Neurol Neurosurg Psychiatry*, **56**, 1259–1264.

(143) De Witte O, Levivier M, Violon Ph *et al.* (1996). Prognostic value of positron emission tomography with [^{18}F]fluorodeoxyglucose in low-grade gliomas. *Neurosurgery*, **39**, 470–477.

(144) Janny P, Cure H, Mohr M *et al.* (1994). Low-grade supratentorial astrocytomas: management and prognostic factors. *Cancer*, **73**, 1937–1945.

(145) North CA, North RB, Epstein JA *et al.* (1990). Low-grade cerebral astrocytomas: survival and quality of life after radiation therapy. *Cancer*, **66**, 6–14.

(146) Philippon JH, Clemenceau SH, Fauchon FH *et al.* (1993). Supratentorial low-grade astrocytomas in adults. *Neurosurgery*, **32**, 554–559.

(147) Reichenthal E, Feldman Z, Cohen ML *et al.* (1992). Hemispheric supratentorial low-grade astrocytomas. *Neurochirurgia*, **35**, 18–22.

(148) Piepmeier JM. (1987). Observations on the current treatment of low-grade astrocytic tumours of the cerebral hemispheres. *J Neurosurg*, **67**, 177–181.

(149) Shaw EG, Daumas-Duport C, Scheithauer BW *et al.* (1989). Radiation therapy in the management of low-grade supratentorial astrocytomas. *J Neurosurg*, **70**, 853–861.

(150) Shibamoto Y, Kitakabu Y, Takahashi M *et al.* (1993). Supratentorial low-grade astrocytoma: correlation of computed tomography findings with effect of radiation therapy and prognostic variables. *Cancer*, **72**, 190–195.

(151) Fazekas JT. (1977). Treatment of grade I and II brain astrocytomas: the role of radiotherapy. *Int J Radiat Oncol Biol Phys*, **2**, 661–666.

(152) Sheline GE. (October 1985). The role of radiation therapy in the treatment of low-grade gliomas. 35th Annual Congress of Neurological Surgeons. Honolulu, Hawaii.

(153) Karim ABMF, Maat B, Hatlevoll R *et al.* (1996). A randomized trial on dose-response in radiation therapy of low-grade cerebral glioma: European Organization for Research and Treatment of Cancer (EORTC) study 22844. *Int J Radiat Oncol Biol Phys*, **36**, 549–556.

(154) Eyre HJ, Crowley JJ, Townsend JJ *et al.* (1993). A randomized trial of radiotherapy versus radiotherapy plus CCNU for incompletely resected low-grade gliomas: a Southwest Oncology Group Study. *J Neurosurg*, **78**, 909–914.

(155) Hoffman HJ, Soloniuk DS, Humphreys RP *et al.* (1993). Management and outcome of low-grade astrocytomas of the midline in children: a retrospective review. *Neurosurgery*, **33**, 964–971.

(156) Packer RJ, Ater J, Allen J *et al.* (1997). Carboplatin and vincristine chemotherapy for children with newly diagnosed progressive low-grade gliomas. *J Neurosurg*, **86**, 747–754.

(157) Prados MD, Edwards MS, Rabbitt J *et al.* (1997). Treatment of pediatric low-grade gliomas with a nitrosourea-based multiagent chemotherapy regimen. *J Neurooncol*, **32**, 235–241.

(158) Bloom HJG. (1978). Management of some intracranial tumours in children and adults. In: Recent Advances in Clinical Oncology. AR Liss Inc, New York, pp. 55–84.

(159) Galanis E, Buckner JC, Burch PA *et al.* (1998). Phase II trial of nitrogen mustard, vincristine, and procarbazine in patients with recurrent glioma: North Central Cancer Treatment Group results. *J Clin Oncol*, **16**, 2953–2958.

(160) Chang CH, Housepian EM, Herbert C Jr. (1969). An operative staging system and a megavoltage radiotherapeutic technic for cerebellar medulloblastoma. *Radiology*, **43**, 1351–1359.

(161) Zeltzer PM, Boyett JM, Finlay JL *et al.* (1999). Metastasis stage, adjuvant treatment, and residual tumor are prognostic factors for medulloblastoma in children: conclusions from the Children's Cancer Group 921 randomized phase III study. *J Clin Oncol*, **17**, 832–845.

(162) Tomita T, McLone DG. (1986). Medulloblastoma in childhood: results of radical resection and low-dose neuraxis radiation therapy. *J Neurosurg*, **64**, 238–242.

(163) Hughes EN, Shillito J, Sallan SE *et al.* (1988). Medulloblastoma at the Joint Center for Radiation Therapy between 1968 and 1984. *Cancer*, **61**, 1992–1998.

(164) Jenkin D, Goddard K, Armstrong D *et al.* (1990). Posterior fossa medulloblastoma in childhood: treatment results and a proposal for new staging system. *Int J Radiat Oncol Biol Phys*, **19**, 265–274.

(165) Silverman CL, Simpson JR. (1982). Cerebellar medulloblastoma: the importance of posterior fossa dose to survival and patterns of failure. *Int J Radiat Oncol Biol Phys*, **8**, 1869–1876.

(166) Deutsch M, Thomas PR, Krischer J *et al.* (1996). Results of a prospective randomized trial comparing standard dose neuraxis irradiation (3600 cGy/20) with reduced neuraxis irradiation (2340 cGy/13) in patients with low-stage medulloblastoma. A Combined Children's Cancer Group-Pediatric Oncology Group Study. *Pediatr Neurosurg*, **24**, 167–176.

(167) Weil MD, Le QT, Sneed PK *et al.* (1994). Pattern of recurrence of medulloblastoma after low-dose craniospinal radiotherapy. *Int J Radiol Oncol Biol Phys*, **30**, 551–556.

(168) Doz F, Kalifa C, Gentet JC *et al.* (1988). Sandwich chemotherapy followed by radiation therapy using reduced dose to the neuraxis in standard risk patients. 8th International Symposium of Pediatric Neurooncology, Rome.

(169) Packer RJ, Goldwein J, Nicholson HS *et al.* (1999). Treatment of children with medulloblastomas with reduced-dose craniospinal radiation therapy and adjuvant chemotherapy: A children's cancer group study. *J Clin Oncol*, **17**, 2127.

(170) Goldwein JW, Radcliffe J, Johnson J *et al.* (1996). Updated results of a pilot study of low dose craniospinal irradiation plus chemotherapy for children under five with cerebellar primitive neuroectodermal tumors (medulloblastoma). *Int J Radiat Oncol Biol Phys*, **34**, 899–904.

(171) Mineura K, Izumi I, Watanabe K, Kowada M. (1993). Influence of O^6-methylguanine-DNA methyltransferase activity on chloroethylnitrosurea chemotherapy in brain tumor. *Int J Cancer*, **55**, 76–81.

(172) Packer RJ, Sutton LN, Elterman R *et al.* (1994). Outcome for children with medulloblastoma treated with radiation and cisplatin, CCNU and vincristine chemotherpy. *J Neurosurg*, **81**, 690–698.

(173) Neidhardt MK (on behalf of the Medulloblastoma Study Committee of the Society of Pediatric Oncology-GPO). (1983). Therapeutic approach to medulloblastoma and results: The Wet German treatment study (interim results). Presented at the 13th International Congress of Chemotherapy, Vienna **208**, 29–33.

(174) Krischer JP, Ragab AH, Kun L *et al.* (1991). Nitrogen mustard, vincristine, procarbazine, and prednisone as adjuvant chemotherapy in the treatment of medulloblastoma. *J Neurosurg*, **74**, 905–909.

(175) Ater JL, van Eys J, Woo SY, Moore B, III *et al.* (1997). MOPP chemotherapy without irradiation as primary postsurgical therapy for brain tumors in infants and young children. *J Neurooncol*, **32**, 243–252.

(176) Duffner PK, Horowitz ME, Krischer JP *et al.* (1993). Postoperative chemotherapy and delayed radiation in children less than 3 years of age with malignant brain tumors. *N Engl J Med*, **328**, 1725–1731.

(177) Geyer JR, Zeltzer PM, Boyett JM *et al.* (1994). Survival of infants with primitive neuroectodermal tumors or malignant ependymomas of the CNS treated with eight drugs in 1 day: A report from the Children's Cancer Group. *J Clin Oncol*, **12**, 1607–1615.

(178) Kühl J, Beck J, Bode U, for the German Pediatric Brain Tumor Study Group. (1995 (abstract)). Delayed radiation therapy (RT) after postoperative chemotherapy (PCH) in chil-

dren less than 3 years of age with medulloblastoma. Results of the trial HIT-SKK'87 and preliminary results of the pilot trial HIT-SKK'92. *Med Pediar Oncol*, **25**, 250.

(179) Fisher PG, Needle MN, Cnaan A *et al.* (1998). Salvage therapy after postoperative chemotherapy for primary brain tumors in infants and very young children. *Cancer*, **83**, 566–574.

(180) Bertolone SJ, Baum ES, Krivit W, Hammond GD. (1989). A phase II study of cisplatin therapy in childhood brain tumours. *J Neurooncol*, **7**, 5–11.

(181) Sexauer CL, Khan A, Burger PC *et al.* (1985). Cisplatin in recurrent pediatric brain tumours. A POG phase II study. *Cancer*, **56**, 1497–1501.

(182) Walker RW, Alleen JC. (1988). Cisplatin in the treatment of recurrent childhood primary brain tumours. *J Clin Oncol*, **6**, 62–66.

(183) Chamberlain MC, Prados MD, Silver P, Levin VA. (1988). A phase II trial of oral melphalan in recurrent primary brain tumours. *Am J Clin Oncol*, **11**, 52–54.

(184) Allen JC, Helson L. (1981). High-dose cyclophosphamide chemotherapy for recurrent CNS tumours in children. *J Neurosurg*, **55**, 749–756.

(185) Duffner PK, Cohen ME. (1986). Recent developments in pediatric neuro-oncology. *Cancer*, **58**, 561–568.

(186) Crafts DC, Levin VA, Edwards MS *et al.* (1978). Chemotherapy of recurrent medulloblastomas with combined procarbazine, CCNU and vincristine. *J Neurosurg*, **49**, 589–592.

(187) Lefkowitz IB, Packer RJ, Siegel KR *et al.* (1990). Results of treatment of children with recurrent medulloblastoma. Primitive neuroectodermol tumours with lomustine, cisplatin, and vincristine. *Cancer*, **65**, 412–417.

(188) Pendergrass TW, Milstein JM, Geyer RJ *et al.* (1987). Eight drugs in one day chemotherapy for brain tumours: Experience in 107 children and rational for preradiation chemotherapy. *J Clin Oncol*, **5**, 1221–1231.

(189) Corn BW, Marcus SM, Topham A *et al.* (1997). Will primary central nervous system lymphoma be the most frequent brain tumor diagnosed in the year 2000? *Cancer*, **79**, 2409–2413.

(190) Pirotte B, Levivier M, Goldman S *et al.* (1997). Glucocorticoid-induced long-term remission in primary cerebral lymphoma: Case report and review of the literature. *J Neurooncol*, **32**, 63–69.

(191) Henry JM, Heffner RR, Dillard SH *et al.* (1974). Primary malignant lymphomas of the central nervous system. *Cancer*, **34**, 1293–1302.

(192) Woodman R, Shin K, Pineo G. (1985). Primary non-Hodgkin's lymphoma of the brain. A Review. *Medicine*, **64**, 425–430.

(193) Loeffler JS, Ervin TJ, Mauch P *et al.* (1985). Primary lymphoma of the central nervous system. pattern of failure and factors that influence survival. *J Clin Oncol*, **3**, 490–491.

(194) Nelson DF, Martz KL, Bonner H *et al.* (1992). Non-Hodgkin's lymphoma of the brain: can high dose, large volume radiation therapy improve survival? Report on a prospective trial by the Radiation Therapy Oncology Group (RTOG): RTOG 8315. *Int J Radiat Oncol Biol Phys*, **23**, 9–17.

(195) Rock JP, Cher L, Hochberg FH, Rosenblum ML. (1996). Primary central nervous lymphoma. In: Neurological surgery, (4th edn). Youmans JR. (YOUMANS).(ed). Saunders, Philadelphia, p. 2695.

(196) Leibel SA, Sheline GE. (1987). Radiation therapy for neoplasms of the brain. *J Neurosurg*, **66**, 1–22.

(197) Brada M. (1995). Central nervous system lymphomas: progress in chemotherapy and radiotherapy. *Int J Radiat Oncol Biol Phys*, **33** (3):769–771.

(198) Chamberlain MC, Levin VA. (1992). Primary central nervous system lymphoma: a role for adjuvant chemotherapy. *J Neurooncol*, **14**, 271–275.

(199) De Angelis LM, Yahalom J, Thaler HT, Kher U. (1992). Combined modality therapy for primary CNS lymphoma. *J Clin Oncol*, **10**, 635–643.

(200) Glass J, Gruber MI, Cher L, Hochberg FH. (1994). Preirradiation methotrexate chemotherapy of primary central nervous system lymphoma: long-term outcome. *J Neurosurg*, **81**, 188–195.

(201) O'Neill BP, O'Fallon JR, Earle JD *et al.* (1995). Primary central nervous system non Hodgkin's lymphoma: survival advantages with combined initial therapy? *Int J Radiat Oncol Biol Phys*, **33**, 663–673.

(202) Sarazin M, Ameri A, Monjour A *et al.* (1995). Primary central nervous system lymphoma: treatment with chemotherapy and radiotherapy. *Europ J Cancer*, **31**, 2003–2007.

(203) Abrey LE, De Angelis L, Yahalom J. (1998). Long-term survival in primary CNS lymphoma. *J Clin Oncol*, **16**, 859–863.

(204) Freilich RJ, Delattre J-Y, Monjour A, De Angelis LM. (1996). Chemotherapy without radiation therapy as initial treatment for primary CNS lymphoma in older patients. *Neurology*, **46**, 435–439.

(205) Cher L, Glass J, Harsh GR, Hochberg FH. (1996). Therapy of primary CNS lymphoma with methotrexate-based chemotherapy and deferred radiotherapy: Preliminary results. *Neurology*, **46**, 1757–1759.

(206) Hoang-Xuan K, Chinot O, Frenay M *et al.* (1997 (abstract)). Chemotherapy alone as initial treatment of primary central nervous system lymphoma in older patients. *Neurology*, **48**, 17.

(207) Neuwelt EA, Goldman DL, Dahlborg SA *et al.* (1991). Primary CNS-lymphoma treated with osmotic blood–brain barrier disruption: Prolonged survival and preservation of cognitive function. *J Clin Oncol*, **9**, 1580–1590.

(208) Posner JB. (1992). Management of brain metastases. *Rev Neurol (Paris)*, **148**, 477–487.

(209) Sze G, Milano E, Johnson C *et al.* (1990). Detection of brain metastases: comparison of contrast-enhanced MR with unenhanced MR and enhanced CT. *Am J Neuroradiol*, **11**, 785–791.

(210) Vecht CJ, Hovestadt A, Verbiest HBC *et al.* (1994). Dose effect relationship of dexamethasone on Karnofsky performance in metastatic brain tumours: A randomized study of doses of 4, 8, and 16 mg per day. *Neurology*, **44**, 675–680.

(211) Weissman DE, Janjan NA, Erickson B *et al.* (1991). Twice-daily tapering dexamethasone treatment during cranial radiation for newly diagnosed brain metastases. *J Neurooncol*, **11**, 235–239.

(212) Hagen NA, Cirrincione C, Thaler HT, De Angelis L. (1990). The role of radiation therapy following resection of single brain metastasis from melanoma. *Neurology*, **40**, 158–160.

(213) Diener-West M, Dobbins TW, Philips TL, Nelson DT. (1989). Identification of an optimal subgroup for treatment evaluation of patients with brain metastases using RTOG study 7916. *Int J Radiat Oncol Biol Phys*, **16**, 669–678.

(214) Patchell RA, Posner JB. (1985). Neurologic complications of systemic cancer. *Neurol Clin*, **3**, 729–750.

(215) Patchell RA, Tibbs PA, Walsh JW *et al.* (1990). A randomized trial of surgery in the treatment of single metastases to the brain. *N Engl J Med*, **322**, 494–500.

(216) Vecht CJ, Haaxma-Reiche H, Noordijk EM *et al.* (1993). Treatment of single brain metastasis: radiotherapy alone or combined with neurosurgery? *Ann Neurol*, **33**, 583–590.

(217) Mintz AH, Kestle J, Rathbone MP *et al.* (1996). A randomized trial to assess the efficacy of surgery in addition to radiotherapy in patients with single cerebral metastasis. *Cancer*, **78**, 1470–1476.

(218) Bindal RK, Sawaya R, Leavens ME, Lee JJ. (1993). Surgical treatment of multiple brain metastases. *J Neurosurg*, **79**, 210–216.

(219) Borgelt B, Gelber R, Kramer S *et al.* (1980). The palliation of brain metastases: final results in the first two studies by the Radiation Therapy Oncology Group. *Int J Radiat Oncol Biol Phys*, **6**, 1–9.

(220) Kurtz JM, Gelber R, Brady LW *et al.* (1981). The palliation of brain metastases in a favorable patient population: a randomized clinical trial by the Radiation Therapy Oncology Group. *Int J Radiat Oncol Biol Phys*, **7**, 891–895.

(221) Eyre HJ, Ohlsen JD, Frank J *et al.* (1984). Randomized trial of radiotherapy versus radiotherapy plus metronidazole for the treatment metastatic cancer to the brain: a Southwest Oncology Group Study. *J Neurooncol*, **2**, 325–330.

(222) Kurup P, Reddy S, Hendrickson FR. (1980). Results of re-irradiation for cerebral metastases. *Cancer*, **46**, 2587–2589.

(223) Hazuka MB, Kinzie JJ. (1988). Brain metastases: results and effects of re-irradiation. *Int J Radiat Oncol Biol Phys*, **15**, 433–437.

(224) Cairncross JG, Kim JM, Posner JB. (1980). Radiation therapy for brain metastases. *Ann Neurol*, **7**, 529–541.

(225) Patchell RA, Tibbs PA, Regine WF *et al.* (1998). Postoperative radiotherapy in the treatment of single metastases to the brain. A randomized trial. *JAMA*, **280**, 1485–1489.

(226) Smalley SR, Laws ER, O'Fallon JR *et al.* (1992). Resection of solitary brain metastasis: role of adjuvant radiation and prognostic variables in 229 patients. *J Neurosurg*, **77**, 531–540.

(227) Lee JS, Umsawasdi T, Barkley HT *et al.* (1987). Timing of elective brain irradiation: a critical factor for brain metastases-free survival in small cell lung cancer. *Int J Radiat Oncol Biol Phys*, **13**, 697–704.

(228) Hoskin PJ, Yarnold JR, Smith IE, Ford HT. (1986). CNS relapse despite prophylactic cranial irradiation in small cell cancer. *Int J Radiat Oncol Biol Phys*, **12**, 2025–2028.

(229) Carmichael J, Crane JM, Bunn PA *et al.* (1988). Results of therapeutic cranial irradiation in small cell lung cancer. *Int J Radiat Oncol Biol Phys*, **14**, 455–459.

(230) Baglan RJ, Marks JE. (1981). Comparison of symptomatic and prophylactic irradiation of brain metastases from oat cell carcinoma of the lung. *Cancer*, **47**, 41–45.

(231) Lishner M, Feld R, Payne DG *et al.* (1990). Late neurological complications after prophylactic cranial irradiation in patients with SCLC: the Toronto experience. *J Clin Oncol*, **8**, 215–21.

(232) Arriagada R, Le Chevalier T, Borie F *et al.* (1995). Prophylactic cranial irradiation for patients with small-cell lung cancer in complete remission. *J Natl Cancer Inst*, **87**, 183–190.

(233) Aupérin A, Arriagada R, Pignon JP *et al.* (1999). Prophylactic cranial irradiation for patients with small-cell lung cancer in complete remission. *N Engl J Med*, **341**, 476–484.

(234) Figlin RA, Piantadosi S, Feld R, and the Lung Cancer Study Group. (1988). Intracranial recurrence of carcinoma after complete surgical resection of stage I, II and III non-small-cell lung cancer. *N Engl J Med*, **318**, 1300–1305.

(235) Caron JL, Souhami L, Podgorsak EB. (1992). Dynamic stereotactic radiosurgery in the palliative treatment of cerebral metastatic tumors. *J Neurooncol*, **12**, 173–179.

(236) Fuller BG, Kaplan ID, Adler J *et al.* (1992). Stereotaxic radiosurgery for brain metastases: the importance of adjuvant whole brain irradiation. *Int J Radiat Oncol Biol Phys*, **23**, 413–418.

(237) Adler JR, Cox RS, Kaplan I, Martin DP. (1992). Stereotactic radiosurgical treatment of brain metastases. *J Neurosurg*, **76**, 444–449.

(238) Mehta MP, Mackie TR, Levin AB *et al.* (1992). Radiosurgery for brain metastases. *Contemp Oncol*, **1**, 12–19.

(239) McKenzie MR, Souhami L, Podgorsak EB *et al.* (1992). Photon radiosurgery: a clinical review. *Can J Neurol Sci*, **19**, 212–221.

(240) Alexander E, Moriarty TM, Davis RB *et al.* (1995). Stereotactic radiosurgery for the definitive noninvasive treatment of brain metastases. *J Natl Cancer Inst*, **87**, 34–40.

(241) Flickinger JC, Lunsford LD, Somaza S, Kondziolka D. (1996). Radiosurgery: its role in brain metastasis management. *Neurosurg Clin North Am*, **7**, 497–504.

(242) Joseph J, Adler JR, Cox RS, Hancock SL. (1996). Linear accelerator-based stereotaxic radio-surgery for brain metastases: the influence of number of lesions on survival. *J Clin Oncol*, **14**, 1085–1092.
(243) Cho KH, Hall WA, Gerbi BJ *et al.* (1998). Patients selection criteria for the treatment of brain metastases with stereotactic radiosurgery. *J Neurooncol*, **40**, 73–86.
(244) Bindal AK, Bindal RK, Hess KR *et al.* (1996). Surgery versus radiosurgery in the treatment of brain metastasis. *J Neurosurg*, **84**, 748–754.
(245) Auchter RM, Lamond JP, Alexander EA *et al.* (1996). A multi-institutional outcome and prognostic factor analysis of radiosurgery for resectable single brain metastasis. *Int J Radiat Oncol Biol Phys*, **35**, 27–35.
(246) Newlands ES. (1985). Chemotherapy for brain metastases. In: Neuro-oncology. Rose FC, Fields WS (eds). Karger, Basle, Switzerland, pp. 167–176,
(247) Logothetis CJ, Samuels ML, Trindade A. (1982). The management of brain metastases in germ cell tumors. *Cancer*, **49**, 12–18.
(248) Rustin GJS, Newlands ES, Begent RHJ *et al.* (1989). Weekly alternating etoposide, methotrexate, and actinomycin/vincristine and cyclophosphamide chemotherapy for the treamtent of CNS metastases of choriocarcinoma. *J Clin Oncol*, **7**, 900–903.
(249) Hildebrand J, Brihaye J, Wagenknecht L *et al.* (1975). Combination chemotherapy with CCNU, vincristine and methotrexate in primary and metastatic brain tumors. *Europ J Cancer*, **1**, 585–587.
(250) Rosner D, Nemoto T, Lane WW. (1986). Chemotherapy induces regression of brain metastases in breast carcinoma. *Cancer*, **58**, 832–839.
(251) Cocconi G, Lottici R, Bisagni G *et al.* (1990). Combination therapy with platinum and etoposide of brain metastases from breast carcinoma. *Cancer Invest*, **8**, 327–334.
(252) Boogerd W, Dalesio O, Bais EM, van der Sande JJ. (1992). Response of brain metastases from breast cancer to systemic chemotherapy. *Cancer*, **69**, 972–980.
(253) Carey RW, Davis JM, Zervas NT. (1981). Tamoxifen-induced regression of cerebral metastases in breast carcinoma. *Cancer Treat Rep*, **65**, 793–795.
(254) Pors H, von Eyben FE, Sorensen OS, Larsen M. (1991). Long-term remission of multiple brain metastases with tamoxifen. *J Neurooncol*, **10**, 173–177.
(255) Postmus PE, Haaxma-Reiche H, Sleijfer DTh *et al.* (1987). High-dose etoposide for central nervous system metastases of small cell lung cancer. Preliminary results. *Europ J Resp Dis*, **149** (suppl):65–71.
(256) Postmus PE, Smit EF, Berendsen HH *et al.* (1992). Treatment of brain metastases of small cell lung cancer with teniposide. *Semin Oncol*, **19**, 89–94.
(257) Giaccone G, Donadio M, Bonardi GM *et al.* (1988). Teniposide (VM-26): an effective treatment for brain metastases of small cell carcinoma of the lung. *Europ J Cancer Clin Oncol*, **24**, 629–691.
(258) Twelves CJ, Souhami RL, Harper PG *et al.* (1990). The response of cerebral metastases in small-cell lung cancer to systemic chemotherapy. *Br J Cancer*, **61**, 147–150.
(259) Kristensen CA, Kristjansen PE, Hansen HH. (1992). Systemic chemotherapy of brain metastases from small-cell lung cancer. A review. *J Clin Oncol*, **10**, 1498–1502.
(260) Ushio Y, Arita N, Hayakawa T *et al.* (1991). Chemotherapy of brain metastases from lung carcinoma: a controlled randomized study. *Neurosurgery*, **28**, 201–205.
(261) Robinet G, Gouva S, Clavier J *et al.* (1991). Chimiothérapie par cisplatine et 5-fluorouracile dans les métastases cérébrales inopérables des cancers bronchiques. *Bull Cancer*, **78**, 831–837.
(262) Jacquillat C, Khayat D, Banzet P *et al.* (1990). Final report of the French multicenter phase II study of nitrosourea fotemustin in 153 evaluable patients with disseminated malignant melanoma including patients with cerebral metastases. *Cancer*, **66**, 1873–1878.

(263) Nakagawa H, Fujita T, Izumoto S *et al.* (1993). Cis-diammine dichloroplatin (CDDP) therapy for brain metastasis of lung cancer. II. Distribution within the central nervous system after intravenous and intracarotid infusion. *J Neurooncol*, **16**, 61–67.

(264) Coakham HB, Kemshead JT. (1998). Treatment of neoplastic meningitis by targeted radiation using ^{131}I-radiolabelled monoclonal antibodies. Results of responses and long term follow-up in 40 patients. *J Neurooncol*, **38**, 225–232.

(265) Adamson PC, Poplack DG. (1996). Leptomeningeal metastases. Pharmacologic approaches to treatment. In: Cancer in the nervous system. Levin VA (ed.). Churchill Livingstone, New-York, pp. 291–301.

(266) Berg S, Balis F, Zimm S *et al.* (1992). Phase I/II trial and pharmacokinetics of intrathecal diaziquone in refractory meningeal malignancies. *J Clin Oncol*, **10**, 143–148.

(267) Ushio Y, Kochi M, Kitamura I, Kuratsu J-I. (1998). Ventriculolumbar perfusion of 3-[(4-amino-2-methyl-5-pyrimidinyl)-methyl]-1-(2-chloroethyl)-1-nitrosourea hydrochloride for subarachnoid dissemination of gliomas. *J Neurooncol*, **38**, 207–212.

(268) Blaney SM, Poplack DG. (1998). New cytotoxic drugs for intrathecal administration. *J Neurooncol*, **38**, 219–223.

(269) Bleyer WA, Pizzo PA, Spence AM. (1978). The Ommaya reservoir: newly recognized complications and recommendations for insertion use. *Cancer*, **41**, 2431–2437.

(270) Chamberlain MC, Kormanik P. (1996). Prognostic significance of [111]Indium-DPTA CSF flow studies. *Neurology*, **46**, 1674–1677.

(271) Shaw E, Evans R, Scheithauer B *et al.* (1987). Postoperative radiotherapy of intracranial ependymoma in pediatric and adult patients. *Int J Radiat Oncol Biol Phys*, **13**, 1457–1462.

(272) Dearnaley DP, A'Hern RP, Whittaker S, Bloom HJG. (1990). Pineal and CNS germ cell tumors: Royal Marsden Hospital experience 1962–1987. *Int J Radiol Oncol Biol Phys*, **18**, 773–781.

(273) Linstadt D, Wara WM, Edwards MSB *et al.* (1988). Radiotherapy of primary intracranial germinomas: the case against routine craniospinal irradiation. *Int J Radiat Oncol Biol Phys*, **15**, 291–297.

(274) Brada M, Rajan B. (1990). Spinal seeding in cranial germinoma. *Br J Cancer*, **61**, 339–340.

(275) Bruce JN, Fetell MR, Stein BM. (1990). Incidence of spinal metastases in patients with malignant pineal region tumors: avoidance of prophylactic spinal irradiation. *J Neurosurg*, **72**, 354A.

(276) Dattoli MJ, Newall J. (1990). Radiation therapy for intracranial germinoma: the case for limited volume treatment. *Int J Radiat Oncol Biol Phys*, **19**, 429–433.

(277) Pinkel D, Woo S. (1994). Prevention and treatment of meningeal leukemia in children. *Blood*, **84**, 355–366.

(278) Schrappe M, Reiter A, Riehm H. (1998). Prophylaxis and treatment of neoplastic meningosis in childhood acute lymphoblastic leukemia. *J Neurooncol*, **38**, 159–165.

(279) Abromowitch M, Ochs J, Piu CH. (1988). Efficacy of high-dose methotrexate in childhood acute lymphotic leukemia: analysis by contemporary risk. *Blood*, **74**, 866–869.

(280) Poplack DG, Reaman GH, Bleyer WA *et al.* (1989). Successful prevention of CNS leukemia without cranial radiation in children with high risk acute lymphoblastic leukemia: a preliminary report. *Proc Am Soc Clin Oncol*, **8**, 213.

(281) Reaman GH, Poplack DG, Wesley R *et al.* (1989). Prognostic factors for central nervous relapse in acute lymphoblastic leukemia. *Proc Am Soc Clin Oncol*, **8**, 218.

(282) Cortes J, O'Brien SM, Pierce S *et al.* (1995). The value of high-dose systemic chemotherapy and intrathecal therapy for central nervous system prophylaxis in different risk groups of adult acute lymphoblastic leukemia. *Blood*, **86**, 2091–2097.

(283) Omura GA, Moffitt S, Vogler WR, Salter MM. (1980). Combination chemotherapy of adult acute lymphoblastic leukemia with randomized central nervous prophylaxis. *Blood*, **55**, 199–204.

(284) Gökbuget N, Hoelzer D. (1998). Meningeosis leukaemia in adult acute lymphoblastic leukemia. *J Neurooncol*, **38**, 167–180.

(285) Steuber CP, Civin C, Krischer J. *et al.* (1991). A comparison of induction and maintenance therapy for acute non-lymphocytic leukemia in childhood: Results of a Pediatric Oncology Group study. *J Clin Oncol*, **9**, 247–258.

(286) Ravindranath Y, Steuber CP, Krischer J *et al.* (1991). High-dose cytarabine for intensification of early therapy of childhood acute myeloid leukemia: A Pediatric Oncology Group study. *J Clin Oncol*, **9**, 572–580.

(287) Recht L, Straus DJ, Cirrincione C *et al.* (1988). Central nervous system metastases from non-Hodgkin's lymphoma: treatment and prophylaxis. *Am J Med*, **84**, 425–435.

(288) Bollen EL, Brouwer RE, Hamers S *et al.* (1997). Central nervous system relapse in non-Hodgkin lymphoma. *Arch Neurol*, **54**, 854–859.

(289) Nkrumah FK, Neequaye JE, Biggar R. (1985). Intrathecal chemoprophylaxis in the prevention of central nervous system relapse in Burkitt's lymphoma. *Cancer*, **56**, 239–242.

(290) Glass JP, Melamed M, Chernik NL *et al.* (1979). Malignant cells in cerebrospinal fluid (CSF): the meaning of a positive CSF cytology. *Neurology*, **29**, 1369–1375.

(291) Siegal T. (1998). Leptomeningeal metastases: Rationale for systemic chemotherapy or what is the role of intra-CSF-chemotherapy. *J Neurooncol*, **38**, 151–157.

(292) Cherlow JM, Sather H, Steinherz P *et al.* (1996). Craniospinal irradiation for acute lymphoblastic leukemia with central nervous system disease at diagnosis: a report from the Children's Cancer Group. *Int J Radiat Oncol Biol Phys*, **36**, 19–27.

(293) Bowman WP, Shuster J, Cook B *et al.* (1996). Improved survival for children with B cell acute lymphoblastic leukemia and stage IV small non-cleaved cell lymphomas: a pediatric oncology group study. *J Clin Oncol*, **14**, 1252–1261.

(294) Young RC, Howser DM, Anderson T *et al.* (1979). Central nevous system complications of non-Hodgkin's lymphoma. *Am J Med*, **66**, 435–443.

(295) MacKintosh FR, Colby TV, Podolsky WJ *et al.* (1982). Central nervous system involvement in non-Hodgkin's lymphoma: An analysis of 105 cases. *Cancer*, **49**, 586–595.

(296) Liang RHS, Woo EKW, Yu YL *et al.* (1989). Central nervous system involvement in non-Hodgkin's lymphoma. *Eur J Cancer Clin Oncol*, **25**, 703–710.

(297) Siegal T, Lossos A, Pfeffer MR. (1994). Leptomeningeal metastases: Analysis of 31 patients with sustained off-therapy response following combined-modality therapy. *Neurology*, **44**, 1463–1469.

(298) Chamberlain MC, Kormanik PA. (1997). Non-Aids-related lymphomatous meningitis: combined mortality therapy. *Neurology*, **49**, 1728–1731.

(299) Hildebrand J. (1998). Prophylaxis and treatment of leptomeningeal carcinomatosis in solid tumors of adulthood. *J Neurooncol*, **38**, 193–198.

(300) Ruff RL, Lanska DJ. (1989). Epidural metastases in prospectively evaluated veterans with cancer and back pain. *Cancer*, **63**, 2234–2241.

(301) Lyons MK, O'Neill BP, Kurtin PJ, Marsh WR. (1996). Diagnosis and management of primary spinal epidural non-Hodgkin's lymphoma. *Mayo Clin Proc*, **71**, 453–457.

(302) Delauche-Cavallier MC, Laredo JD, Wybier M *et al.* (1988). Solitary plasmacytoma of the spine. Long term clinical course. *Cancer*, **61**, 1707–1714.

(303) Vecht CJ, Haaxma-Reiche H, Van Putten WLJ *et al.* (1989). Initial bolus of conventional versus high-dose dexamethasone in metastatic spinal cord compression. *Neurology*, **39**, 1255–1257.

(304) Maranzano E, Latini P, Checcaglini F, Ricci S *et al.* (1991). Radiation therapy in metastatic spinal cord compression. A prospective analysis of 105 consecutive patients. *Cancer*, **67**, 1311–1317.

(305) Cobb CA, Leavens ME, Eckles N. (1977). Indications for nonoperative treatment of spinal cord compression due to breast cancer. *J Neurosurg*, **47**, 653–658.

(306) Findlay GFG. (1984). Adverse effects of the management of malignant spinal cord compression. *J Neurol Neursurg Psychiatry*, **47**, 761–768.

(307) Martenson JA, Evans RG, Lie MR *et al.* (1985). Treatment outcome and complications in patients treated for malignant epidural spinal cord compression. *J Neurooncol*, **3**, 77–84.

(308) Gilbert RW, Kim JH, Posner JB. (1978). Epidural spinal cord compression from metastatic tumor: diagnosis and treatment. *Ann Neurol*, **3**, 40–51.

(309) Chamberlain MC, Kormanik PA. (1999). Epidural spinal cord compression: a single institution's retrospective experience. *Neurooncol*, **1**, 120–123.

(310) Loblaw DA, Laperriere N. (1998). Emergency treatment of malignant extradural spinal cord compression: an evidence-based guideline. *J Clin Oncol*, **16**, 1613–1624.

(311) Siegal T, Siegal T. (1993). Spinal epidural metastases form solid tumors. In: Neuro-oncology. Twynstra A, Keyser A, Ongerboer de Visser BW (eds). Elsevier, Amsterdam, pp. 283–291.

(312) Schiff D, Shaw EG, Cascino TL. (1995). Outcome after spinal reirradiation in malignant epidural spiral cord compression. *Ann Neurol*, **37**, 583–589.

(313) Wong ET, Portlock CS, O'Brien JP, De Angelis LM. (1996). Chemosensitive epidural spinal cord disease in non-Hodkin's lymphoma. *Neurology*, **46**, 1543–1547.

(314) Young RF, Post EM, King GA. (1980). Treatment of spinal epidural metastases. Randomized prospective comparison of laminectomy and radiotherapy. *J Neurosurg*, **53**, 741–748.

(315) Schiff D, O'Neill BP, Suman VJ. (1997). Spinal epidural metastases as the initial manifestation of malignancy. Clinical features and diagnostic approach. *Neurology*, **49**, 452–456.

(316) Sundaresan N, Krol G, Digiacinto GV, Hughes JEO. (1990). Metastatic tumors of the spine. In: Tumours of the spine, diagnosis and clinical managment. Sundaresan N, Schmidek H, Schiller A, Rosenthal A (eds). Saunders, Philadelphia, **30**, pp. 305–315.

(317) Harrington KD. (1984). Anterior cord decompression and spinal stabilization for patients with metastatic lesions of the spine. *J Neurosurg*, **61**, 107–117.

Index

muscle disorders and fatigue *contd*
  main aetiologies 185–93
  therapy 197–8
muscle invasion by malignant
    tumours 186
muscle metastases 186–8, 197, 198
mutism 28
myasthenia gravis 184, 189, 191,
    197
  investigations 185, 191–2, 196
myelomas 25, 137, 161, 164
myoclonus 71, 108
myopathy
  carcinoid 193, 196
  glucocorticosteroid 189, 195, 197
  necrotizing 144, 147

nasopharyngeal carcinoma 114,
    211
necrotizing myelopathy 144, 147
necrotizing myopathy, acute 193,
    196
Nelson's syndrome 218, 219
neoadjuvant treatment 225
  chemotherapy 236–7, 242, 246
neomycin 189
neoplastic lesions
  altered consciousness 5–10
  cerebellar dysfunction 62–5
  cognitive and behavioural
      disorders 30–2
  cranial nerve and brainstem
      lesions 103–16
  diffuse PNS lesions 154–6, 163
  endocrine disorders 206–10
  epileptic seizures 49–51
  focal PNS lesions 170–4
  muscle disorders and fatigue
      185–8
  spinal cord lesions 132–41
  visual alterations 80–91
neoplastic meningitis *see*
    leptomeningeal metastases 5
nerve sheath tumours
  focal PNS lesions 170–1, 176,
      181
  spinal cord lesions 133, 134,
      145–7, 148
  see also neurofibromas;
      schwannomas
neuroblastomas 70, 71
neurofibromas 133, 147, 148,
    170–1
neurofibrosarcomas 148

neuroleptics 12, 52, 53, 68
  see also named neuroleptics
neuromyopathy, carcinomatous
    161–2
neuromyotonia 117
neurosurgery, *see* surgery
nitrogen mustard 11, 52
nitrosureas 232
  altered consciousness 11
  brain metastases 261
  cranial nerve and brainstem
      lesions 122
  epileptic seizures 52
  glioblastomas and anaplastic
      astrocytomas 237
  medulloblastomas 248
  visual alterations 91
  see also named nitrosureas
Nocardia asteroides 13, 24, 68
Nocardia sp. 43
non-bacterial thrombotic
    endocarditis (NBTE) 14
non-convulsive status epilepticus
    47, 48, 57–8
non-fluent aphasia 28
non-Hodgkin's lymphoma
  altered consciousness 12
  cranial nerve and brainstem
      lesions 118
  diffuse lesions of the PNS 156,
      162
  epidural metastases 270
  leptomeningeal metastases 265,
      266
  muscle disorders and fatigue 191
  visual alterations 94
non-opioid analgesics 180
  see also named non-opioids
non-steroidal anti-inflammatory
    drugs 181
  see also named NSAIDs
nortiptyline 43
numb chin syndrome 112
nutritional disorders 185
nystagmus 61

octreotide 198, 216, 217–18
ocular metastases 98
olfactory groove meningiomas 87
oligodendrogliomas
  altered consciousness 5, 17
  prognostic factors for survival
      226
  therapy 232–3, 239–42, 243–4

Onuf's nucleus 130
ophthalmoscopy 94
opsoclonus 70–1, 103, 108, 120
optic atrophy 92, 95, 96
optic gliomas 82–3, 84, 97–8
optic nerve
  infiltration 94–5
  ischaemia 92
  meningiomas 86–7, 88
optic neuritis 93
orbit metastases 87–90, 98
orthostatic hypotension 131
osmotic diuretics 22, 24
  see also named diuretics
osteolytic myeloma 161, 164
ovary cancer 70, 71, 176, 192–3
oxacillin 24

paclitaxel (Taxol®) 153, 156, 157,
    158, 164
pain 169, 172, 173, 180–1
PALA 65–6
pancerebellopathy 62
Pancoat's syndrome 172, 173
panic attacks 30
papilloedema 3, 90–1, 95, 96
papovavirus, *see* progressive
    multifocal leucoencephalopathy
paracetamol 180
paranasal sinus carcinomas 114
paraneoplastic lesions
  altered consciousness 6, 14, 25
  cerebellar dysfunction 62, 68–72,
      74, 75
  cognitive and behavioural
      disorders 30, 37–8, 42
  cranial nerve and brainstem
      lesions 103, 107–8
  diffuse PNS lesions 156, 160–2,
      164
  endocrine disorders 206
  epileptic seizures 50, 53–4
  focal PNS lesions 170, 177
  muscle disorders and fatigue 188,
      190–3
  spinal cord lesions 132, 144–5
  visual alterations 81, 93
paraneoplastic opsoclonus without
    anti-Ri antibodies 14
paraneoplastic vasculitis,
    neuropathies caused by 162
parathyroid-hormone-related
    peptide 14
parenchymal brain lesions 54

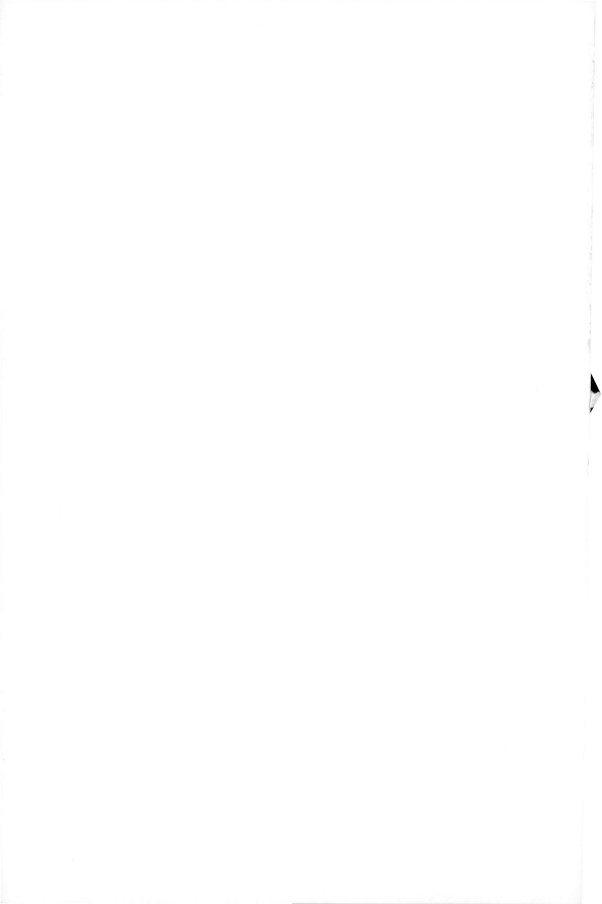